Psychology for Musicians

Psychology for Musicians

Understanding and Acquiring the Skills

ROBERT H. WOODY

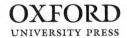

OXFORD
UNIVERSITY PRESS

Oxford University Press is a department of the University of Oxford. It furthers
the University's objective of excellence in research, scholarship, and education
by publishing worldwide. Oxford is a registered trade mark of Oxford University
Press in the UK and certain other countries.

Published in the United States of America by Oxford University Press
198 Madison Avenue, New York, NY 10016, United States of America.

Library of Congress Cataloging-in-Publication Data
Names: Woody, Robert H., author.
Title: Psychology for musicians : understanding and acquiring the skills /
Robert H. Woody.
Description: New York : Oxford University Press, 2022. |
Includes bibliographical references and index.
Identifiers: LCCN 2021029415 (print) | LCCN 2021029416 (ebook) |
ISBN 9780197546598 (hardback) | ISBN 9780197546604 (paperback) |
ISBN 9780197546628 (epub)
Subjects: LCSH: Musicians—Psychology. | Music—Psychological aspects.
Classification: LCC ML3838 .L464 2021 (print) | LCC ML3838 (ebook) |
DDC 781.1/1—dc23
LC record available at https://lccn.loc.gov/2021029415
LC ebook record available at https://lccn.loc.gov/2021029416

DOI: 10.1093/oso/9780197546598.001.0001

Paperback printed by LSC Communications, United States of America
Hardback printed by Bridgeport National Bindery, Inc., United States of America

Contents

Foreword   vii
Preface   ix

PART I. MUSICAL LEARNING

1. Introduction to Music Psychology   3

2. Development   21

3. Motivation   46

4. Practice   66

PART II. MUSICAL SKILLS

5. Learning and Remembering Musical Works   95

6. Expressing and Interpreting   116

7. Composing and Improvising   138

8. Managing Performance Anxiety   169

PART III. MUSICAL ROLES

9. The Performer   195

10. The Teacher   221

11. The Listener   240

12. The User   265

References   291
Index   345

Foreword

Some 17 years ago, Robert H. Woody invited us to spend a week's "retreat" with him at the School of Music at the University of Nebraska–Lincoln, where he has been a music educator and researcher for nearly 20 years. Out of that retreat was crafted the structure and main content areas of a book that we then cowrote and published in 2007 as *Psychology for Musicians: Understanding and Acquiring the Skills*. Our intention was to fill a gap in the textbook and teaching literature that was positioned between psychology, musicology, and music education. In particular, we wanted to provide a resource for musicians, music learners, and those that support them. This was not to be a checklist of "dos and don'ts" for musicians and teachers, nor a scholarly treatise for researchers, but something that drew on the voluminous research literature and structured it in a way designed to inform musicians and lovers of music about the scientific underpinnings of music making and assist them to think more deeply about this remarkable and ubiquitous practice.

Each of us took major responsibility for 4 of the 12 chapters, although contributing to all. We were gratified that the book seemed to fill a niche that complemented the growing range of more specialized and scholarly oriented books that have given shape to the very diverse range of research endeavors that have mushroomed since the 1980s. Somewhat surprisingly, ours was the first book with the title *Psychology for Musicians* since the 1940s, when the British music educator Percy Buck wrote a monograph with the same title, long before the "cognitive revolution" of the 1960s that shaped much of modern scientific music psychology. We are particularly pleased that our book got translated into a number of languages other than English. Addressing more diverse audiences (and musical cultures) is an important priority in our field, as Robert H. Woody rightly acknowledges in the preface to this second edition.

The field has moved on apace since our cowriting efforts, and Woody has taken on the herculean task of completely revising and updating each of the 12 chapters with a wealth of more recent references. In doing so he has also brought his long and varied experience of using the first edition as a teaching resource in a range of contexts, tailoring the content and the study materials more closely to the recurrent concerns and questions of those he has taught.

As an experienced music educator, Robert H. Woody wants research findings to be applied in various musical settings. He clearly has target audiences in mind, which he addresses specifically with interactive side boxes. These are labeled "Taking the Stage" for aspects surrounding performance and "Leading Learning" for issues related to teaching/coaching. Furthermore, study questions invite all readers to reflect on important issues communicated in the respective chapters. The language is deliberately accessible, engaging, and carefully selected to introduce terms and findings that musicians and music lovers at large might find interesting and useful.

We salute this sequel to the 2007 *Psychology for Musicians* as a significant milestone in the body of resources designed to help musicians and music teachers understand more about the powers they possess and how to productively develop them. For those who do not perform but love music and want music and musicians to prosper, this book explains how music functions in our lives and why it is so important to pass on our love of music to future generations.

Andreas C. Lehmann & John A. Sloboda

Preface

For over 20 years now in higher education, I have had the privilege of sharing the psychological perspective with musicians. During this time, I am sure I have learned from them just as much as they have learned from me. The many music psychology classes and seminars I have led have attracted many kinds of persons: exceptionally talented performers already making a living as professionals, university music majors deciding whether to pursue a career as a teacher or working musician, and some not defining themselves as "musicians" per se or even as particularly musically inclined.

I was one of three authors who wrote the first edition of this book published in 2007. When the three of us collaborated to plan, write, and edit that text, I was very much the junior partner. Andreas Lehman was a dear mentor of mine from graduate school who had become a good friend. John Sloboda was, well, quite likely the world's foremost authority in music psychology. Now nearly 20 years later, I can hardly consider myself a junior anything. Andreas and John are still important contributors to the field of music psychology, of course, but have prioritized other ventures over the effort required for another round of transatlantic communication and coordination in revising a book much in need of an update. But because they remain such valued mentors and inspirational role models to myself, I am delighted that they entrusted the writing of this second edition to me. I am also extremely grateful to them for providing a foreword to this edition.

What may have begun in my mind as a revision project grew into much more. It is cliché to say it, but this book became a labor of love for me. I have always found the psychology of music fascinating, and years of sharing it with others only increased my interest and dedication. As I carefully examined the first edition, I quickly realized that what was needed was much more than an update. Therefore, this second edition is truly a new edition, indeed, a "retelling" of the story of music psychology, to borrow a phrase from the television and film industry.

At some point during the last 20 years, my perspective changed from considering music psychology an interesting field of study to an essential one. Given that music is created *by people* and performed *for people*, I now maintain that musicians cannot afford to ignore psychology, which, after all, is essentially the study of *people*. And as I have made this case to musicians I have interacted with—through classes taught, workshops presented, and other publications written—they have clearly responded to this message. On the whole, musicians have indicated that they want to know what psychology has discovered about how human thought and behavior intersect with music.

In this book, I offer the insights of the field in a way that combines the rigor of empirical research with the need for practical application demanded by musicians. In writing these chapters, I have aimed to retain the first edition's coverage of foundational concepts of music psychology and to meaningfully add important ideas that have emerged since then. The overall organization of the book is very similar to that of the first edition, but I have reimagined each chapter in a way to optimally communicate with musician readers. No doubt my efforts were guided by my experiences over the years working with real musicians via classes, workshops, and publications, including blog posts that drew musicians' immediate and honest comments.

I am especially pleased that this second edition includes the kind of breadth and diversity that is needed in advanced music study today. Like much of the music professorate in North America, I was swayed by the College Music Society's 2016 publication of their "progressive manifesto" titled *Transforming Music Study From Its Foundations*. Among its recommendations was a call for college- and university-trained musicians to grow in cross-cultural musical awareness and experience a greater diversity of creative and artistic influences. This book, while affirming the rightful place of Western classical music in higher education study, includes the perspectives of other cultures and music traditions. The College Music Society's manifesto also called for greater consideration of human learning and cognition, which obviously is a focus of this volume.

Perhaps the most important diversity accomplished by this book is the broad readership. These pages do not speak to any one type of musician. I, myself, have benefited greatly from interacting with many different kinds of musical people in my life. In addition to performing in a variety of styles and settings, I have taught music: as a teacher of private lessons, a middle school music teacher, and now a professor of music and music education. I have also been a "music parent" to children in my own home. My music students over the years have been wonderfully diverse in many musical and personal characteristics. My aim in this book is to reach all who read it in ways that will help them make their musical lives more meaningful and rewarding.

PART I
MUSICAL LEARNING

1

Introduction to Music Psychology

On the surface, psychology and music may seem like disparate topics, but they do in fact make quite complementary fields of study. After all, psychology is the study of the amazing human mind, and it seeks to understand people's behavior. And music, for its part, comprises some of people's most fascinating behaviors, which allow expression and understanding of what it means to be human. So there is actually a strong connection between psychology, a social science, and the art of music, a highly social form of human expression.

Psychology offers insights into humankind that can be very useful to musicians. Psychology promotes understanding of people: how they perceive and process the world around them, how they feel emotion, how they learn, and how they can skillfully perform certain behaviors, just to name several areas of interest. Music is made *by* human beings *for* human beings. Musical instruments (including the voice) are important components of our musical world. They produce the pitches and rhythms that make up sounded music. Accordingly, advanced music students receive much instruction in music theory and technical training on how to operate instruments. Although performance technique and knowledge of music theory are essential to musicians, *people* are the most important elements of music. People are responsible for the emotion in music. Therefore, aspiring musicians really cannot optimally advance their craft without considering the insights offered by psychology.

For decades, British psychologist John Sloboda has been one of the most influential researchers in the psychology of music; he was responsible for advancing the field greatly in the late 20th century and was one of the authors of the first edition of this text. In his seminal book *The Musical Mind* (1985), he eloquently explained:

> If emotional factors are fundamental to the existence of music, then the fundamental question for a psychological investigation into music is *how* music is able to affect people. Seen with the cold eye of physics a musical

Psychology for Musicians. Robert H. Woody, Oxford University Press. © Oxford University Press 2022.
DOI: 10.1093/oso/9780197546598.003.0001

event is just a collection of sounds with various pitches, durations, and other measurable qualities. Somehow the human mind endows the sounds with significance. They become symbols for something other than pure sound, something which enables us to laugh or cry, like or dislike, be moved or be indifferent. (p. 1)

Readers should find practical value in this book's coverage of psychology regardless of whether they focus their musical energies on performance, music teaching, or creative production (e.g., as composers, songwriters, recording engineers/producers), or just as hobbyists who make music as a leisure activity. Although the title of this book indicates it is "for musicians," it also embraces a broad definition of what *musicians* are. This term, of course, includes people who make a career of music and those who receive advanced training in it. The term *musician* can also be applied to people who lead musically active lives, even if only in their spare time. Regardless of whether they use the label musician to describe themselves, most people would like to be more musical. This book offers insights that can help all people advance their musical lives beyond a current level.

This first chapter introduces the psychology of music as a field of study. Readers can expect to learn about these major points:

1. Although music is *not* a universal language (as is commonly said), it is a universally human phenomenon. Truly understanding a particular piece or style of music, however, necessarily requires cultural familiarity.
2. In people's most meaningful musical experiences, the three broad contributors are (a) the music, (b) situational factors, and (c) the people themselves.
3. Insight into human thinking and behavior, as provided by a psychological perspective, can be beneficial to musicians of all kinds.
4. Musicianship is best understood as a skill set that is acquired. As such, all music making is governed by underlying cognitive and psychomotor processes. Improving one's musicianship necessarily involves psychological skill building.

Insight into Music and Humankind

Music psychology may sound like a highly specialized field of study, and strictly speaking it is. Psychologists who choose to focus on exploring human musical behaviors are surely specializing their research efforts. On the other hand, though, music psychology can address some rather "big picture" issues. Considering the origins of psychology and music as fields of study, it is easy to see why music psychology can approach some profound topics related to the human experience and the most meaningful moments in life.

Psychology as a discipline emerged as an offshoot of philosophy, which is understood to be the study of knowledge, reality, and existence. It cannot get more "big picture" than that. Much early psychological study centered around understanding human beings in terms of temperament and consciousness. As the field evolved through the 20th century, psychologists took greater interest in developing theories to explain broad phenomena such as human behavior, emotion, thought, and memory.

Music also is an extraordinarily human field of study. Music is an important branch of the arts, and one that in one form or another is extremely popular—even beloved—among people worldwide. The arts are understood to be concerned primarily with creative expression of the human experience. Those who have studied music from a distinctly psychological perspective have called it a "human obsession" (Levitin, 2006) and a phenomenon that "reveals what it means to be human" (Williamson, 2014).

Music is an integral part of virtually all human cultures. Anthropologist Alan Merriam (1964) was one of the first to conduct research toward explaining why music is so important to human beings worldwide. His work led him to create a cross-cultural and comprehensive list of functions that music plays in human societies, which comprised the following:

1. Emotional expression
2. Aesthetic enjoyment
3. Entertainment
4. Communication
5. Symbolic representation
6. Physical response
7. Enforcing conformity to social norms
8. Validation of social institutions and religious rituals
9. Contribution to the continuity and stability of culture
10. Contribution to the integration of society

Surely, in the 1960s, no one could have foreseen how digital technology and telecom transmission of information would result in our musical world changing as it has. Although people now make and share music with each other in vastly different *ways* than in the mid-20th century, the *functions* of music are remarkably similar. Over a half century later, Merriam's list still holds up well.

Music is more ubiquitous in the modern world than ever before. It is so readily accessible that often people may use it simply out of habit, with their musical choices serving as something like a soundtrack to their lives and an expression of identity. With music occupying so much of their leisure time and accompanying diverse activities such as traveling, house-cleaning, exercising, and socializing (Clark et al., 2010; North et al., 2004), people use music to express "who they are" to both themselves and others. Having a clear and secure sense of identity is critical to psychological health and socioemotional well-being. Without question, for many people, music is a substantial contributor to identity development, whether they interact with it somehow as consumers or music makers.

Strangely, music's power and prevalence in society have been viewed by some as reasons not to invest more into its conservation (Njoora, 2015) but to devalue it, including as curricular matter. Kelly (2002) suggested it is a curious paradox that "widespread availability makes many people take music for granted as just another commodity" (p. 41). Some musicians seem to unwittingly acquiesce to this perspective by focusing their efforts exclusively on musical forms that are esoteric and presenting music education as a special opportunity, of which relatively few students are worthy.

Of course, an activity that is native to a culture does not disqualify it from a valued place in formal education. For example, in the United States virtually all children who enter formal schooling with English as their native language still receive years of English education, usually for the entirety of their elementary and secondary school experiences. Music need not be any different. The fact that music is so pervasive and universally human can be viewed as reason that it *should* necessarily be included in school curricula, and that all children should be afforded opportunity for music learning. Psychological research supports the perspective that *all* people have the capacity to become musical.

Music and Language

The previous example of native English speakers benefiting from English education is but one example of similarities between language and music.

Before discussing those similarities further, however, it must be clearly stated here that *music is not a universal language* as has been said by many. Music is language-like—it can be used for purposes of communication—but it is *not universally understood*. To *understand* a kind of music that is heard, a listener must first *know* it.

In other words, music can sound foreign to a listener. As with a language, to understand some music that is heard, a listener must have some familiarity with the culture from which it originates. Native English speakers need not be *fluent in* Spanish to know the meaning of some Spanish phrases they hear, but they must have some familiarity with the language to understand. The same is true for music. Even people who are highly experienced with Western music can find themselves thoroughly bewildered when hearing non-Western music. A language psychologist made this point when he explained that music and language systems vary widely from culture to culture, recalling having once "overheard Western-trained music scholars dismiss Javanese gamelan as 'clanging pots' and traditional Chinese opera as 'cackling hens'" (Ludden, 2015).

The main similarity of music to language is that people can use it to communicate with each other. Of course, music and language do not use the same constituent elements to accomplish their communication. Language uses vocalized sounds (phonemes), which are put together to form words that have meaning (morphemes), and the combination of words to express ideas is guided by a set of rules (syntax). Sound is also the "stuff" of music, but it is used differently. The meaning expressed by musical sounds is not as specific and literal as it is with language. Rather than combining words, musicians organize and combine expressive sounds to use their properties (e.g., pitch, rhythm, loudness, tempo, timbre) to communicate. The difference in communicativeness between language and music can account for why some artists choose language as their primary medium—for example, poets, authors, and storytellers—while others choose music. And some artists use both: singers, songwriters, choral and opera composers.

Music is also like language in that it is naturally learned (McMullen & Saffran, 2004). Just as young children typically gain command of their native language before they ever start formal schooling, most young people have many formative experiences with music in informal settings before they ever start deliberately learning it through school or other lessons. Informal learning processes start very early for people; this is especially true with cultural staples like language and music. With their native language, infants *hear* the words spoken by the people around them and come to *identify patterns* in the sounds they hear. At some point, they begin to *vocally imitate* what they have heard. Their first speaking attempts may sound like rough approximations and may overpatternize words they have heard (e.g., "daddy" becomes "da-da" and "bottle" sounds like "bah-bah"). Gradually, their baby talk becomes more recognizable speech, and eventually they string words together to make phrases to express themselves. Once this process has taken place with a few favorite words, then more are learned, and typically quite quickly. Children are then on their way to achieving *speech fluency* with their native language, and with it they take part in the enjoyable language activities of childhood, all of which further fast-track language development. They recite memorized texts (e.g., nursery rhymes or the words of picture books read to them), retell known story materials (e.g., folktales and personal stories told to them by caregivers), and eventually spontaneously create original stories of their own.

These rather sophisticated language abilities are all learned *by ear* and as a result of everyday interaction with other people. Once children possess these ear-based speech competencies, they are ready to understand the written symbols that are used to represent their native language. They learn these symbols (called letters for the English language) as they are linked to the sounds that the children already know so well as speakers of the language.

This developmental sequence of language learning can transfer quite well to informal music learning too. The musical development of children starts early as they first have opportunity to *listen to* the sounds of their native music culture and come to *identify patterns* in what they hear. They then try to *imitate* what they have heard. Over time, their rough approximations of music give way to recognizable melodies and rhythms. Soon they achieve a degree of musical fluency and can sing music material from memory (e.g., lullabies or play songs sung to them), reproduce known songs and rhythms (learned from other people and recordings), and even improvise original musical ideas.

People need not be born "highly intelligent" or otherwise specially gifted to become a fluent speaker of their native language and eventually to learn to read and write it. The same is true with music. The development described previously is typical for language acquisition and also for music development when children grow up hearing music and have the opportunity to playfully make it themselves.

Enculturation and Acculturation

The process by which people learn elements of their native culture—like language and music—is called *enculturation*. Communities of people have certain values, customs, and activities that they share with each other. Growing up in their native communities, children gradually take on for themselves their group's characteristics and norms. The learning accomplished through enculturation is understood to occur unintentionally and to take place in informal social settings rather than through any kind of formal educational means.

Enculturation has been described as the "process of socialization to and maintenance of the norms of one's heritage culture, including the salient values, ideas, and concepts" (Kim & Alamilla, 2017, p. 28). The fact that ideas, concepts, and customs are among the elements transmitted through enculturation tells us that *learning of knowledge and skills* is culturally constrained. *Constructivism* is a prominent theoretical school in psychology: it states that through interaction with their social environments, people construct individual versions of knowledge (because psychomotor skills reside in the mind, they are best understood as a type of knowledge too—*procedural knowledge*). Knowledge is constructed in people's minds as they find meaning in their experiences. There is a certain cumulative effect indicated by constructivism: people are selective in what they attend to, process, and learn, and that selectivity is influenced by prior personally constructed knowledge. Through repeated exposure and interaction with certain values and activities, people can attain impressive expertise of complex knowledge and sophisticated skills; the knowledge and skill that make up that expertise, however, are culturally limited.

Most relevant to musicianship, skill development is greatly impacted by cultural context, with respect to both time and place. A child born in 18th-century Europe likely had greater opportunity and interest to become a skilled violinist, certainly in comparison to someone born in 20th-century New York City. That American child would have been more likely to aspire to become a skilled musician of a different kind, perhaps a freestyle rapper, hip-hop singer, or jazz musician.

The cultural nature of musical skills can also be seen in the fact that the proficiency of young instrumentalists has soared over the past century as expectations have risen and competition has grown (Lehmann & Ericsson, 1998). For example, Franz Liszt's Transcendental Étude No. 5 in B♭, "Feux follets," once considered to be performable only by the world's top concert pianist masters, can now be heard at national junior piano competitions (teenage pianists). Moreover, there are pieces for nearly every instrument that were deemed practically unplayable at the time of their composition, such as Beethoven's Hammerklavier Sonata, that are today part of the standard repertoire. Performance skill expansion is particularly tangible when, technologically, modifications of instruments emerge (e.g., electric guitar). Thus, certain musical skills can increase or decrease over time depending on the demand for them in society. After Benjamin Franklin invented the glass harmonica in 1761, the instrument enjoyed significant popularity well into the 19th century, with prominent composers writing for it (e.g., Mozart, Beethoven, and Berlioz) and numerous musicians aspiring for and attaining virtuoso-level performance on it. In modern times, however, despite occasional use by creative musicians looking for an unusual and ethereal sound, the glass harmonica is largely unknown and virtually extinct. Nobody would assert that some people are just born with a natural talent for playing the glass harmonica, like so many do for players of current prevalent and popular instruments, such as piano and drums.

Of course, culture can be defined beyond obvious characteristics of geographic location, nationality, ethnicity, and religion. Demographic factors can be so prominent that they practically define a culture of which a young would-be musician is a member. A community's educational values can greatly affect musical development. In one cultural community, it may be the norm to encourage children to pursue musical growth through formal education, such as school music involvement or instrumental/voice lessons with a one-to-one "private teacher." If a different community, however, has a general low regard for schooling and formal lessons, an aspiring young musician may develop through more informal settings.

Those people whose musical involvement takes place predominantly in formal instructional settings tend to gain entry into a different culture, in this case one that is essentially defined by its values and practices having to do with music. In many cases, these musical values and practices differ significantly from those gained through enculturation in people's general heritage cultures. Thus, if a formal music instructional setting becomes the context in which most of a person's musical involvement occurs, it can become a dominant culture, at least musically. Psychological *acculturation* is the process by which people assimilate to a dominant culture that is different from their original one (Kim & Alamilla, 2017). Although the term *acculturation* is often used to describe the cultural adjustment that immigrants undergo after relocating to a new country, this process surely happens with people whose music experiences occur mostly in formal educational settings. The value system of formal music education includes a high regard for Western art music (i.e., classical music) over all others. This musical culture values the use of music notation over exclusively ear-based musicianship (e.g., playing music by ear, improvising) and values sophistication and innovation in compositional structure, which necessitates the study of music theory and the elevation of "masterworks" written by celebrated Western composers.

Another interesting example of how historical/cultural context affects musicianship is how different music notation systems have developed in the Western music world. The standard notation used in formal music education is quite different from the tablature, or TAB, used by guitarists in the popular music world. Standard music notation evolved in Europe before sound recording had been invented. Thus, music notation was the only means that composers had to capture their musical ideas. In that time and place in history, notation was needed to transmit to musicians *what* to perform. In contrast, TAB has existed in a time and place in which sound recordings of music have been readily available. Accordingly, instrumentalists in this musical culture are adept at learning music by ear. From their avid listening to music, they know *what* the music is supposed to sound like, so they look to TAB to inform them of *how* to perform it.

Music and culture are inextricably linked. This is certainly seen in the aforementioned list of musical functions offered by 1960s anthropologist Alan Merriam. More recently, Clayton (2016) proposed that human beings use music for four broad purposes:

1. Regulation of emotional, cognitive, or physiological state. This includes using music in ways we typically call entertainment (e.g., to amuse or captivate). It also includes less common uses of music—at least less common in some cultures—such as using music to induce trance. It also includes people's use of music to manage mood, whether it be the everyday way to "help pass the time" during household chores or using music for therapeutic means to reduce pain, anxiety, and stress (Nilsson, 2008).

2. Mediation between self and other (e.g., communication, worship). Music commonly serves as a tool for human interaction. Such music-facilitated interactions may be between people, as when artists use

the expressiveness of sound to communicate their emotional states to others. People also use music to get in touch with feelings or "voices" within themselves and to interact with the spiritual (e.g., God, ancestral spirits).

3. Symbolic representation (e.g., advertising; nationalism). Although in many cases the message of a piece of music is ambiguous (allowing it to be relatable by a larger number of people), nonetheless music can effectively signify objects and ideas outside of itself. Musical motifs as brief as a few pitches or a single chord have been used in commercial advertising, and many nations and heads of state have officially designated musical anthems that signify them (e.g., "Hail to the Chief" as a musical symbol of the office of the president of the United States).

4. Coordination of action (e.g., dancing; social movements). Human beings seem to have a natural tendency for entrainment, the synchronization of physical action to external stimuli, including music. It can be seen in the cross-cultural ubiquity of dance and other individual physio-musical movements, such as swaying and foot-tapping to music.

It is interesting to note that in addition to using music in a sociocultural context, people use it for more individual and personal purposes. That is, music is often used—or perhaps it is most visible when it is used—for *interpersonal* functions, such as sharing emotions and conveying other expressive "messages" to others, and bonding with other people; music is also used for *intrapersonal* means (e.g., meditation, affirming identity to oneself, emotional catharsis).

Meaningful Moments

Indeed, *emotion* seems to be the most important aspect of music (and many would say of all the arts more generally). Among those who identify as musicians, *emotional expression* usually is considered to be the paramount quality of performed music. And among music listeners, at both the casual and connoisseur levels, having an *emotional response* to music is often the primary criterion by which they judge their liking or appreciation of it.

The experience of powerful emotion largely explains why people often speak of the "magic of music." Profoundly emotional moments have been the subject of psychological study for decades. Humanistic psychologist Abraham Maslow in the 1960s emphasized the importance of "peak experiences" as deeply moving moments that have an exhilarating, elevating, or even mystical-like effect on people. Later in the 1980s and 1990s, the idea of "flow experiences" was advanced by Hungarian-American psychologist Mihaly Csikszentmihalyi (1990). Flow is characterized by immersive feelings of energizing focus, a loss of self-consciousness and worry, and even an altered sense of time.

Not surprisingly, the emotional power of music has been frequently cited in psychological discussions of peak experiences and flow. Research specifically studying the psychology of music has concluded that strong emotional experiences with music are multifaceted and can be categorized as physical, quasi-physical, perceptual, cognitive, and emotional (Gabrielsson, 2010). Often, the most powerful music experiences take place at live performance events, occur in the company of others, and are perceived by people to be emotionally positive (Lamont, 2011b). The research indicates that strong experiences with music result from the interaction of three broad factors: (1) *the music*, (2) *the person*, and (3) *the situation* (Gabrielsson, 2010).

The sound properties of *the music* that make it emotionally expressive include timbre, rhythm, pitch, tempo, dynamics, and articulation. It is perhaps the most important role of composers and performers to create the sound properties that will effectively communicate emotionally with a listening audience. Listeners can be quite good at decoding emotion from musicians' sound properties, especially when it comes to basic emotions such as happiness, anger, and sadness (Akkermans et al., 2019). Although some research has shown musicians *can* effectively convey emotions to listeners, other studies have shown that they sometimes fail to do so reliably. Even among advanced musicians, expressive intentions may not translate into the sound properties of performance without applying explicit attention to the process (Juslin & Laukka, 2000; Woody, 2002a, 2003).

The other two factors of strong experiences with music are *the person* (i.e., the listener/audience member) and *the situation*, and these two factors can be difficult to distinguish from each other. For example, audience members' judgments about what they hear in live performances tend to be affected by what they see. This bias likely results both from audience members' personal ideas about physical beauty and from nonmusical situational factors, such as the performance venue, performer wardrobe, and stage behavior. Quite a few research studies have confirmed that what people hear—or *think* they hear—can be heavily influenced by the ideas they bring into a musical experience and by nonmusical factors around a performance situation. Listeners who believe a musician is a prestigious performer are likely to judge the music heard to be of higher quality. Similarly, judgments of *musical sound* quality can be greatly influenced by *visual* judgments of performer attractiveness (Griffiths, 2010).

By acknowledging the two nonmusical factors that contribute to strong emotional experiences, music performers need not feel weakened. On the contrary, they may be in a better position to create powerful performances with a realistic awareness that factors beyond their sounded performance affect how listeners perceive their music. Instead of passively accepting performance conventions that may not benefit the experiences of modern audiences, musicians may decide to assert some decision-making power around the nonmusical situational aspects of their performances. More broadly, musicians may choose to be more deliberate in building a public image and in selecting the enterprises to which they lend their music making. Indeed, musicians should recognize that among potential future audience members, past personal associations or reminiscences will affect responses to presently heard music (Gabrielsson, 2010).

Contributions of Psychology

Gaining actionable insight into people's strong emotional experiences with music (described earlier) is just one example of how understanding psychology can empower musicians to carry out their craft better. Of course, the term *psychology* can mean very different things to different people. Especially outside of the academic world, the word *psychology* is often used to describe the mental makeup of people: one might say that a good youth coach needs to understand the psychology of preteen kids. Among others, *psychology* is a section in a bookstore that is filled with self-help publications. Even within the academic world, *psychology* can refer to different fields of scholarly work. Some psychological inquiry reflects the field's early origins in philosophy (mentioned earlier in this chapter), relying on scholarly introspection and examination and questioning of cumulated knowledge and theories of human mind and emotion.

Subdisciplines that would fall under the heading of philosophy-oriented psychology include phenomenology, psychoanalysis, and humanistic psychology.

The type of psychology that is central to this book is best described as scientific psychology. This type of psychological inquiry places a premium on careful observation of human behavior as indicators of internal mental processes, and on using scientific methods to test theories seeking to explain human behavior, emotion, and thought processes. Subdisciplines that tend to be scientific include experimental, developmental, social, and educational psychology.

The science of psychology values *objectivity* in its research methods. That is, psychological researchers are expected to take measures to reduce as much as possible the threat of bias or personal beliefs influencing accurate observation and assessment of behavior studied. Objectivity in a research study's methods is key to its results being trustworthy. For specific research results to be dependable and useful to the larger field of psychology, those results are expected to be testable and reproducible by others. This points to another important value of scientific psychology, namely *generalizability*, or the ability of research results to be applied to other contexts that are similar to that of the original research study.

A third important value in scientific psychology is *explanation*. In other words, it is not enough for music psychologists to discover through research that, say, a certain practicing strategy results in better musical performance quality. In disseminating their research in scientific circles, the music psychologists would be expected to offer a *theory to explain why* the certain practice strategy was so effective. In fact, the best psychological research of this type would have been designed to test a previously developed theory and to gather evidence that either supports or refutes it.

In our science-exposed modern society, the value of explanation can seem well accepted. If you really *understand* something, it seems obvious that in addition to knowing "what works," you should also know *why* it does. But this scientific mindset may not be so well accepted in certain musical circles. Science has long been pitted as an adversary of the arts. In fact, when people cannot or will not offer an explanation of a skill of theirs, they may just insist that what they do is "more of an art than a science." Even among the most dedicated and hard-working musicians, some still seem to prefer to attribute their musicianship to unknowable supernatural or mystical factors than to explainable actions of their own.

Obviously, some musicians doubt that science can provide any useful insights into the arts. In fact, they may fear that by explaining musical phenomena in objective, scientific terms, the magic of music may somehow be ruined. Such an unfounded fear could actually be interpreted as reflecting a low regard for music. A music psychologist's perspective is that the processes of music need not remain mysterious for its power to be remarkable. Indeed, the more musical discoveries that are made by scientific psychology, the more music is shown to be an amazing human phenomenon.

Those involved in the research enterprise of scientific psychology (and the other human sciences) are usually quite careful to communicate the details of their work clearly and to be cautious in applying their results. For example, good scientific researchers will never assert that their research has "proven" anything. They will, however, present their research findings as evidence that is supportive of psychological theories they seek to advance. When research results are presented in overly bold ways—for example, headlines such as "Playing a Musical Instrument Shown to Relieve Stress" or "Statistics Show Music Students Score Better on Standardized Tests"—the claims are usually oversimplifications and overgeneralizations not made by the researchers themselves. Well-intentioned writers and media members may paraphrase the research to make it more accessible to the general public, who want to avoid wading through academic jargon. Other times, though, people may cite research simply to bolster their own position on an issue, using authoritative phrases such as "Research proves . . . " or "Statistics show . . . ." As a result, what began as good scientific research can end up being mishandled and its findings applied too broadly. One of the worst music examples of this came in the 1990s with the so-called Mozart effect. The original study found that college undergrads (not music majors) did better on a spatial reasoning task after listening to a 10-minute Mozart piano piece, as compared to spending the same amount of time sitting in silence or listening to a relaxation tape. Yet the results in this very specific context somehow morphed into a simplistic movement, "music makes you smarter," which was embraced by far too many in the field of music education.

Good psychological research can share much in common with artistic creativity in that it is often stimulated by a human spirit of curiosity and exploration. The fascinating power of music is not spoiled by careful consideration of its component processes and effects. Rather, greater study of the phenomenon of music typically leads to enhanced appreciation of it.

Music as Acquired Skill

This book considers musicianship as the result of the processes of *skill acquisition*, and not the result of the endowment of innate talent. Recall that in the discussion in this chapter's earlier "Insight into Music and Humankind" section, music compares similarly to language in how it is learned. Just as no newborn baby ever appeared in the hospital delivery room already speaking its native language, no baby has ever been born already displaying recognizable musical abilities. Thus, in a sense, we all know that musical ability—like language fluency—is acquired. And though few people would contend that speaking one's native language requires special talent, many people do express the belief that being musical requires some extra capacity that some people just do not possess. They often point to cases of musical prodigies and virtuosos to support their certainty that inborn musical talent must be real.

In the enduring nature-nurture debate (on how to explain advanced human abilities), this book favors the nurture explanation, because the best psychological research supports this. It must be acknowledged, however, that the nature explanation remains heavily preferred among many musicians. There are a number of reasons the talent explanation has been perpetuated. The psychological phenomenon of availability cascade is a self-reinforcing process by which a collective belief gains more and more plausibility through its increasing repetition (see Tversky & Kahneman, 1973, for a seminal psychological study, and Wang et al., 2016, for more recent neuropsychological coverage). Although concepts of inborn musical talent may have once only been a common belief, it grew closer to becoming a well-accepted fact because it was proliferated through repetitious cultural transmission.

Instead of attributing it to innate talent, advanced musicianship is better understood as the acquisition of a set of musical skills. The concept of acquired skills is a robust and scientifically supported explanation of how people become musical. This explanation of musicianship cannot be reduced to simplistic adages that point to a single factor of supreme importance, such as "hard work wins out," "practice makes perfect," or "nothing breeds success like a positive mental attitude."

Many factors contribute to the acquisition of musical skills. They include physiological traits, cultural influences, childhood exposure and experiences, opportunity and support, a variety of motivational sources, education, and practice (both formal and informal). A thorough explanation of these factors comprise the contents of the remaining chapters of this book.

Musicians of all kinds can benefit from insight into the processes of musical skill acquisition. With increased understanding of how people become musical—even to the point of attaining advanced musicianship—music performers and creatives can better manage their own activities toward greater fulfillment, and music teachers can maximize the effectiveness of the learning experiences they provide their students.

The notion of innate talent is not just misguided; it can be educationally harmful to would-be music learners (Hoffman, 2015; Lamont, 2011a; Ruddock, 2012). Some 20 years ago, eminent music psychologist John Sloboda (2000) lamented that talent remained as one of the favorite concepts in the "folk psychology of the musical world" and explained that by invoking the concepts of "talent" and "inspiration," the underlying processes of music making are kept shrouded in mystery. "They have no explanatory power," he wrote, "but their power in the lives and motivations of individuals can be disproportionate. The number of people who disengage from musical activity based on the belief that they 'lack musical talent' constitutes a continuing cultural and educational tragedy" (p. 398).

Acquiring musical skill (this book's recommended alternative to the talent account of musical ability) is a decidedly psychological undertaking. A specifically cognitive perspective is helpful because the skills that a musician possesses are stored in the mind and learning is understood to be adding new skills to one's mental storage. Accomplished musicians' skill sets are composed of conceptual knowledge (information or ideas) and physical skills. Conceptual knowledge is sometimes called "declarative knowledge" because it is usually readily defined in words; skills are sometimes called "procedural knowledge" because they refer to what someone knows *how to do*.

One certain conclusion derived from psychological consideration of music is the perspective of skill development. That is, all people *become* musical. Musicianship—even the advanced musicianship of virtuoso performers—is best understood as a skill set that is developed.

Taking the Stage: Plan and Practice Emotional Expression

Each chapter in this book contains a "Taking the Stage" sidebar box, which focuses on a particular research finding and offers a practical application of it for performing musicians. For example, recall the research finding presented earlier in the chapter that musicians' expressive intentions do not always reliably translate into the sound properties of performance that listeners depend on to move their emotions. Instead of dwelling on their own inner intentions and trusting that their emotions will naturally infuse their music, some performers may significantly improve their expressiveness by paying more conscious attention to the sound properties they produce—and critically evaluating how listeners perceive them. Consider a pianist who wishes to communicate joy and frivolity in a melody she is performing. To play the melody expressively, she may simply recall a very festive and joyful occasion in her past and try to muster up the feelings she had then. This strategy may not be the most effective one to take. In fact, the process of emoting could divert her attention from accurately hearing whether her sounded music contains expressive properties that are perceptible to listeners, and her own felt emotion could wrongfully convince her of the expressiveness of her music. Instead of merely dwelling on her own felt emotions, a better approach may be to generate an explicit plan for the sound properties (i.e., expressive variations in loudness, tempo, and articulation) of the melody she is performing.

Leading Learning: Advocate Music for Its Unique Benefits

Each chapter in this book contains a "Leading Learning" sidebar box, which applies a research finding to the practical context of music teachers' work with students. The text earlier mentioned the inclination of some to devalue music as a school curricular subject, in part because music is already so prevalent in human cultures. This perspective can appear occasionally when school districts face budget shortfalls and are forced to re-examine the value of their offerings to students. It seems that nobody debates the necessity of schools providing instruction in language literacy or math, but some inevitably wonder if schools can afford to have music programs. Music teachers can effectively dispel a "music as frill" perspective by accepting the responsibility of educating other parents, school administrators, and other stakeholders—along with their students—about the unique contribution of music learning in the educational enterprise. Also, they can more easily defend music's place in the curriculum if their modus operandi more resembles that of a "core" academic subject rather than an extracurricular activity. Music course offerings should have clearly stated student learning objectives that center around music's unique ability to provide people with a means of artistic creativity and self-expression. Their teaching efforts should focus on guiding every individual student to attain those objectives, with publicly shared group performances as a by-product of this learning (not vice versa). With these things in place, music teachers can more easily and honestly promote the value of music based on its own merits.

Chapter 1 Discussion Questions

1. Recall the "Taking the Stage" box earlier in the chapter. Have you ever been in the audience when a performer onstage acted as though his or her music making was emotionally intense, but you just did not hear much expressiveness in the musical sounds being produced? What could have led to that performer being so misguided?
2. Would you say that emotional experience has been at the heart of your most meaningful moments with music? Can you share a specific occasion that illustrates this in a powerful way?
3. Recall the "Leading Learning" box earlier in the chapter. Thinking back on your own musical development, were you ever told that you were "gifted"? If so, did you then expect things to come more easily to you?

2

Development

Although few adults in the general population call themselves musicians, the vast majority say they like music very much. Many people are musically active as listeners and concertgoers despite possessing little skill as music makers themselves. While all too aware of this divergence, some express regret at not learning more about music earlier in life when they could have. Others describe being musical as a dream that was never realistically attainable because they were not born with the innate talent required. Can all children become musical? How can they (and their parents and teachers) know if they have "what it takes" to become a musician?

These kinds of questions are best answered with an understanding of the developmental psychology of music. In the previous chapter, psychology was described as a discipline that seeks to explain human behavior, emotion, thought, and memory. The subfield of *developmental psychology* is concerned with the human being's lifelong process of change. In studying the changes—physical, mental, and behavioral—that human beings typically undergo, psychologists have identified that people's development across the lifespan is affected by a variety of biological, socioemotional, and environmental factors. Traditionally, developmental psychologists have focused their efforts on the maturation process by which children become adults. This has served the field of music education well because most music teaching has been directed toward children and adolescents. In more recent years, however, both developmental psychology and music education have paid greater attention to various stages of adult life, from emerging adulthood to old age (Hargreaves & Lamont, 2017).

Perhaps the greatest contribution of developmental psychology is the explication of the growth and increasing capabilities that emerge across childhood. Changes in physical development are often obvious; most people would realize it impractical to have four-year-olds begin instrumental music studies on the tuba. Not so evident, however, is the emergence of other cognitive and fine motor skill capability in young people. When can we expect young children to have the aural perception and voice control needed to

Psychology for Musicians. Robert H. Woody, Oxford University Press. © Oxford University Press 2022.
DOI: 10.1093/oso/9780197546598.003.0002

musically match pitch and sing accurately? At what age can most children begin instrumental music studies and expect to have a successful and rewarding experience?

The ability to answer such questions highlights the practical value of developmental psychology. Historically, one of the most important contributors to the scientific study of human development was Swiss psychologist Jean Piaget. He was the first to provide a systematic account of children's development in terms of a fixed sequence of stages through which most children pass in the same order at comparable ages (Piaget, 1958). To identify the sequence of developmental stages, he devised a set of tasks presented to children as games or puzzles, which most children would invariably get wrong or answer randomly at one age but which the same children would almost invariably get right a few months later.

In the mid-20th century, a number of researchers explored how musical development may fit with Piagetian stage theory. This included Pflederer (1964), who sought to find a musical equivalent of Piaget's conservation tasks, in which the key to children solving a puzzle was their ability to understand that a particular property of something can stay constant even while elements around it change. More recently, music psychologist David Hargreaves proposed a phase model of artistic development that indicates five age-related phases through which developing musicians pass; though the model borrows some of Piaget's terminology (e.g., "sensorimotor" is the earliest phase, and "conservation" of melodic properties is an indicator of a later developmental phase), it also was designed to "avoid the Piagetian connotations of logical-scientific thinking, which may well be quite inappropriate in the arts" (Hargreaves & Lamont, 2017, p. 18).

Psychological research suggests the following principles about human musical development, which will be elucidated throughout this chapter:

1. Human beings are "hardwired" to be musical. Rather than a special gift endowed upon only a few, musical *talent* is best understood as a skill set that is acquired as the result of a number of powerful contributing factors.

2. There is a predictable progression in which children typically develop musical abilities. This development is more an outcome of enculturation and experience than education.

3. Children can quickly assimilate the musical system that they are exposed to early in life and come to hear and understand music much

like adults do. Children who become particularly interested in and committed to music can rapidly build their musical abilities to impressive levels.

4. Music activities—both formal and informal—can be extremely important in the lives of adolescents and young adults. Music can become a primary context in which young people develop cognitively, emotionally, and socially, and for some artistically and professionally.

5. The experiences and education received as a child typically are very consequential in determining the level of musical expertise a person attains later in life.

Musical Humanity

A commonly held view is that musical ability is somewhat rare within the population. According to this view, only a few talented individuals can become musicians, and so a key task for the music profession is the early detection of talent so that it may be properly encouraged and nurtured. Music teachers may consider their educational efforts best used if they focus on those young people with the requisite musical talent, rather than haphazardly spreading their teaching among all children.

Over the centuries, Western culture's preferred explanation for the exceptional ability of certain people has shifted from the theological (e.g., "a gift from God") to the metaphysical/supernatural (e.g., "otherworldly" abilities and "mad genius") and more recently to the scientific. A shift to the scientific has largely eluded the arts, within which subjectivity and creative inspiration are considered hallmarks, and thus supposedly poorly suited to be explained rationally. This is unfortunate because researchers have done well explaining how exceptional music performance skill results from a combination of physiological traits and environmental catalysts (McPherson & Williamon, 2016). Still, many within the music world embrace and proclaim innate talent as the chief determinant of musicianship.

Talent: Aptitude or Skill?

Modern broadcast media may have contributed to the perpetuation of the innate talent account of musical performance ability. The discovery of an exceptional child performer—"the next Mozart" is a common label—makes for a much better story than reporting how advanced musical learning has resulted from an unusually plentiful combination of environmental, educational, and economic factors. Beyond simple media sensationalism, however, the belief in talent offers other appealing effects. Giving the musically talented person the designation of specialness can turn the experience of a concert into a fantastic, even supernatural, happening. Plus, musicians themselves can benefit from the "gifted" label. Feeling special—or even divinely blessed—can contribute to musicians' self-esteem and motivation; consequently, many "talented" musicians feel an obligation to nurture their gift, which allows them to approach their musical activities with confidence and the expectation of success (see Chapter 3).

From the perspective of scientific psychology, however, there are many reasons to doubt the existence of inborn musical talent and to challenge attempts to identify and measure it. Talent is defined and understood to be a "special natural ability or aptitude" or a "natural capacity for success" ("Talent," 2021). Educational researchers have aspired to measure aptitude and have designed some sophisticated measurement instruments; some of the tests commonly used by educators and researchers to measure musical aptitude include the Seashore Measures of Musical Talents (Seashore, 1960), the Wing Standardised Tests of Musical Intelligence (Wing, 1981), and the Gordon Measures of Music Audiation (Gordon, 1986a, 1986b, 1989). In general, these are tests of musical ability but are considered measures of aptitude because the musical abilities measured do not result from formal music instruction or training on specific instruments. They tend to test perception, rather than performance, and the most common type of test involves listening to two short musical sequences and judging whether they are the same as or different from each other with regard to pitch and rhythm. The ability to detect smaller differences is interpreted as indicative of greater musical aptitude.

Not all people accept this interpretation and the general assumption that more finely tuned music perception is innate. While some may believe greater musical skill is the result of being born with a brain well suited for music, an alternative explanation is the converse, that a different (more musical) brain results from engagement in music perceptual activity. The latter explanation appears to find support from brain research. For example, differences in brain structural neuroplasticity between highly trained pianists and nonmusicians has been linked to their sustained musical training; furthermore, the pianist structural brain characteristics are more pronounced in those who began piano study early in childhood as compared to those with a later onset of piano playing (Vaquero et al., 2016). There are many studies showing how the brain is altered by experience (Kolb, 2018).

The practice of music aptitude testing has been criticized by many in the fields of music psychology and music education, in part for formal definitions of aptitude being far from real-world musicality and the tests themselves having poor validity (Karma, 2007; Law & Zentner, 2012). It is problematic to measure a human capacity—whether it is intelligence, musicality, or athletic potential—when a definition usually borrows much from concepts of physical capacity. For example, people in sports often talk about a particularly talented athlete having a "higher ceiling" than others. Or in music, a young singer with much potential may be said to have a lot of room in which to fill out as a performer. However, talk of ceilings and room to develop depends on the metaphor of physical capacity, which breaks down quickly when it comes to psychological measurement. The capacity of a physical structure, say, the seating capacity of the main auditorium of Carnegie Hall, is measurable because the structure of the building and seats are physically present and fixed. To measure the capacity, simply count the seats or otherwise measure the floorspace limited by the extant walls. The task of measuring how much musicality a human being can someday possess is far more difficult, and some would say impossible. After all, how can any tool measure what is not there (yet)?

Seemingly undaunted by this conundrum, advocates of aptitude testing take the approach of measuring current musical ability present in people and interpreting it as an indicator of capacity rather than learning. This approach has led to peculiar definitions of the term *aptitude*. One enduring book about psychological measurement in music education defines aptitude as "including the result of genetic endowment and maturation plus whatever musical skills may develop without formal musical education" (Boyle & Radocy, 1987). Gordon (2003) defined music aptitude as both a person's inborn musical potential and a function of informal and formal music environment during childhood. Given these definitions that encompass learning, aptitude testing has little to contribute to the nature-nurture debate. Such efforts to measure aptitude necessarily deviate from a plain-language understanding of talent. Aptitude tests cannot actually measure a natural capacity because researchers' and test designers' definitions of aptitude *add nurture to the nature*. At best, aptitude testing is a predictive endeavor that measures what can be done currently, and results are used to forecast the level of achievement that lies ahead (evidence for "predictive validity" is commonly reported with published aptitude tests).

Rather than accepting musical ability as a special endowment received by the gifted few, it is better understood to be a set of musical skills that people develop. Research has identified a number of factors that are powerful contributors to musical skill acquisition. It can be a difficult and overly academic exercise to categorize the many factors that contribute to the development of musicality. The subsections that follow offer but one way to organize such. They include Physiological Traits, Opportunity and Support, Motivational Sources, Learning, and Practice. McPherson et al. (2012) have presented a more detailed taxonomy of factors in their developmental explanation of human musicality. Theirs is a particularly insightful model in that it emphasizes the *transactional* nature of musical development. That is, as people interact with their environments, not only do the environments affect the people, but also the people affect the environments, which, of course, affect other people within them. When a person develops to be particularly musical, this result derives from the "alignment of key and often wide-ranging transactions—across social, biological, psychological, and environmental spheres—that create promotive conditions for significant musical growth" (p. 183).

Physiological Traits. Individual differences in physiological human characteristics constrain the development of musicality. Some physical traits, such as muscularity and motor control, affect musical development, including with performance skills on musical instruments. Physiological traits also include perceptual capabilities. In a most plainly evident example, children born deaf will surely come to understand music very differently from those born with typical hearing. It also has been suggested that children whose neurological makeup includes a particular sensitivity to sound may be especially attentive to and attracted to musical stimuli in their environments; such a trait would likely aid musical development (McPherson & Williamon, 2016). Finally, some theorists have posited that certain psychological traits relevant to musical development, such as creativity, emotionality, and achievement orientation, are inborn; however, results of other research suggest that temperament and personality traits are more environmentally determined and situationally displayed.

The existence of physiological and psychological traits does not denote a "music gene" that predestines someone to accomplish significant musicianship in life. Even those who advance the role of hereditary characteristics in human abilities acknowledge the complexity of establishing genetic influence, which "does not denote the hard-wired deterministic effect of a single gene but rather probabilistic propensities of many genes in multiple-gene systems" (Gagné, 2013, p. 13). Most importantly, research indicates that the physiological traits required for musical development are present in the vast majority of people, rather than being "gifted upon" a fortunate few. In answering the question of whether some children are more gifted for music than others, Sloboda (2005a) decided:

> The most consistent and educationally sound conclusion to adhere to at the present time is that if there is such a thing as musical talent (interpreted as an inborn capacity for and predisposition towards musical activity), then it exists to equal measure in the vast majority of the population, and in no way accounts for the very wide range of adult musical accomplishment that exists in the populations of industrialized societies such as ours. (p. 301)

It is incorrect to assume that all physiological attributes are genetically determined. With the exception of height and body size, people's physiological attributes are generally affected by the conditions and experiences of their lives.

Opportunity and Support. Simple exposure to music typically marks the beginning of people's musical development. Surely, children can experience very different levels of musical exposure in their lives, ranging from musically rich environments—perhaps where music is very often heard, and parents, siblings, and other caregivers frequently sing and play instruments as part of leisure time—to environments where music is virtually never present. Greater exposure leads to a better understanding of music, which amounts to better mind and brain readiness for additional growth and learning (Hallam, 2016). For young people whose early environments include much opportunity surrounding music, their development can quickly snowball. That is, musical opportunities that seem small on the surface—say, an infant having parents sing lullabies before every nap and bedtime—accumulate over time and make young people better equipped to benefit from subsequent opportunities, perhaps when the then-toddler's own music making is greeted with praise and encouragement by parents. Positive environmental factors precipitate the emergence of basic human musical behaviors and contribute to greater development of musicality.

Young people who are fortunate enough to grow up in musically rich and supportive homes are likely to have greater musical *access* too. "The opportunities to make music during childhood often require support (practical, moral, and financial) from parents, so parents' own conceptions of their children's abilities and aptitudes are clearly important" (Lamont, 2017, p. 183). Musical opportunities typically are common with parents who believe in the value of music and who believe in their children's ability to become musical. Music teachers also are providers of musical growth opportunities. Thus, two children who seem very similar on the surface can experience very different levels of exposure, opportunity, and support when it comes to music. These differences can exponentiate (snowball) and become highly consequential in development and the levels of musicality attained. The accumulation of opportunities and support helps determine people's *musical agency*, that is, the sense that they can be musical (Wiggins, 2016), with agency being a critical factor in achieving more advanced levels of musicianship.

Motivational Sources. Since musical development in children tends to co-exist with enjoyment when engaged in musical behaviors, one might conclude that a love for music is what ultimately impels people through musical development. When they get older, however, high-achieving musicians-in-training often demonstrate keen commitment to long hours of individual practice and acceptance of other challenges; these actions suggest that a strong will and work ethic are key motivational contributors to musical development.

In reality, few people become accomplished musicians as the result of any single source of motivation. Most musical development stories have as plotlines a variety of shifting and combining motivational factors. As such, understanding motivation can be complex. "Being motivated" to achieve musically also can be quite elusive, even to the most well-intentioned music-loving person. The multidimensional nature of motivation can be seen in this paradox: playing a musical instrument is intrinsically rewarding; yet, attaining the necessary skill level to enjoy the greatest musical rewards demands time, effort, and sacrifice, none of which are inherently appealing. As challenging as it is, motivation is not an unsolvable mystery. The next chapter of this book is devoted to the subject of motivation.

Learning. The general public often equates the concept of learning with schooling and teaching. Indeed, formal education can be a positive and powerful contributor to musical development. Throughout human history, however, people have acquired much knowledge and skill through informal means. This continues today, both through modern mass communication technology and through old-fashioned face-to-face social learning. Whether in a formal or informal context, some learning can occur without learners devoting conscious attention; this is surely the case with very young children, who are not yet capable of metacognition (the awareness of one's own thinking). More advanced knowledge and skill acquisition, however, requires learners to consciously apply deliberate attention and effort.

In simple terms, learning represents a *change* in knowledge or skills. Both cognitive (knowledge) and psychomotor (skill) learning are stored in the mind. Accomplished learning is the result of anything that adds to what is in the mind. Whether it takes place in a formal or informal context, learning requires *experience*, and levels of experience can vary greatly. Although a course instructor can deliver an information-packed lecture and a musical role model can demonstrate virtuosic performance technique, learners will benefit most when their experience goes beyond merely observing a lecture or model performance. With an ability-based domain such as music, learning is enhanced when students have opportunity to personally apply knowledge they have been told and to practice skills that have been demonstrated for them.

Practice. Individual practicing and ensemble rehearsing are time-honored staples of the musician's life. It is practically common sense that before performing something—especially publicly before an audience—people will want to practice it. As it is colloquially used, the term *practice* simply refers to repeatedly carrying out an activity in an effort to learn to do it more easily or accurately. In the fields of music and psychology, the term *practice* conveys very special meanings. Although musicians can differ dramatically in what they consider to be good practice and they may not always articulate it clearly, researchers in cognitive psychology have endeavored to precisely define practice in the context of skill acquisition. The type of practice that has emerged as the most important is *deliberate practice*, which is defined as the solitary practice a performer does with the specific purpose of improving skill (Ericsson & Harwell, 2019). Obviously this type of practice involves more than mere repetition. Deliberate practice also differs from group "rehearsal" and from an individual musician's work or leisure music-making activities.

Chapter 4 in this book offers very thorough consideration of the practice of musicians. It will show that musicians' practicing can vary greatly in terms of efficiency or productivity, which can greatly affect musicians' motivation, skill development, performance success, and career advancement. Musicians—even those who have been "practicing" for years—may learn that with better organization, goal setting, and in-practice self-evaluation, they can actually improve their skills more with fewer hours spent in solitary practice, thus providing more time for other music-enhancing and life-enriching activities.

Regarding the general factors outlined earlier—physiological traits, opportunity and support, motivational sources, learning, and practice—in real life, these interact and overlap to compose the life stories of those who become musical people. Consider jazz great Louis Armstrong. Being born and growing up in the jazz-rich culture of 20th-century New Orleans provided him special musical opportunities. In addition to hearing much music around him, he received his first cornet as a child and learned to play it under the tutelage and mentoring of experienced jazz musicians willing to work with him. Armstrong, a passionate music learner, was thought to have honed his skills by "playing and practicing jazz constantly" (Bergreen, 2012). The particulars of Armstrong's biography could fit under the headings of opportunity and support, motivational sources, learning, and practice.

Typical and Atypical Musical Development

Obviously, not all people have the same developmental opportunities and experiences, so children—even before the age of 10—can come to differ from each other quite widely in what they can do musically. To some extent, however, most people are more *similar* to each other than they are *different*. All humans share a common genetic heritage—that is, each human being is genetically more similar to each other than to any nonhuman animal. All humans share a common environment—we all live on the surface of the same planet, surrounded by similar objects, plants, animals, and humans, which affect us in broadly similar ways; and the way in which the environment affects our bodies and brains to bring about physical and psychological change is determined jointly by our genetic makeup and the specific characteristics of our shared environments. Accordingly, it is possible to see a number of broad patterns emerging that seem to characterize typical musical development.

First, *receptive skills precede productive skills*. Musicality is first manifested through perceptual (primarily aural) ability before music making. Children are able to perceive characteristics in music they hear significantly earlier than when they are able to reliably produce those characteristics in their own performing of familiar music or creating original musical ideas. In this, music is exactly similar to other symbolic skills, such as language.

Second, *spontaneity precedes control* in productive skills. Children begin with free, somewhat undisciplined experimentation and then naturally move to more ordered and controlled use of elements. Mature creativity arises when models and patterns that are well learned are departed from for explicit and motivated reasons. Many (perhaps most) people never acquire this higher level of creativity.

Third, *concrete operations precede abstract ones*. Early conceptualizations are holistic. Only later can children acquire the capacity to break down musical objects into their component parts and transform and recombine them (going from global to local features). For example, the ability to imagine musical objects appears relatively late in the developmental sequence.

One of the most comprehensive models of musical development is the spiral model of Swanwick and Tillman (2016), illustrated in Figure 2.1. This model was developed to account for observed changes in children's performed compositions in classroom contexts. The model proposes four main levels of operation, with two sequential modes nested within each level, reflecting, respectively, the child's internal motivation and more external cultural features of music. We will consider this model in greater detail later in this chapter while discussing musical developmental characteristics of people in various age groups.

Developmental psychology has identified broad patterns and explicates characteristic behaviors of human beings at various stages of life. Although these contributions can offer great insight into typical human development, it is also important to acknowledge that every human being is a unique individual, and some develop *atypically*. Although music is typically a built-in capacity of the human brain, there are cases in which people's brains struggle to process music at all. *Congenital amusia*, a disorder that prevents individuals from perceiving music, is associated with abnormalities of the gray and white matter that relate the auditory cortex to the inferior frontal region of the brain. Although many people may describe themselves as "tone deaf" or not at all musical, the best estimates are that only 3% to 5% of the general population are people with congenital amusia (Nan et al., 2010; Vuvan et al., 2015; Wong et al., 2012).

This finding indicates that the vast majority of people can successfully engage with music in more or less typical ways. This includes individuals with

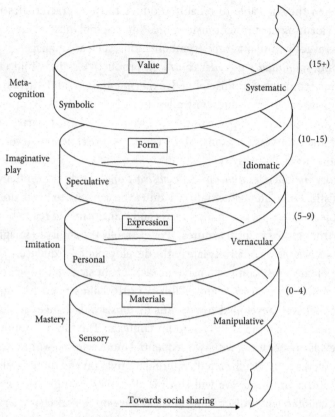

Figure 2.1 Swanwick and Tillman's spiral model of musical development.
From Swanwick & Tillman (2016). The sequence of musical development: A study of children's composition. In A developing discourse: The selected works of Keith Swanwick (pp. 68–98). London, UK: Routledge, p. 92. Reproduced by permission of Taylor & Francis Group through PLSclear.

various physical, sensory, and cognitive disabilities. Most children with disabilities are very much like all other children in that their musical development is best advanced with ample opportunity for musical engagement of a variety of types, and with consistent yet flexible support of the people around them (Jellison, 2016; Ockleford & Welch, 2018).

The term *atypical development* might also be used to describe the small number of *mono-savants* who excel in very specific skills, often at an early age and in the absence of formal instruction. Such musical savants often can quickly commit classical piano pieces to memory by ear, and do so despite evident intellectual or social-emotional disabilities. The impressive musical ability, seemingly acquired quite differently than normal, leads some observers to conclude that savants are rare examples of supernatural giftedness. From a psychological perspective, however, a less fantastic explanation is likely. Mono-savants' disabilities do not prevent them from perceiving music, but often do cause the people around them to have generally low expectations of them; because they are perceived by many as being incapable of normal behavior, their highly skilled musical behaviors seem that much more amazing. In fact, the full nature of some disabilities may actually *facilitate* savants' musical development. Many savants exhibit a language that includes struggling to talk about their music making. The underlying deficit with respect to language may ultimately aid an individual in "tuning out" the spoken conversations in the environment and devoting more focused attention to and processing of music heard; "the savant will spend all available time on the activity, without ever tiring of it" (Sloboda, 2005e, p. 251). That savants' musical ability is the result of a developmental process—rather than an unexplainable gift—is also seen in the common reports of their early attraction to musical stimuli, as well as attempts to reproduce sounds at an early age (Miller, 2014).

Like savant performance, the ability called *perfect pitch* has long fascinated those interested in the psychology of music. Usually called absolute pitch (AP) by those who have researched it, this feat of memory is reportedly found in only 1 in every 10,000 individuals (Levitin & Rogers, 2005). Those who claim AP is a sign of innate talent are often refuted by musicians who consider it of little advantage—or even a disadvantage—in real-life musicality (Marvin et al., 2020; Parncutt & Levitin, 2001).

Prenatal and Early Childhood Development

One of the difficulties in determining what if any musical talent is inborn is that opportunities for musical development begin very early in life, well before children could be expected to demonstrate any feats of natural musicality. In other words, separating the nature from the nurture is practically impossible. In fact, opportunity for humans to develop musically appears to begin *before birth*. Fetal hearing begins about halfway through gestation and gradually improves until birth. In the environment of the womb, hearing is likely the dominant sensory modality and the one that can best detect differences in stimuli available (Parncutt, 2016a). Research has documented human fetuses responding to music (via heart rate changes and motor responses), especially in the third trimester of pregnancy (Parncutt, 2016b).

To the extent that music is concerned with tonal and rhythmic patterns and emotional associations, evidence suggests that musical development begins prior to birth. Although a fetus certainly cannot perceive music like people do after birth, the prenatal environment allows for perception of physiological happenings within the mother. In addition to being exposed to sounds and movements of the mother, the fetus is also exposed to maternal emotional states via hormonal changes that reach the placental environment. It is possible, then, that what the mother experiences, the fetus does also through sound and movement patterns, as well as emotionally via blood hormone levels. "The fetus may associate these with each other, giving emotional connotations to patterns of sound and movement" (Parncutt, 2016a, p. 371).

Infant Musicality

Lying beneath their helpless appearance, human babies typically possess an astonishing array of musical perceptual abilities. Psychologists have established this fact thanks to some innovative research techniques. Because infants are not able to simply tell a researcher when they perceive a difference between musical tones played for them, a special procedure has been used to identify when a baby can detect differences in musical stimuli. Infants as young as 5 months have participated in an experimental procedure in which behavioral conditioning is used to "train" babies to perform a certain physical movement—typically a head turn—when they detect a change in musical patterns they hear. In a small room, an infant sits on the lap of his or her mother. To one side of the infant is a loudspeaker playing a musical pattern over and over again; directly in front of the infant is a research assistant manipulating a puppet (Figure 2.2). In this setup, the infant quickly loses interest in the repeated pattern coming from the speaker and looks at the puppet show straight ahead. The researcher can then change the music being sounded. When an altered musical pattern is sounded, infants tend to turn their heads to look at the speaker where it came from. Upon turning their heads, a remote-controlled animated toy—previously undetectable in a darkened cabinet next to the speaker—lights up and moves. This stimulus brings great pleasure to the infant, thereby reinforcing the behavior of head turning when changes occur in a musical pattern. Infants come to associate

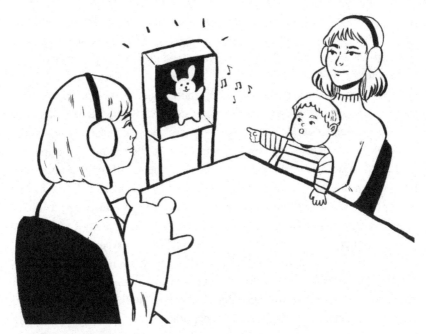

Figure 2.2 Conditioned head-turn procedure used in music research with infants.
Original drawing by Annie Wang.

the animated toy presentation with a change in the sounded music. They are soon conditioned to turn their head toward the loudspeaker when they detect a change. This conditioning allows researchers to investigate the acuity of infants' music perception.

The results of this research suggest that these very young children have surprisingly strong listening skills. By the age of 5 months, babies can show an understanding that in music, perceiving melodic contour is more important than listening pitch to pitch. For example, going from a C major melodic triad (C-E-G-E-C) to a C augmented triad (C-E-G#-E-C) is perceived as a stimulus change by infants (Trehub & Degé, 2016). Infants are much less likely, though, to perceive as a stimulus change a C major triad transposed to an F major triad (note, going from a C major triad to a C augmented triad changes only one pitch, and transposing the C major triad to another key changes all of the pitches). Thus, we can see that infants, like adults, hear melody according to pitch relation (contour pattern), rather than as a sequence of discrete tones (Trehub & Hannon, 2006).

It appears that infants learn a lot about melodic contour from singing and speech directed to them by their mothers (Trehub, 2017). Maternal vocal communication features a baby's most familiar—and likely most preferred—voice, and as such can easily capture the infant's attention. As useful as mothers' *infant-directed speech* is at regulating infant emotion (e.g., calming before a nap) or arousal (e.g., a game of "peekaboo"), *infant-directed singing* has been shown to be even more effective. Mothers and other caregivers can make significant contribution to babies' musical development through the rhythmic and melodic content of vocalizations, the meter concepts experienced through bounces and pat-a-cake games, and the expressiveness learned visually through face-to-face interactions with an emotionally engaged music-making adult (Trehub, 2017).

As important as musical exposure is in infancy, babies are not merely passive recipients of musical information. In addition to responding to music they hear through swaying, bouncing, and clapping (nonrhythmically), they typically use their voices in distinctly musical ways. Long before they are able to produce recognizable speech, babies experiment with their voices, playing with the elements that will later be incorporated into speaking and singing. This *babbling* includes cooing, gliding, and music-like repetition of specific pitch and vowel-consonant patterns (e.g., "ba-ba-ba-ba-ba"). Much of this experimentation takes place through interactions between infant and caregiver (usually the mother) that feature vocal imitation that is two-way: Just as babies imitate their caregivers' vocalizing, the caregivers tend to incorporate their babies' vocal sounds into their infant-directed speech and singing. In fact, when speaking to their babies, many parents change their voice use to make their speech more musically expressive, including through the properties of pitch contour, loudness, and even vocal timbre—research has identified that a mother's smiling at her baby can alter the shape of her vocal tract, giving her voice a special quality described as warmth, intense emotional engagement, or a "smiling sound." Such changes make for effective infant-caregiver communication as they have been shown to increase and better sustain infant attention to a caregiver's vocalizations (Trehub et al., 2010).

Musical Childhood

Toddlers, roughly age 1 to 3 years old, encounter their world at a stage of development when human brain plasticity (the "rewiring" into more interconnected networks) is at its peak. Young children at this age typically experience rapid growth in physical, cognitive, and socioemotional development. All of these relate to musical development.

Singing is a common and preferred activity in early childhood. Toddlers imitate melodies they hear, typically first approximating melodic contour, then exact pitch content. Their music making also features spontaneous singing, including personally made-up songs, the content of which develops to reflect consistent meter and recurring rhythms. The spiral model of musical development (Figure 2.1) identifies the "Materials" level occurring from birth through age four. In the *sensory mode* of this level, children explore the pleasantness of sound through spontaneous vocalizations and soundings of instruments and other objects. Experimentation focuses particularly on loudness and timbre. In the subsequent *manipulative mode*, children acquire greater ability in handling musical instruments and their music making reflects simple conventions of music, including repeated rhythmic and melodic patterns.

The spiral model specifies the "Expression" level taking place from age 5 to 9. This begins with the *personal mode*, during which children convey emotions and stories with their music, particularly through singing; their expressiveness concentrates on changes in tempo and dynamics. In the *vernacular mode* that follows, children show greater conformity to established musical conventions. Their music making is marked by the presence of melodic and rhythmic patterns, regular meter, and standard phrase lengths.

The gradual development from child to adolescent, called middle childhood, can be a period of great change. It also can be a time during which young people's connection to music is solidified. Middle childhood can also bring a narrowing of musical tastes, as many children begin to like only the styles of music preferred by their peers (Louven, 2016). This decline in "open-earedness" may be especially unfavorable toward classical music (Hargreaves & Bonneville-Roussy, 2018; Kopiez & Lehmann, 2008). Ideally, musical experiences during middle childhood—including formal music education—help to build a musical foundation within children, upon which additional musical development can be built. This seems to depend on children beginning to incorporate music into their developing self-concept, such that they can envision their future selves being musical (Evans & McPherson, 2015).

Adolescent and Adult Development

Those whose early childhood takes place in a musically rich environment can build a robust foundation for greater musical achievement in later stages of childhood and as adults. The Swanwick and Tillman spiral model (Figure 2.1) indicates the "Form" level occurring from age 10 to 15 years old. In its first *speculative mode*, young musicians show growing interest in deviating from musical conventions they have learned of. They experiment with ways of varying patterns and adding contrast to their music, often at the expense of larger structural cohesion. In the next *idiomatic mode*, they are better able to integrate their imaginative ideas into recognizable styles. Musical authenticity becomes important, as does technical, expressive, and structural control. There also is greater emphasis on fitting their music into existing musical styles, often popular ones.

Significance of Music to Teens

Over the last century, advancements in electronic and communications media have made it possible to hear music virtually any place and at any time. Many adolescents particularly avail themselves of technology to pursue their musical interests. Even those who in no way consider themselves to be "musicians" declare music as a very important part of their lives. Having choice in the music they listen to is important to young people (Greasley & Lamont, 2011). Adolescents' desire to choose the music they hear is also quite understandable considering the importance music can have in social and emotional development; their musical involvement affects not only their personal development but also their social group formation. Especially after entering adolescence, the vast majority of young people show preference for a narrow range of popular music styles (Hargreaves et al., 2016).

Preoccupation with popular music leads some adolescents to go beyond listening in order to learn to sing or play it (Kamin et al., 2007). Historically, this learning has occurred outside of schools. The jam sessions of garage bands provide the setting for much personal and social development and musical growth (Davis, 2005). Such groups routinely engage in creative ventures, including improvising together and collaborating to compose, perform, and record original songs. In summary, popular music is a significant part of most adolescents' lives. For those who are engaged in out-of-school music making, the recommendation of Pitts (2005) is appropriate, namely that "music teaching in schools needs to be compatible with, but distinctive from, the musical learning in which students are engaged beyond the classroom" (p. 128). Others have asserted that by looking to popular and vernacular music making, school music programs can diversify their curricular offerings to improve the music learning afforded to students (Woody & Adams, 2019).

Identity Development in Adolescence into Adulthood

Adolescence is typically an eventful stage of development. As young people go through this period, experiencing expanded privileges and encountering greater responsibilities, they also become increasingly capable of adult-like skills. Such skills, when combined with youthful enthusiasm and competitive drive, can produce extremely impressive young prodigies in the arts, athletics, and other domains as varied as chess and the medical field. Musical prodigies tend to develop their exceptional skills through enriching and intense development opportunities afforded to so-labeled "gifted" children including *hothousing*, being brought up in an unusually stimulating environment designed to encourage rapid skill growth (Gabor, 2011; McPherson & Williamon, 2016; O'Connor, 2012). This kind of intense musical upbringing can have some real drawbacks (the subject of burnout is addressed in Chapter 3).

Even among nonprodigies, music typically is a very important part of adolescent life. It can contribute greatly to another type of human development yet to be mentioned in this chapter: *identity development*. Although the process of identity development begins before adolescence (likely around age 7 or 8), many consequential experiences typically occur during the years of adolescence (Parker, 2020). In the adolescent search to discover, understand, and express "who I am," music making and listening are "especially pertinent" (Elliott & Silverman, 2017, p. 27). Although not many will readily admit it, teenagers rely heavily on important others in their lives, including adults like parents and teachers. In the process of developing their identity, adolescents consider—perhaps for the first time for themselves—how they think and feel about themselves and elements of their lives. This can include thoughts and feelings about their own ability to be musical. Largely based on input and feedback they get from key individuals in their lives, adolescents formulate beliefs about how musical they are and can become. Such beliefs lead to their decisions about what music involvement, if any, they engage in when opportunities arise, whether coming in the form of school music, private lessons, community music experience, or musical leisure activities with peers. Greater involvement can be key when young people build a belief in their musical agency (Wiggins, 2016) and find a sense of belonging and acceptance in a subculture of musicians (Dagaz, 2012; Evans & Liu, 2019; Parker, 2010). The development of a musical identity (or lack thereof) can have lifelong consequences (Lamont, 2017). Adolescents' development of musical identity appears to be a dynamic process built around their coming to feel musical; Parker's (2020) conceptualization of this is presented in Figure 2.3.

Until fairly recently, most people conceived of adolescence as the transition into adulthood, at which point young people are then ready to take on the responsibilities and expectations of being "grown up." That conception changed when a body of psychological research indicated that a stage of *emerging adulthood* immediately follows adolescence and is passed through before becoming a full-fledged adult (Arnett, 2016). Rather than a universal life stage, emerging adulthood is theorized as a developmental stage that has

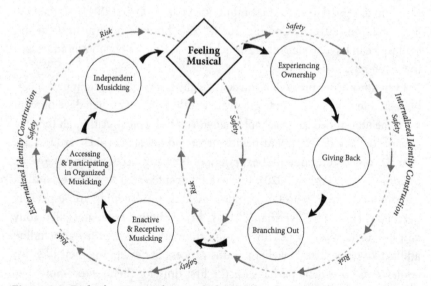

Figure 2.3 Parker's process of musical identity development.

From Parker, E. C. (2020). Adolescents on music: Why music matters to young people in our lives. New York, NY: Oxford University Press. Reproduced with permission of Oxford University Press through PLSclear.

appeared in certain industrialized societies in which social and economic changes have delayed the onset of traditional adult roles, such as marriage and parenthood. It is a time of life exploration (unaccompanied by parents) and consideration of future possibilities (Syed, 2015). Music can be particularly important for emerging adults as it can serve as a basis for continued identity development, social interaction, and romantic relationships (Coyne et al., 2015). The transition to postschooling life—whether with or without college—is typically a process of "ups and downs, back and forth, exhilarating leaps forward, crushing falls backward, and everything in between" (Marshall and Butler, 2015, p. 330). This description is likely apt for emerging adults who choose music as an occupation.

Toward Lifelong Musicianship

Some young adults further their musical development by studying it at a college or university, and others by working as musicians. For others, music becomes a serious avocation, an important activity that they intentionally pursue in their leisure time. Across these different musical categories of people, musical development will continue well into adulthood.

The highest level of development indicated by the Swanwick and Tillman spiral model (Figure 2.1) is called "Value." It can begin as early as adolescence, but is also attained later in life, or never attained at all by some. In its initial *symbolic mode*, musicians become more personally committed to music, especially related to its affective power. There is greater interest in broad compositional qualities (e.g., orchestration, harmonic progressions). In the final *systematic mode*, advanced musicians begin to approach music in especially innovative or sophisticated ways, perhaps by employing novel compositional systems or seeking to understand music from various intellectual or philosophical perspectives.

The goal of attaining the highest levels of musicianship leads some people to study at a college or university as music majors. In this context, advanced music students grow through mentoring relationships with expert musician role models and influential peers. These social interactions, coupled with extensive curricular experiences, allow music majors to construct an occupational identity focused on music, most frequently as a music teacher or professional musician (Austin et al., 2012; Creech, 2016; Mills, 2006). Those who eschew advanced study in higher education may instead try to start a career as a "gigging musician" in a popular music scene. Identity development for these musicians may center around prioritizing artistry over economic concerns and building a sense of professionalism defined by dedication and demeanor (Scarborough, 2017).

Of course, few people choose music for work or study in higher education. As for the greater majority of those who do not, research has shown that most discontinue music activities upon their entry into adulthood. This may be especially true of those whose music learning experiences have come exclusively in formal educational settings, in which music teachers have assumed the primary role of support, structure, and direction to students and demand compliance and invested time from them. The resulting lack of *musical independence* may produce people who, postschooling, believe that "they are simply unable to make music without a leader to select music, organize rehearsals, and instruct them on how to perform" (Woody & Parker, 2012, p. 201). For such graduates of formal music education, finding a nonauditioned community ensemble is perceived to be the *only* opportunity they have to participate in music making as adults because they may consider themselves unable to be musical outside of that narrow context (Isbell & Stanley, 2011).

People who do continue organized musical involvement into adulthood often do so because the social, emotional, and artistic rewards hold particular value to them (Pitts & Robinson, 2016). Musical involvement can play a special role in enjoyment of life and search for meaning (Lamont, 2012). One thing is certain: Musical development need not only be a process of childhood and adolescence. Music can provide adults important ways to understand and develop identity, bond with others, experience and express spirituality, and maintain a sense of well-being late in life (Hays & Minichiello, 2005; see also Perkins & William, 2014).

Importance of Early Experience in Developing Musical Expertise

Children who have opportunities to participate in musical activities in their everyday lives develop musical skills and abilities faster than those whose main experience is one of passive consumption. Because the first and most prevalent aspect of everyday life is the home, the level of musical activity in the home, and particularly that instigated by the parents, is likely to be a major influence on musical development. Early enrichment leads to acceleration of skill acquisition, and parental involvement and support is a strong correlate of young people's later musical motivation and achievement (Evans, 2015).

Those who attain the highest levels of music performance expertise, especially in classical music, usually receive specialized instruction beginning fairly early in childhood. Their musical development is also hastened by engaging in deliberate practice, as assigned by teachers and monitored by parents. Theirs is often a musical environment that is effectively well organized by the adults in their lives and one in which musical activity is consistently made available and encouraged. Notwithstanding the formality of lessons, classes, and organized enrichment programs of modern Western society, there is nothing inherently unnatural about early musical learning and development. Cross-cultural data suggest the opposite. In many cultures around the world, children acquire a wide repertoire of songs and dances at an early age, often at a level of complexity and skill that exceeds Western norms (Campbell, 2016).

As a whole, psychological research supports a clear and coherent account of the development of musicality. Most children are born with the full capacities to engage with music. As such, music learning should be seen as a birthright for all children. Although many do not experience the confluence of factors needed to reach the expertise of professional musicians, virtually all people can develop musically and enjoy the rewards that music listening and participation can provide.

Taking the Stage: Embrace the Social in Music Making

Music is a well-known means by which people socialize, interact, and feel connected to others. This is especially common among music fans. Performers too can gain much by embracing the natural sociality of music. Musical people who are active as performers usually find themselves as members of certain musical subcultures, perhaps built around the styles of music they perform or instruments played. Certainly, this provides opportunities for friendships with people of similar backgrounds, interests, and lifestyles. Such "offstage" relationships can be even more rewarding when performers also collaborate in their music making. This deserves explicit mention because some musicians who especially appreciate the value of solitary practicing and music study may unwittingly relegate themselves strictly to solo work when they are not involved in large ensemble activities that are carried out under the direction of a conductor/leader, in which talking between musicians can be perceived as "time wasted." Unlike solo and large ensemble experiences, smaller group "chamber music" activity provides ample opportunity for performers to interact and bond around music creation. As people for whom music is deeply important, this kind of collaboration can provide a meaningful context for forming personal friendships and productive professional relationships.

Leading Learning: Give Children Age-Appropriate Enrichment

Music teachers must know their students very well to best plan and deliver effective instruction. To realistically "chart a course" ahead into the future, teachers must have a clear idea where they currently are and where they can progress to, in terms of learning. To truly understand their students and know how to nurture their musical growth, teachers not only need to have an accurate assessment of their current levels of knowledge and skills but also factor into account students' preferences for certain musical styles and for types of music-making activity. While there is no substitute for getting to know a student as an individual (through discussing music and interacting musically together), it can be helpful for teachers to know something about human developmental psychology. This is why some training in educational psychology is a standard requirement in teacher preparation programs. Music teachers should avail themselves of the many resources—in print and online—that describe in detail the developmental progression of young people through music learning of various types (e.g., rhythmic development, vocal development). Additionally, teachers should remember that the musical experiences that are age appropriate for students are the experiences that are developmentally best and most facilitative of learning. Some music educators, like many proud parents, yearn to be told that their students/children are "advanced." In reality, however, even if it is possible to get children to do adult-like musical things, it is doubtful that it will be good for their musical development in the long run.

Chapter 2 Discussion Questions

1. When you were a child, were you told you were *gifted* in some way? Did it motivate you to give greater effort and commitment, or did it have an opposite effect—perhaps because you thought the nature of the gift would allow you to achieve without working at it? What do you think now?

2. What are your earliest musical memories as a young child? Looking back, does it seem like certain early music experiences laid a foundation for subsequent experiences with music and perhaps even your musical orientation today?

3. In your experience, how many of your musical friends from childhood and adolescence continued their musical involvement into adulthood? Regarding those who did not, what factors likely prevented them from developing a lifelong musicianship?

3

Motivation

Consider this true account of a real young musician:

> Damien loved music from an early age, especially rhythm. After a few years of hearing him beatbox with his mouth and drum out rhythms with pencils, spoons, and whatever else he could get his hands on, Damien's parents arranged lessons with a private drum teacher. He thrived in his private lessons and in school music too. In high school, he was the leading percussionist, including as set drummer in the top jazz band and section leader of the marching band's drumline. An outstanding student all around, he earned a full-ride academic scholarship to a nearby Big Ten university. But his passion was music, and when he was not busy with the school music program and doing homework to keep up his excellent grades, he spent his free time mixing beats on his laptop computer, often recording original raps to them. His songwriting became his primary means of coping with the stresses of adolescent life as a high-achieving student and a bit of a creative oddball (as he considered himself).
>
> Damien was heavily recruited by the university's music school and declared as a music major. In his first year, however, he realized he did not fit in with the other percussion students who, unlike Damien, concentrated almost exclusively on marching percussion during the fall semester, and on symphonic playing (i.e., timpani and mallet percussion) in the spring. Damien saw no hope for focusing on his interest in set drumming and felt he had to hide his passion for rapping and beat-mixing. At the end of his freshman year, Damien changed his major to business. He would continue to be musical, but he would do it on his terms.

To clearly explain what allowed Damien to achieve so much with music and then change life direction so abruptly, we turn to the psychology of motivation, a critical consideration for those trying to improve their own musicianship or for teachers and parents of young musicians. Although aspiring performers may know what they need to do to improve their skills,

Psychology for Musicians. Robert H. Woody, Oxford University Press. © Oxford University Press 2022.
DOI: 10.1093/oso/9780197546598.003.0003

it is quite another thing to actually do it. Similarly, it is easy for a teacher to write down a list of exercises to be practiced, but much more difficult to get students to carry them out. Often, musicians and teachers talk about motivation as a feeling or inner desire. But to study motivation, we have to look to its manifestations as behaviors, such as a young child who insists on learning to play the trumpet, a teenager who continues music studies in school when others have dropped out, or a collegiate musician who employs special strategies to maximize practice time (Linnenbrink-Garcia et al., 2011).

Multiple sources of motivation exist in the lives of musicians. One simple way to understand these many sources is to categorize them as intrinsic versus extrinsic. Intrinsic motivation comes from the activity itself and the enjoyment experienced from engaging in it. In general, human beings make music because of the enjoyment and fulfillment they get from doing it. However, because acquiring musical skill takes much time and effort, developing musicians also rely on extrinsic motivation, which is the secondary nonmusical reward that comes with musical participation. This is seen when young musicians respond to the support and encouragement of people close to them, including parents, teachers, and peers. At any one time in their development, musicians may be drawing on several intrinsic and extrinsic sources simultaneously (Hallam, 2011; Woody, 2020b). Some performance experiences include both intrinsic and extrinsic elements. The pleasure of group music making is intrinsically rewarding, and additional extrinsic motivation comes from the applause of an audience. It is sometimes difficult to distinguish between extrinsic and intrinsic motivation (see the later section on beliefs and values).

Although a great many people get involved with music as children (either intrinsically or extrinsically, as in the case of parental coercion) and set out to learn an instrument, relatively few of them achieve a satisfying level of proficiency. Building a skill of any kind necessarily involves effort. In music, the effort can include a lot of concentrated time repeating musical exercises. Even among professional musicians, practice is not seen as an enjoyable activity and many "maintain an ambiguous relationship with it" (Lehmann & Jørgensen, 2018, p. 126). But music learning need not be an unpleasant undertaking. A better understanding of motivation may allow musicians to approach rigorous practicing with a positive perspective and to supplement practice with other musical activities that are more immediately and personally rewarding.

Based on the research that has examined motivation and music achievement, this chapter explains the following principles:

1. Music is intrinsically motivating. Early pleasurable experiences with music draw children into pursuing greater involvement, including formal training. Maintaining an intrinsic love of music can ultimately determine how long musicians will continue in the field and how rewarding it will be for them.
2. The support of parents and teachers can be the difference between a young student's benefiting from music training and dropping out altogether (see Chapter 2). Motivating a child musician to do the practice necessary for skill development requires the supervision of parents and the encouragement of respected teachers.
3. Social relationships with musical peers prompt many teenagers and young adults to strengthen their commitment to music. Musical subcultures can exert very strong influences on the motivation of music students.
4. Young musicians' beliefs—about music and about themselves—can greatly influence motivation going forward. They can build positive mindsets when music has met certain psychological needs and when they envision music being an integral part of their future selves.

Intrinsic Motivation for Music

Human beings have a "love affair" with music. Virtually everyone claims to like music, at least some kind of music, and most people would say they *love* music. Generally speaking, listening to and making music are intrinsically motivating activities. People are naturally attracted to them because the activities themselves are emotionally rewarding experiences. Attraction to music is not acquired (although tastes for certain styles of music certainly are) but is something inherently human.

Childhood Experiences

Although a person may not begin to study music until school age, the motivation for that involvement has likely been built earlier in life. Young children's

home environments can differ greatly in opportunities for musical exploration and discovery. Later musical skill development is facilitated by early
home environments that include playful, fun-filled, and spontaneous musical behavior (Forrester & Borthwick-Hunter, 2015). Toddlers' first music-
making experiences can involve singing and experimenting with musical
instruments, suggesting that active participation (music making) at home,
rather than passive experience (listening, watching), promotes later musical
involvement.

Although a child's everyday playful music making can build lasting positive associations, more exceptional musical events can also capture musical
interests for life. Many music lovers recall having highly emotional "peak
experiences" in childhood, characterized by feelings of wonder, awe, or surrender (Gabrielsson et al., 2016). The great classical guitarist Andrés Segovia
recounted how, as a young child, he first became captivated by the instrument when a strolling flamenco guitar player came to his town:

> At the first flourish, more noise than music burst from the strings and,
> as if it had happened yesterday, I remember my fright at this explosion
> of sounds. . . . [R]earing from the impact, I fell over backward. However,
> when he scratched out some of those variations he said were *soleares*, I felt
> them inside of me as if they had penetrated through every pore of my body.
> (Segovia, 1976, p. 3)

This is but one example of how emotionally meaningful peak experiences,
particularly early in life, may produce children who are "more likely to pursue
a high level of involvement with music in later life" (Sloboda, 2005d, p. 185).

Enjoyment and Exploration in Learning

A basic fascination with music and enjoyment-oriented discovery can be
powerful motivators beyond childhood. Whereas some young people soon
turn to formal music instruction to build on their early experiences, many
others stay on a more exploratory path. In her book *How Popular Musicians
Learn*, music education researcher Lucy Green (2002) attracted much scholarly attention to the informal learning of popular or "vernacular" musicians.
Research has identified several key learning practices that draw on intrinsic
motivation for music (Woody & Adams, 2019). The music that vernacular

musicians work on is of their choosing. They practice their preferred songs or parts of songs (e.g., guitar solos or shorter "licks"), as opposed to technical exercises and études. In their group learning sessions with musical peers, they collaborate to reproduce popular songs, create new compositions, or "jam" (improvise) for fun. In addition to the social rewards of this group setting, the music making itself can be tremendously gratifying. Some music scholars have asserted that classical music performing ability comes through discipline but popular music skills happen through osmosis. Green (2002), however, has provided evidence that popular musicians expend similar time and effort as their classical counterparts, and that the real difference between these realms is whether the investment is experienced as pleasant or unpleasant. Popular musicians describe their learning process as voluntary, enjoyable, and what they love to do.

The phrase *intrinsically motivated* is often mistakenly used by people to describe any strong desire felt inside themselves. This reflects a common misperception that intrinsic motivation is that which comes from within a person. In fact, it is more accurately understood as motivation that comes from *within an activity*. This is why it is accurate to say (as earlier) that many vernacular musicians operate largely out of intrinsic motivation. This is not because they feel so much passion to do music, but because the musical activities they engage in are primarily done for the rewards provided by the activities themselves. They jam with friends because it is what they want to do (not out of a belief that it will help them accomplish some later goal). They create and perform original music because that experience provides them personal rewards in and of itself.

As this explanation shows, being passionate about one's musical endeavors does not necessarily make a musician intrinsically motivated. In fact, recent research has shown that musician passion comes in two broad types: harmonious passion and obsessive passion. *Harmonious passion* is characterized by unpressured choice to engage in musical activity, and the experience of positive emotions during and as a result. *Obsessive passion*, in contrast, is typified by an unmanageable compulsion to carry out an activity, even through negative consequences (Bonneville-Roussy et al., 2011). Harmonious passionate musicians show a flexible persistence and ability to balance their music activities with other aspects of life. Obsessive passionate musicians' compulsive practicing and performing are largely done to gain the approval of people in their lives or to maintain a self-esteem that is contingent upon success, and it often comes at the expense of their health and wellness (Bonneville-Roussy

& Vallerand, 2020). Although harmonious passion and intrinsic motivation are different psychological constructs, they clearly share some similar characteristics.

While intrinsic motivation may be more linked to the activities of vernacular musicians (as described earlier), it is also very important for those who undergo formal training (Woody, 2020b). Music students of all ages benefit from learning experiences that provide them moments of personal enjoyment. Making music "just for the fun of it" and engaging in creative experimentation can also help sustain students' intrinsic motivation. Although these activities may not contribute to skill improvement as directly and effectually as deliberate practice, they can still reinforce students' commitment to music study and involvement.

Research suggests that freedom and choice are conditions that maintain and enhance intrinsic motivation. Music students practice more conscientiously when they are working on pieces of music they have chosen for themselves. In addition, when assigned repertoire by teachers, music students more wholly invest themselves in practicing the pieces that they are most interested in and enjoy (Austin & Berg, 2006; Burwell & Shipton, 2011; Oare, 2012). The effect of choice on motivation can be great, as shown in Renwick and McPherson's (2002) case study of a beginning clarinetist: the young musician spent 12 times as much time practicing self-selected music than repertoire assigned to her; her practice behavior also showed "increased use of advanced strategies" (p. 185). Having choice in their musical activities adds to musicians' sense of autonomy, which has been shown to predict the amount and quality of practice they will engage in (Evans & Bonneville-Roussy, 2015). A lack of autonomy can cause many young people to opt out of organized music involvement altogether and pursue music learning in informal settings (Feichas, 2010; McPherson & Hendricks, 2010; Rusinek, 2008).

As important as choice is, choosing well is also a factor in maintaining intrinsic motivation for music. Young musicians seem to develop best when they take on challenges, but ones that are attainable in light of their current ability level (Diaz & Silveira, 2012; Evans & Bonneville-Roussy, 2015; Valenzuela et al., 2018). Balance between a person's perceived skill and the demands of an activity has been identified as a condition for experiencing *flow*, an immersive state of optimal enjoyment that can contribute to people's commitment to music activity moving forward into the future (Csikszentmihalyi, 1990; Miksza et al., 2012). Flow is most likely to occur in an activity that is highly challenging for a person, but for which the person possesses a high

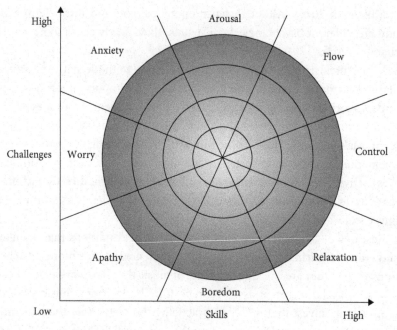

Figure 3.1 Model of flow state.

From Nakamura & Csikszentmihalyi (2009). Flow theory and research. In *Oxford handbook of positive psychology*. Reproduced with permission of the Oxford University Press Ltd. through PLSclear.

skill level. An imbalance produces unmotivating results: anxiety results when a challenge exceeds one's skill level, and a feeling of unstimulating relaxation results when one's skill is much greater than the challenge presented. Figure 3.1 illustrates the interaction of skill and challenge.

Music-Involved Goal Orientation

The act of performing music itself can be an intensely powerful experience for musicians. Making music is fundamentally pleasurable. In addition to the rewards of making music alone and with peers in informal situations, public performance can be an intrinsically motivating factor (Hallam et al., 2016; Lamont, 2012). The presence of a live audience may provide a heightened emotional experience for performers. Communicating with the people in the audience and "losing oneself in the music" can add to the aesthetic enjoyment musicians feel while onstage (Lacaille et al., 2007, p. 247).

Musicians' perspective on performance is an important variable in motivation. Those with a *task-involved* orientation see performance primarily as an opportunity to make music (i.e., something that is personally important to them) and, in the case of music students, a chance to demonstrate their skill development; their thoughts leading up to a performance focus on "the task at hand," namely performing up to their ability level. Those with an *ego-involved* orientation, however, are primarily concerned about how their performance will be judged by others. Task-involved orientation has been associated with intrinsic motivation, the experiencing of positive emotions, and the seeking of performance challenges. Ego-involved orientation, however, has been linked to negative emotions such as anxiety and choosing performance activities on the basis of what will help them be viewed as successful and not a failure (Hatfield, 2016; Smith, 2005). In an intervention study that provided psychological skills training to European conservatory students, one participant described the move from an ego-involved perfectionistic mindset to a more resilient and adaptive task-oriented one:

> I would say that the main difference consists of not being too egocentric before concerts. This is not about me, and how great I want others to believe that I am to play the instrument. It is all about being satisfied and accepting that one is in the middle of a process that takes time, and that every outcome is just fine. (Hatfield, 2016, p. 11)

Additional psychological evidence from performance research outside of music suggests that task-involved orientation facilitates the optimal flow state during performance (Stavrou et al., 2015) and that an ego-involved orientation may make performers more likely to engage in unethical actions to attain success (Ring & Kavussanu, 2018).

As this explanation shows, identifying intrinsic motivation (versus extrinsic motivation) is much more than an academic exercise. Intrinsic motivation can be quite predictive of whether young people's musical lives are sustainable in the long term or whether they will be especially susceptible to performance anxiety and possibly burn out from music altogether.

Extrinsic Motivation for Musical Young People

The aforementioned intrinsic sources of motivation can provide a foundation for lifelong musical involvement. However, they also can prove ineffective by negative experiences with music. People who at a young age were

told that they were not "musical" seldom enjoy a childhood of growing musicianship (see the section on beliefs and values later in the chapter). This
fact indicates the critical importance of extrinsic sources of motivation in
a person's musical development. The most primary sources are parents,
teachers, and peers.

Important Others

Within Western cultures, parents are a main source of motivation and support in the beginning stages of their children's music development (see
Chapter 2). A parent's praise and encouragement are meaningful rewards
for young children as they demonstrate their developing musical abilities
and express interest in learning more about music. With children who begin
formal music study, parents are especially important. In addition to simply
paying for lessons and providing transportation, parents also offer support
by sitting in on lessons and supervising their children's beginning practice
efforts (McPherson, 2009). Parents need not have extensive musical training
or experience themselves for their supervision to be beneficial (Davidson &
Burland, 2006). Children can also be influenced by siblings who play musical
instruments (Leung & McPherson, 2011). In addition to simply making a
younger child aware of music, an older sibling may serve as a musical role
model. It is common for a younger child to look up to older brothers and
sisters and aspire to be like them and learn to do what they can do. This phenomenon applies to music endeavors and may prompt a child to learn to
play the same instrument as an idolized sibling or wish to take music lessons
(even if on a different instrument).

Support at home seems to be a basic requirement for children to continue
their musical involvement. A lack of parental support is widely recognized
as a deciding factor when children drop out of music training. There can
be, however, a negative side of parental involvement. Parents who are too
pushy (or try to "hothouse" their child) face the risk that their child may
lose intrinsic enjoyment of music and eventually wish to drop out. Some
parents may believe that, however negative the experience, the child will
thank them later for making them take piano lessons. Research suggests,
though, that among those who enjoy music success later in life, the children
themselves initiated the onset of formal lessons or at least were agreeable to
the idea.

Teachers—especially first teachers in a new area of interest—are naturally very influential in the lives of young students. Initial music teachers contribute to a positive foundation of motivation by being warm, playful, and friendly (Hallam & Burns, 2018; Leung & McPherson, 2011; Moore et al., 2003). Not many children will thrive musically if rushed into demanding lessons and rigorous practice assignments. In contrast to such a work-like approach, *play* is a natural way of life for young children and seems to be the context in which they learn best (Marsh & Young, 2016).

Subsequent teachers are also important. Once a student has begun a committed musical involvement, the teacher is a primary source of motivation, but in a slightly different role. This person will have great influence in the young musician's developing belief system concerning the value of music involvement, and he or she can also provide encouragement to achieve. As critical as it is for an initial music teacher to be warm and friendly, subsequent teachers of more advanced students offer musical leadership that inspires and challenges them, mobilizing them to stretch their musical commitment in a positive way (Hewitt & Allan, 2013).

One of the primary ways that teachers can challenge young musicians concerns practice. Music students must learn *how* to practice and often rely on teachers for this (Miksza, 2011; Oare, 2012). The teacher is an integral cog in a motivational cycle of practice, reward, and achievement: with better practice comes greater and more rapid skill development, which supplies young musicians with important self-motivating rewards—musical, social, and otherwise.

Social Environment

As young musicians enter adolescence, their peers become increasingly important. The extrinsic motivation provided by peers can eclipse the influence exerted by parents and teachers; it can lead a child to either quit music instruction or continue. Social pressure can have a direct positive or negative effect, such as when young instrumentalists decide whether to join the school band based on whether they perceive the "band kids" as a socially good group or "not cool." More indirectly, adolescent peer groups assert their identity through the kind of popular music they like. A young music student may come to realize that the music he or she plays at school does not match the music of his or her peer group.

Peer relationships help sustain interest in music involvement and guide decisions made by young musicians (Cantero & Jauset-Berrocal, 2017; Evans et al., 2012). For many teenagers, their music activities essentially provide them with a social life (Hallam et al., 2016). It is common in American high schools for musical subcultures to exist in the form of close-knit groups of "band kids" or choir students (Abril, 2013; Parker, 2010, 2016; Rawlings & Young, 2020). Social recognition within these groups is linked to the members' musical abilities. Proficient young musicians are often motivated to excel musically to maintain their standing among their peers. Usually, music students enjoy the support and encouragement provided by their peers, and they value joint music-making opportunities. An adolescent in one research study described his relationship with musical peers as "like a family bond," explaining, "We just know that we've got people you can rely on when you need them" (Parker, 2020, p. 109).

Immersion into a musical social structure can confirm a student's commitment to music. Participation in organized music activity allows young people to make friends and socialize with them as they work together on an artistic venture. Multiple socially related positive outcomes increase confidence and provide an important sense of belonging (Hewitt & Allan, 2013). Unfortunately, some social dynamics can instead have a harmful effect if the environment is highly judgmental or competitive. While intense music training can effectively prepare young people for a career in classical music, it can also lead to maladaptive behaviors, mental health problems, or dropping out of music altogether (Bernhard, 2010; Gabor, 2011; Kingsbury, 2010; O'Bryan, 2015).

Internalizing Extrinsic Motivation

As young musicians become adults, it becomes problematic to depend on parents, teachers, and peers to provide the motivation to practice and carry out the necessary activities to advance musically. Ideally by then, musicians have begun to internalize the sources of extrinsic motivation that previously existed. This means that the influence and values of parents, teachers, and musical peers have gradually become part of the self, that is, internalized. They now have the extrinsic motivations within themselves. They have personally adopted a certain work ethic with their music and value the rewards they can enjoy if they apply themselves and become better musicians.

The internalization of extrinsic motivation is an important component of the very prominent self-determination theory (SDT; Evans et al., 2012;

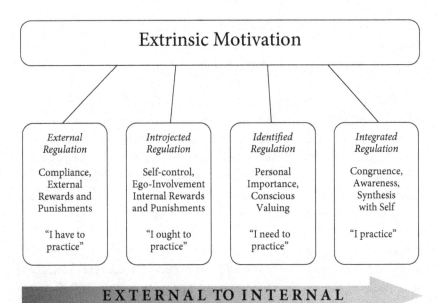

Figure 3.2 Process of internalizing extrinsic motivation, according to self-determination theory, as applied to practice.
Based on Woody (2019), adapted from Ryan and Deci (2002).

MacIntyre et al., 2017; Ryan & Deci, 2002). SDT explains people's goal-oriented behavior as being regulated by three psychological needs: competence, relatedness, and autonomy. The theory indicates that extrinsic motivation has four levels, varying primarily in how the motivation is experienced. As greater autonomy is felt with a certain activity, the more internally situated the motivation feels. This dynamic, illustrated in Figure 3.2, is useful in explaining how developing music students come to accept the hard work of practicing. When young musicians are first introduced to practicing, they typically carry it out only if they are made to by a parent or teacher (external regulation); they practice because they feel like they *have to*. As their initial practicing efforts yield skill improvement and they better understand practice as a useful activity, they engage in it because they feel they *ought to* (introjected regulation). When greater development has further convinced musicians of the value of practicing and success in music activities has become personally important to them, they feel that they *need to* practice (identified regulation). And finally, when the motivation to practice has been fully internalized, musicians simply do it (integrated regulation), likely with little deliberation about whether they want to, need to, or otherwise should. This progression can be seen in comments once made by concert pianist André Watts (SDT regulation type added in brackets):

> I wouldn't be a pianist today if my mother hadn't made me practice [external regulation]. . . . On days when I wasn't exactly moved to practice, my mother saw to it that I did. Sometimes she tried coaxing me to the piano by relating the careers of famous musicians, hoping perhaps to inspire me to practice [introjected]. At thirteen, however, I realized the necessity of practice [identified]. I still don't really "like" it all the time, but by now it has become second nature [integrated]. (Mach, 1980, p. 182)

Autonomy is but one of the three psychological needs specified by SDT, along with the need for relationship and need for competence. These three needs have been theorized to impact people's overall disposition toward life (i.e., "global motivation"), as well as impact their perspective on music in general ("domain-specific motivation") and more particular activities within music ("situation-specific motivation"). At each level, the extent to which people's needs are met affects their thoughts, emotions, and behavior. An illustration of this, offered by Evans (2015), is shown in Figure 3.3.

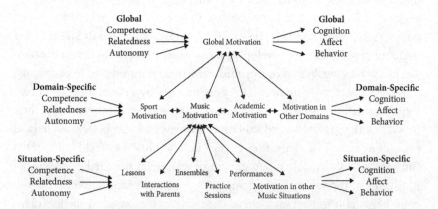

Figure 3.3 Hierarchical model of motivation in music learning.

From Evans, P. (2015). Self-determination theory: An approach to motivation in music education. *Musicae Scientiae, 19*(1), 65–83. doi:10.1177/1029864914568044

Beliefs and Values

Components of the SDT model (Figure 3.3)—specifically the feelings of competence, relatedness, and autonomy and the outcomes of cognition, affect, and behavior—point to the contents of the mind as critical in understanding motivation. Thoughts and feelings affect the motivation people have. More specifically, what they believe (about music and about themselves), how they think, and how they explain their past musical experiences greatly determine the kind and intensity of musical engagement they will pursue.

Self-Efficacy: What You Think You Can Do

As explained earlier, young musicians rely on the people in their lives in building a belief system about music. Based on the feedback they receive from parents, teachers, and peers, music students begin to solidify ideas about how good they are in certain pursuits, including music. The term *self-efficacy*, first advanced by American psychologist Albert Bandura (1977), refers to people's judgments about their abilities to achieve in a specific domain. Belief in one's musical competencies can affect young people's decisions about the direction, intensity, and persistence of their future musical activities.

Much educational research has shown that student self-efficacy is highly predictive of achievement, including in music (McPherson & McCormick, 2006). Musical self-efficacy can be thought of as self-confidence in music, provided "confidence" refers to trust musicians have in their skills, rather than an air of greatness they put on. True confidence is based on expectation. To realistically expect to achieve their goals—that is, to have confidence in themselves—musicians must get their skills to a reliably high level. This usually requires investing a good deal of time and effort, including through effortful deliberate practice. As shown in Chapter 4, achieving skill mastery usually involves explicit planning, thoughtful execution of practice, and careful monitoring of progress (Mornell et al., 2020). True mastery of a task allows musicians to not only be *able to perform* it but also have *full confidence in the ability*.

It is important to remember that self-efficacy is inextricably linked to competence. It is not built by simply getting people to believe that they are good at music when, in fact, they are not. Self-efficacy is not the result of "positive thinking" or getting musicians to believe "I think I can" in the manner of the children's story of the little engine that could. Rather, expectations of future attainment are based on past successes of accomplishment, or "mastery experience" (Zelenak, 2015). Formal music education experiences do not always result in music students building self-efficacy, perhaps because of teachers "requiring students to perform music beyond their ability level" (Zelenak, 2015, p. 400). In contrast, the self-efficacy built through successful and enjoyable music-making experiences can impact people's musical self-appraisals going forward (Woody et al., 2019).

Mindset: Self-Theories of Ability

In recent years, one of the most popular theories of human motivation for learning is the powerful and practical mindset framework (Dweck, 2006). It characterizes people's self-theories of ability according to two broad frames of mind. People with a *fixed mindset* believe ability (of a certain kind) is innate and unchangeable; they may see it as a genetically determined trait or an inborn talent. On the other hand, those with a *growth mindset* believe ability is malleable and can be improved through learning.

Mindset theory can be understood as an extension of the earlier *attribution theory* of motivation, which explains learners' motivation for future activity and achievement as being largely determined by how they explain past successes and failures (Weiner, 2004). Students make decisions about continuing in music based on their beliefs about their own prospects for success in it. Generally speaking, success breeds more success; early successes in music will encourage children to pursue greater music engagement, but failures can bring discouragement. *Attribution theory*, however, maintains that learners' motivation and achievement are affected not only by prior successes and failures but also by how they explain those outcomes. In other words, they ask themselves, "*Why* did I do well or do poorly in my last attempt?" In explaining a successful performance, musicians may rely on attributions of ability/talent ("I've always been good at sight-reading"), effort ("My months of practice really paid off"), luck ("I got lucky and played well this time"), or task difficulty ("I couldn't go wrong with that easy music"). Studies of music students show that ability/talent and effort are common causal attributions (Grings & Hentschke, 2017). Of particular interest to music educators is a possible trend across childhood in which as students get older, they believe less and less that effort determines musical success, and instead favor innate talent instead as the main determining factor. Research suggests that music teachers can be influential in students' building a self-concept that includes a belief in their capability to be musical (Shouldice, 2020). Learners' motivation seems to be best sustained when they attribute success to effort or strategy use (Hallam et al., 2016).

Music learners' mindset will affect the amount of *resilience* they show as they face challenges in their music activities (O'Neill, 2011). A growth mindset facilitates bouncing back from adversity and persevering through challenges. A fixed mindset, in contrast, undermines resilience. Resilience in learners is associated with inquisitiveness, a sense of personal autonomy, and a *mastery orientation* in skill development.

Musical Identity: Taking a Long-Term View

Resilience to setbacks and commitment to continuing musical involvement are much more likely to be shown in people who consider music part of their identity. Identity—that sense of *who one truly is*—is informed by beliefs about oneself and the world; values can be understood as beliefs that are especially influential in decision-making (Evans, 2016). The *expectancy-value theory* of motivation emphasizes the importance of personal values regarding an endeavor, and expectations about the benefits of achievement versus the costs required to attain it (Eccles & Wigfield, 2020). Students who especially value music typically do so for its intrinsic rewards and its ability to meet certain psychological needs (for competence, relatedness, and autonomy according to SDT), as well as for its more practical benefits (e.g., providing a social group, making one appear artistic or "well rounded" on college/scholarship applications). Those who come to value music are more likely to continue studying it, even when forced to choose between it and other elective subjects of study (Freer & Evans, 2018; Kingsford-Smith & Evans, 2019).

The original researchers of SDT labeled the upper levels of this internalization process as *identified regulation* and *integrated regulation* (Ryan & Deci, 2002). These terms reinforce the idea that among advanced musicians, the beliefs and behaviors that make them musicians have been integrated into their very identity. Those musical characteristics define who they are. Research has linked the construction of a musical identity—or lack thereof—to students' electing to continue or drop out of formal music study, as well as older people's decisions about whether to pursue music participation in adulthood (Evans & McPherson, 2015). Unfortunately, it appears that constructing a musical identity is no easy building project. It appears that many young people make decisions about their own musicality by comparing themselves to others, including what they are exposed to via mass media, and may too readily come to consider themselves not good at music or even "unmusical" (Shouldice, 2014). The majority of the general public considers themselves to not be musical, including many who have received multiple years of music education (Woody et al., 2020; Zhang et al., 2020). Further, the specific characteristics built into a musical identity can be very consequential in decisions about exactly how to be musical in life (Lamont, 2017). Also, as seen in the story of Damien at the very beginning of this chapter, simply considering oneself a musician for life does not necessarily lead to choosing it as a profession (Zhang et al., 2020).

Establishing a musical identity can be viewed as a positive outcome of a musical childhood that featured ample motivation from a variety of sources. An alternative way to look at musical identity is as a key contributing factor to ongoing musical learning (Evans & McPherson, 2015). It appears that young people having a long-term identity goal involving music enables them to show greater persistence in their future music studies and to enjoy more productive practicing toward skill development (Evans, 2016).

In conclusion, the research provides clear guidance to music performers and teachers about the kinds of motivation that are most likely to contribute to a rewarding and healthy musical life. Unfortunately, the most positive contributing factors are not always easily attainable. Not all children's early environments are playful and encouraging. Some music teachers still promote a fixed talent explanation of musical ability over a growth mindset about the learnability of music for all people. And many musicians depend on looming performance to propel them to practice and take the stage with no expectation of enjoying the shared expressive experience with an audience.

Perhaps the most important application musicians can take from a study of motivation relates to the importance of goals. Musicians would do well to articulate their goals, remind themselves of them frequently, and use them to guide their musical lives. And when it comes to goal setting, aspiring to accomplish something positive is very different from seeking to avoid something negative (Hatfield, 2016; Smith, 2005). Musicians need to be honest and realistic about their goals. For example, a perfectionist mindset is not really about attaining a high performance goal for oneself.

Perfectionism is not only musically unrealistic, it usually takes the practical form of trying to avoid mistakes. Recall the previous explanations of task-and ego-involved orientations to performance; whereas a task-involved goal orientation allows musicians to focus on improving their skills and make performance about sharing their music with others, an ego-involved goal orientation often reduces performance to avoiding errors and failure. Cellist Yo-Yo Ma once recounted an early performance situation:

> While sitting there at the concert, playing all the notes correctly, I started to wonder, "Why am I here? I'm doing everything as planned. So what's at stake? Nothing. Not only is the audience bored but I myself am bored." Perfection is not very communicative. However, when you subordinate your technique to the musical message you get really involved. Then you can take risks. It doesn't matter if you fail. (Blum, 1998, pp. 6–7)

Taking the Stage: Adopt a Music-Involved Orientation

Musicians can take an active role in shaping their own motivation. Performers too often find themselves primarily responding to the expectations of others such that they unwittingly learn to ignore their own goal orientation. The chapter text mentioned a research study with music conservatory students in which one described a move from ego-involved to task-involved orientation to performance. Musicians should consider whether there is room for such movement in their own performance orientation. With honest musical soul searching, some performers may need to acknowledge that their performance experiences are too often characterized by anxiety, concerns about failure, and a preoccupation with how they will be judged by others. To reorient themselves to more of a task-involved approach, performers can try to exert more autonomy in their music-making activities. They can look for ways to include more of their musical "true loves" in their practicing and performing. They also can seek out opportunities to perform musical favorites in informal settings. With these steps, they gain more musical experiences that are personally meaningful to them and benefit from sharing music with friends, family members, and others in more naturally human settings. Then the next time they do return to the stage, perhaps they can more readily think of formal performance similarly: as a simple artistic sharing of emotional expression between human beings.

Leading Learning: Praise the Progress, Not the Person

Would-be musicians develop a fixed or a growth mindset primarily through enculturation. Children build beliefs about how musical they are—and how musical they could become—from what they learn about themselves from the important people in their lives, including teachers. Music educators should choose their words carefully when providing verbal instruction and feedback to their students, with the goal of nurturing a growth mindset and promoting resilience in young musicians. Telling a student "you are awesome" or "you are such a talented musician" may be well intentioned and may seem like the kind of compliment that will encourage a music student. The impact of such simple praise can, however, unintentionally signal to the recipient—as well as other music students in earshot—that music ability is a fixed aptitude that people either have or do not. Such a concept of music ability does not propel many students toward the motivation and achievement in music. In contrast, teachers can empower their learners by directing their feedback to students' music-making efforts, such as, "Your breath support has gotten so much better and now your tone sounds great" or "I'm so impressed with your singing improvement this semester. Your hard work is really paying off." Such feedback gives learners something to take with them into their future music making and reinforces their capability to accomplish musically what they set their minds to.

Chapter 3 Discussion Questions

1. Do you know a story of a promising young person who burned out or dropped out of an activity, like the account of Damien that started the chapter? If not a promising musician, then perhaps you recall a similar story about a gifted young athlete or prodigious student in another subject matter. Can you explain their burning out or dropping out in terms of some of the motivational principles in this chapter?

2. Thinking back on your own musical development, can you trace a progression of parents to teachers to peers to self, in terms of who provided extrinsic motivation? Was there another person or social dynamic that extrinsically motivated you to improve your musical abilities?

3. What elements of your mental makeup—thought patterns, beliefs, values—do you credit for allowing you to become the musician you are today? What mental elements are you working on improving?

4

Practice

This chapter concludes the book's Part I on Musical Learning. Note that the first two chapters addressed the natural musicality of human beings and the musical development that they typically experience in life. Chapter 3 explored why some people may become especially devoted to music, such that they end up committing many hours of their lives to serious study of music. This chapter focuses on an activity that accounts for the highest levels of musical expertise, but one that most people do not typically—or at least consistently—carry out, practice.

It is likely that readers of this book have done some music practicing in their lives, or at least engaged in practice-like athletic training or studying for school. Of these kinds of pursuits, people often encourage practice by saying, "You've got to put in the time" or offering the old joke "How do you get to Carnegie Hall? Practice, practice, practice." Platitudes like these seem to indicate that *quantity* of practice is the critical factor in skill acquisition. Unfortunately, popular handling of psychological research largely reinforced this misconception (discussed later in this chapter) and specifically propagated a "rule" that becoming an elite-level performer requires 10,000 hours of practice. More careful consideration of the research, however, shows that although developing musicians certainly must make time for practice, the efficiency and deliberateness of time spent is of critical importance.

Musicians need a comprehensive understanding of practice to enjoy the results that it can provide. This chapter addresses the following:

1. The word *practice* can have quite disparate meanings among different groups of people. Within performance psychology, however, practice refers to very specific activity, the definition of which should be instructive for musicians.
2. Through practice, musicians' skills gradually progress from being highly conscious and effortful to being more fluently and automatically executed. This process of skill acquisition is carried out as various physiological, perceptual, and psychomotor adaptations are made.

Psychology for Musicians. Robert H. Woody, Oxford University Press. © Oxford University Press 2022.
DOI: 10.1093/oso/9780197546598.003.0004

3. Although some musicians practice only as preparation for a particular performance, the most valuable function of practice is to build (or
maintain) proficiency in skills deemed important in one's musicianship. Outwardly observable performance is made possible by underlying cognitive skills that reside in the mind.

4. Rather than striving to simply amass hours of practice time, musicians
can be more productive and efficient by strategically planning, executing, and reflecting on their practice.

The Importance of Defining Practice

Practice is a concept that is common in many music cultures, as well as
other areas of skilled performance and professional training. Performers in
the arts, athletics, and other fields consider practice a standard part of their
preparations before showing their skills in a public event. The concept of
practice is also well established in the professional training of schoolteachers
and health care providers, among others. These programs include significant
"practicum" components, in which professionals-in-training demonstrate
and refine their developing skills in a real-world context under the supervision of experienced mentors.

Among Western classical musicians and those who have developed primarily
in a formal educational context, practice is usually carried out alone; preparation for group performance is known as "rehearsal." Rehearsal, but not practice,
is likely to have a teacher or director there structuring and leading the activities. This, of course, does not apply to the world of sports, in which the word
"practice" more typically refers to team (group) preparatory activity. Athletic
"practices" are almost always carried out under the leadership of coaches.

Not surprisingly, across the wide range of cultures and domains that exist,
there is great divergence in the purposes, structure, and strategies that characterize practice. The concept of practice that will guide this chapter (and
book) is that of *deliberate practice*, defined in psychology as a structured and
effortful activity, done in isolation, that is designed to improve performance
skill in certain specific and carefully chosen ways (Ericsson & Harwell,
2019; Lehmann & Jørgensen, 2018; Miksza, 2007; Platz et al., 2014). The
components of this definition are drawn from the best research on musical
expertise and performance skill acquisition and adapted to be readily applicable to musicians.

Also important in defining and understanding practice is distinguishing it from paid work and recreational activities. Whereas deliberate practice requires concentrated physical and psychological effort, work and recreation consist of behaviors that can be carried out at a more comfortably functioning level. When musicians are hired to work, they are expected to (and paid to) reliably perform what they already can do, not to push their limits, and to find and correct performance flaws in the process. When making music for recreation, musicians do the activities that will give them enjoyment, not those that reveal areas needing improvement. In both work and recreation, the activity can be sustained for very long times without psychological and physiological overload. The overload—which results from trying to do what has never been done before—is important to practice because the recovery from it produces the desired increase in skill.

Unfortunately, the defining and distinguishing characteristics of deliberate practice have not always been well understood and used by those interested in the attainment of performance expertise. After the 1993 publication of the seminal research study "The Role of Deliberate Practice in the Acquisition of Expert Performance" (Ericsson et al., 1993), a number of best-selling books cited it heavily in promoting the merits of intentional learning and hard work (rather than innate talent) in the pursuit of "greatness" (Colvin, 2008; Coyle, 2009) and "world-class status" (Syed, 2010). Perhaps the most popular of these, *Outliers: The Story of Success* offered the "10,000 Hour Rule," which presented this figure as the amount of practice required to achieve the true mastery of a world-class expert performer; "ten thousand hours is the magic number of 'greatness'" (Gladwell, 2008, p. 40). One of the author's prime music examples was the early rock band the Beatles, who, prior to their mass popularity in the 1960s, worked as a live band in strip clubs in Hamburg, Germany. These gigs reportedly lasted five to eight hours per night and helped the Beatles amass roughly 10,000 hours of time. The problem, however, is that a band's performance time together fails (in multiple ways) to meet the definition of deliberate practice. Frequent loose handling of the definition and research on deliberate practice eventually prompted the lead investigator of the hallmark 1993 study to confront it directly, even specifically addressing Gladwell's example of the Beatles: "An hour of playing in front of a crowd, where the focus is on delivering the best possible performance at the time, is not the same as an hour of focused, goal-driven practice that is designed to address certain weaknesses and make certain improvements" (Ericsson & Pool, 2016, p. 111).

Deliberate Practice as a Predictor of Expertise

It was not just popular nonfiction writers who were imprecise with the original deliberate practice research. The Ericsson et al. (1993) study became the target of some scholars who sought to advance an alternate explanation of musical skill resulting from factors other than practice (Macnamara et al., 2014; Mosing et al., 2014). Such research efforts tended to use estimations of practice times without specific attention to the defining characteristics of *deliberate* practice and concluded that practice "is important, but not as important" as argued by Ericsson and colleagues (Macnamara et al., 2014, p. 1). Similar research approaches that adhered to the proper definition of deliberate practice, however, have corroborated the primacy of deliberate practice in explaining expert performance in music (Ericsson & Harwell, 2019; Platz et al., 2014).

Although it can be easy to refute such tropes as "practice makes perfect," it is quite another thing to disregard the well-established finding of psychology that performers who engage in deliberate practice attain higher levels of performance expertise than those who practice less. Authentic deliberate practice is evident when musicians have explicit goals and can focus on feedback received about performance attempts. More advanced musicians can provide feedback for themselves in a practice session and use it to progress toward improved performing. Less advanced students, however, require the feedback assistance from a listening teacher, parent, or peer, or may benefit from audio recording their performances so they can subsequently listen when not distracted by the effort of performing.

Deliberate practice necessitates effort and concentration. These are needed to support the typically circular nature of practice: play → evaluate → play differently → re-evaluate and so forth. Practicing requires sustained focus on specific goals, detailed and attentive listening, and identifying problems and applying solutions. Obviously, carrying out these processes makes practice very effortful (and frankly beyond the capability of many young musicians without the supervision of an adult). The effortful nature of deliberate practice also means that it can be sustained for only limited amounts of time every day before psychological or physiological fatigue makes it an unproductive activity.

Although the development of the Beatles may not be a valid example of deliberate practice, the figure of 10,000 hours was derived from good psychological research. The seminal study of Ericsson et al. (1993) found this number from data collected from advanced music students who had attained various levels of performance expertise. In one study, violin students from a German music academy were compared with regard to the amount of time they had spent practicing over their lifespans. Accomplished students were rated by their teachers as being among either the "best" or the "good" students, and a third group consisted of aspiring students music teachers judged to be the "least accomplished" performers (all three groups were matched for age and sex). Also, to ascertain whether the "best" students were comparable with current professionals, members of professional orchestras in Berlin were also studied. Through an in-depth interview process, participants reported on current durations of solitary effortful practice and also estimated retrospectively how long and how many days per week they had practiced in a given year since the start of their training. Those estimates were later summed to a total duration of accumulated practice. A second study carried out a similar procedure with pianists, including a sample of amateurs. When comparing the lifetime accumulated practice durations among these various groups of musicians, the data indicated that the professionals and most advanced student performers had practiced significantly more than the other groups, approximately 10,000 hours by the age of 20. These data, presented graphically in Figure 4.1, offer compelling evidence for the importance of deliberate practice and against the existence of innate talent; if talent actually gives inherent advantage to the best musicians, one would expect them to be able to practice similar amounts (or even less) compared to others yet still achieve more.

The second study with pianists also involved their performing several motor skill tasks. The results indicated that accumulated deliberate practice correlated with motor skill speed and complex movement coordination. A few years later, the results of Ericsson et al. (1993) were corroborated by the research of Sloboda et al. (1996), which studied a large sample of student musicians, age 8 to 18, similarly grouped by levels of performance achievement. Data were collected in a carefully constructed practice diary, and results showed a strong positive relationship between performance achievement and deliberate practice, called "formal, task-oriented practice" by these researchers (p. 306). Perhaps more importantly, their data showed that the best students needed as many hours to progress from one level to the next as did the less proficient students, suggesting that there is no "fast track" to performance expertise.

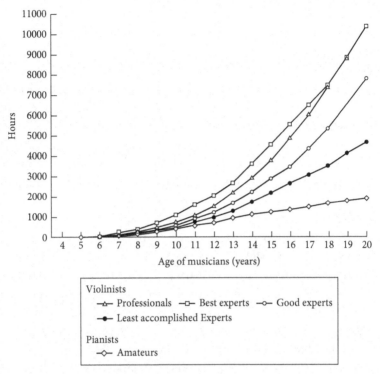

Figure 4.1 Relation between accumulated deliberate practice and attainment of instrumental music performance expertise.

Learning With and Without Deliberate Practice

As important as deliberate practice is to skill acquisition in classical music and similar genres, we must acknowledge that throughout history and all around the world, many people have become proficient music makers without that kind of practicing. Members of some musical cultures learn very sophisticated performance skills and huge song repertoires almost exclusively through enculturation and oral/aural transmission of music (i.e., person-to-person musical interactions including from generation to generation). Ear-based musicianship is the norm worldwide and is often developed and maintained in informal social settings.

Sloboda (2005e) referred to this kind of learning as the "acquisition of musical expertise in noninstructional settings" and pointed to folk music cultures and early New Orleans jazz musicians as examples (p. 248). Additionally, some non-Western music traditions include teaching and practice activities that differ considerably from Western music education. For example, in traditional Balinese gamelan, student instrumentalists are taught by a music leader, but only in a context of full ensemble rehearsal. The teaching is based on a demonstration and imitation process in which the leader offers a performance model and observing students attempt to reproduce it immediately. Many repetitions of this model-and-copy cycle take place with virtually no accompanying verbal instruction or slowing down, though the teacher may occasionally use head or hand signals to coordinate the music making with students (Bakan, 1999; McIntosh, 2018). One-on-one teaching is not part of this learning tradition, nor is solitary personal practice.

As mentioned in the previous chapter on motivation, popular or "vernacular musicians" develop their skills in contexts that differ greatly from the solitary technique-intensive practice that formally trained students are often asked to do. Vernacular musicians learn primarily through listening to and copying music they hear, and they usually practice informally in more socially enjoyable group settings with peers. Recall the point made earlier that deliberate practice is distinct from musical work and recreational activity. It must be noted, however, that vernacular musicians who are especially committed to their skill development may come to adopt elements of deliberate practice in their learning activities. They may be motivated to do solitary goal-driven practice upon seeing a more skilled peer carry out an impressive playing technique in a group rehearsal or after hearing a particularly captivating riff in a recording (Davis, 2005). They also may take up deliberate practice on the advice of famous musicians shared in published books, musician magazine articles, and websites (Green, 2002).

Similarly, performing musicians engaged in a work activity can make the opportunity more practice-like. Especially if the music being performed is not particularly challenging and includes considerable repetition, musicians may choose to use their music making during a gig to try out yet-to-be-mastered performance techniques. If they are able to set explicit goals and carefully monitor their attempts during this time, the deliberateness applied can yield performance skill improvement.

By no means should readers come away from this portion of the text concluding that practice is somehow optional. In music contexts where music education is prevalent, musicians who participate in informal music making only, that is, without deliberate practice, rarely attain a high level of performance expertise. The rare musicians who do seem to engage in inordinate amounts of informal rehearsing and performing and enjoy an unusually high level of motivational support that sustains the many long hours and sacrifices required in other areas of life (perhaps like the Beatles, as described previously). Some music researchers have referred to informal and nonde-liberate practice as a "suboptimal" learning activity (Lehmann & Jørgensen, 2018; Mornell et al., 2020). Such activities can indeed be helpful—especially for motivation—but all other things being equal, practicing music with the mind focused on improvement will always triumph in skill acquisition over less deliberate music-making endeavors.

Learning Accomplished Through Practice

For many musicians, what ultimately drives them to practice is a looming public performance. With this mindset, the goal of their practice at any given moment is to become better able to perform pieces of music for the coming concert or recital. However, the immediate behavioral goal (i.e., per-forming specific pieces of music) is best understood as merely an indicator of the broader and more long-term outcome of musicians' practice: the overall skill level of their performing musicianship. For instance, many people learn to play "Chopsticks" on the piano, but that does not make them pianists. Similarly, a person can learn to speak a sentence in a foreign language without really understanding what it means. In essence, productive practicing not only enables performance of given pieces of music but also establishes ge-neric mental representations (or cognitive skills) that support musicianship going forward, that is, music performance skills that transfer from one piece and difficulty level to the next. Quality practicing yields powerful under-lying cognitive skills that allow musicians to more readily learn subsequent pieces of music, because certain note combinations and other music material encountered can be anticipated, and much of the motor execution required will have already been experienced. In sum, new learning pathways rely on previously acquired mental structures.

The power and efficacy of practice comes from deliberately employing the mind. After all, the mind is where learned knowledge and skills reside. This is why truly productive practice can elude even well-intentioned musicians. Those practicing amid potential distractions (e.g., friends, a television, or a smartphone loaded with social media and game apps) will be able to log prac-tice time but fail to register any lasting skill gain. Similarly, musicians who push themselves to practice in time blocks of several hours at a time invariably lose concentration and attention to detail as the time passes; all human beings are subject to fatigue, which usually sets in well before practicing musicians care to admit.

Practicing allows musicians to build new mental representations: of music, of performance skills, and of beliefs in one's own musicianship. This kind of mental construction is no easy task. While components may be built gradually (and covertly) through enculturation and mere "time on task" with music, the mental representations that support expert music performance are constructed more expeditiously and permanently via deliberate practice.

Progressing Through Stages of Skill Acquisition

Of course, the mental representations associated with deliberate practice are not acquired instantly but, rather, through a process over time. The field of cognitive psychology has established that fully learned skills first begin as mentally effortful, but with enough practice, they progress to where they can be done without thinking. Even abilities that people take for granted, such as walking or driving a car, first began as deliberate and highly conscious. Obviously babies cannot verbally articulate their thought processes, but the effort is usually written all over their face when they try taking those first steps. And many drivers can recall the thoughts racing through their heads as teenagers when they first sat behind the wheel.

The process of skill acquisition is thought to pass through three stages: cognitive, associative, and autonomous (the first presentation of these stages is usually attributed to Fitts & Posner, 1967; see Hallam, 2010, for a music-focused application). With a new skill in the cognitive stage, music learners rely on *knowledge* about how to physically perform a task, for instance, knowing that a particular fingering pattern will work best for a scalar passage on the piano. Using this knowledge, they essentially instruct themselves deliberately or methodically to carry out the bodily movement required. With proper repetition, learners can pass into the associative stage, in which procedural knowledge is attained. Using the piano example, musicians in the associative stage no longer need to mentally draw upon the factual knowledge about the fingering; they now associate the "feel" of the performed pattern and can consciously apply it. With continued repetition, the skill enters the autonomous stage. Procedural memory is solidified to allow performance to become faster and more fluent. Pianists in this stage can play an entire scalar passage in various musical contexts, devoting virtually no conscious attention to carrying out the movements.

Music performance skills in the autonomous stage are said to have reached a level of *automaticity*, which is particularly empowering to performers because it frees up their cognitive resources to deal with musical matters other than the skill itself. This achievement can allow them to attend to and musically interact with coperformers, to respond to an audience's feedback, or to spontaneously add expressive elements in the moment. The automaticity produced by practice leads to a consistent reproducibility of performance. That some performers can demand large sums of money for their performances attests to the fact that they deliver the same high-quality "product" every time—within small margins of error that are imperceivable to the audience. Small variability in performance is a hallmark of expert performance. On the contrary, amateur musicians display much greater variability in performance; they may have "good nights" and "bad nights" in their music making.

Although the cognitive, associative, and autonomous stages are best understood as outlining the learning and mastering of specific skills, this three-stage model can also be applied to the lifespan development of musicians (Hallam & Bautista, 2018). Figure 4.2, taken from Papageorgi et al. (2009), shows this: As beginners, musicians spend a lot of time in the cognitive phase as they initially explore the domain of music and begin musical study and practicing. Later, much of their skill acquisition is in the associative phase as they make a greater commitment to music and aspire for high levels of performance achievement. Subsequently, with most of their musical skills in the autonomous phase, musicians can devote attention to other pursuits, including mentoring or teaching younger musicians.

Among performing musicians, the fluency of the autonomous stage is a much-desired outcome of practice. With it, fast scalar runs, "licks," and genre-specific embellishments can be performed without thinking. Such programmed movement sequences allow the performer to attend to more important aspects of performance. Without this automaticity, novice musicians must divide their attention between multiple performance aspects—including simply producing the physical movements required—which can limit the overall performance quality. It should be noted, additionally, that acquired skill in the autonomous stage is very different from a

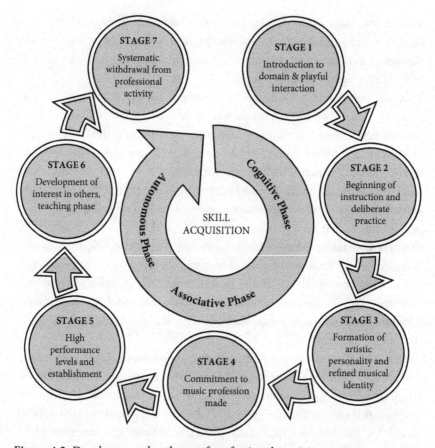

Figure 4.2 Developmental pathway of professional musicians.

From Papageorgi, I., Creech, A., Haddon, E., Morton, F., De Bezenac, C., Himonides, E., Potter, J., Duffy, C., Whyton, T., & Welch, G. (2009). Investigating musical performance: Perceptions and prediction of expertise in advanced musical learners. *Psychology of Music, 38*(1), 31–66. doi:10.1177/0305735609336044

motor process that has become incidentally automatized through mere repetition, such as bad habits that performing musicians are not aware of. Such unintentionally automatized behavior (i.e., not supported by underlying mental representations) can become a liability during performance. This effect can sometimes be observed among young musicians who repeatedly play a piece of music from start to finish (always and only start to finish), but if experiencing a memory lapse—say, in the big year-end recital—the result is catastrophic because, without a good mental representation of the piece, they are unable to restart anywhere in the middle of the piece.

Physiological Adaptations

Practicing music is just one of many regular occurrences in musicians' lives, and their bodies and minds respond to it in the same way that they do to recurring demands of other kinds. The human body is extremely responsive in this way. For example, farmers may have rough hands as a result of their time spent working the land, and weightlifting fitness buffs are often easy to spot because of their muscle-bound physiques. Musicians also display such telltale physical characteristics: calluses on the fingertips can be indicative of a string instrument player, and a violinist may have a discolored spot on the neck where the instrument contacts the player's skin. Not all physiological adaptations are as obvious. For example, pianists have been found to possess greater finger coordination (flexibility and isolated finger movement) across multiple joints and muscles of the hand, as compared to nonpianists (Furuya & Altenmüller, 2013, 2015). Wind instrument players have shown greater pulmonary function (lung capacity and respiratory strength) than nonplayers (Dhule et al., 2013).

Brain research has indicated that the physiological changes made are related to the amount and intensity of musical training and practice. For a long time, scientists believed that the brain remained anatomically unchanged except for pathological or aging symptoms. That is no longer the case as brain adaptations have been revealed by neurophysiologists using sophisticated imaging techniques (Münte et al., 2002; Oechslin et al., 2018). This kind of research has shown some interesting things about the brains of musical performers. For example, in string players, the area of the brain's cortex responsible for the left hand (which works the strings on the finger board) was enlarged compared to that of the right hand (which merely plucks, strums, or holds a bow). This kind of cortical reorganization tends to be more pronounced for persons who started their musical training at an earlier age. Other studies have shown that this reorganizing in the brain is not restricted to performing music but also appears when listening to music: larger areas of the cortex are activated when musicians listen to tones of their own instrument as opposed to instruments they do not play. Finally, research has found differences in the volume of gray matter in the motor, auditory, and visuospatial brain regions of professional musicians compared with amateur musicians and nonmusicians. It appears that training and deliberate practice induce far-reaching changes in musical brains.

Perceptual and Psychomotor Adaptations

What types of adaptations might be expected to coincide with growth in performance skill? These include perceptual and psychomotor adaptations. Note the word *psychomotor* is used instead of *motor performance* because human beings' skilled physical movement (including in music making) is mediated by mental processes, which also trigger further mental activity. It is also possible to talk about perceptual-motor skill when motor skills are interconnected with hearing and vision (as in reading music notation).

Musicians develop enhanced listening skills, which include greater sensitivity to pitch (frequency), timbre, loudness, and timing, as compared with nonmusicians (Kraus & Chandrasekaran, 2010). The improved discrimination of timbres and tones by musicians can be so specific that it does not always transfer even to speech sounds (Wallentin et al., 2010). Also, musicians playing instruments that require fine-tuning of individual notes during performance develop a more accurate discrimination for pitch height, whereas percussionists acquire an improved perception of durations (Rauscher & Hinton, 2003). Ensemble conductors develop the ability to preattentively monitor an unusually large auditory space (e.g., from first violin to cellos and basses) in which they can detect wrong notes or other inaccuracies (Nager et al., 2003). Similarly, pianists acquire superior tactile perception, and the gains made in this perceptual acuity can be linked to the amount of practice completed (Ragert et al., 2004).

Practice also appears to develop a special connection between motor activity and auditory perception for a variety of musicians. Percussionists have been shown to have better rhythmic perception when they tap along to the music with a drumstick (Manning & Schutz, 2016). Similarly, professional club DJs, who routinely engage in complex timing tasks with music in their work, have demonstrated superior rhythmic perception when free to move (e.g., head bobbing, silent foot tapping), compared to when sitting still (Butler & Trainor, 2015). Brain scans have shown coactivation of motor and auditory parts of the brain when musicians carry out certain sensory-singular tasks. When violinists silently (with no music playing) tap out the rhythm of a well-known concerto, the auditory part of the brain is coactivated (Lotze et al., 2003), and when pianists listen to familiar piano music, the motor parts of the brain coactivate (Bagert et al., 2006).

Cognition Underlying Practice

The adaptive changes made in the body and brain are obviously important in the acquisition of musical skill. From the standpoint of cognitive psychology, however, what happens *in the mind* is even more critical. Recall that the previous section laid out three broad stages of skill acquisition and made the point that musicians progress through these stages by building mental representations of their musical experiences. These structures of the mind are built more readily and permanently through deliberate practice. Consider, for example, a beginning bassoonist who, at the encouragement of her music teacher, is striving to play with a "good tone" in a practice session. She will first need to have in mind some idea of what that tone actually sounds like. Then she must be able to accurately hear her own attempts to produce a good bassoon tone herself. And only when she can mentally represent both the goal and her own sound can she compare the two to evaluate her progress.

Building mental representations is no simple undertaking, which is why good practice is so effortful and why it can be so difficult to get music students to do it. This challenge also explains why there is no substitute for the power of deliberate practice. Should our young bassoonist engage in some consistent practicing, in time she will become much better able to imagine a good bassoon tone and physically execute one on the instrument. She then goes into her future music-making activities equipped with the skills of being able to imagine music, produce it on the bassoon, and monitor her own performing. These new skills are newly built mental representations that reside in the mind.

Learning as Encoded Memory

Memory is best understood as mental function or capacity, rather than a personal account of a past happening in someone's life. All of the knowledge and skills that an individual possesses are stored in that person's memory. All that a musician has come to understand (factual knowledge) and has learned to do (procedural knowledge) has been encoded or "written" into his or her memory. This includes physically playing a musical instrument, which is best categorized as psychomotor skill rather than just motor skill. The popular term *muscle memory* is a good one for describing automatized physical skill, but only if it is understood as residing not in the muscles but in the memory (i.e., the mind).

Because deliberate practice is effortful, at one point or another fatigue becomes a factor for all musicians. Although more advanced musicians can build up a practicing stamina that allows them to carry out longer practice sessions, they too are susceptible to fatigue that reduces mental focus and concentration. Fatigue can lead to mistakes one would not otherwise make, failing to identify errors, and being too tired or distracted to use a strategy to correct them. In such conditions, practicing becomes subject to a law of diminishing returns; that is, the amount of energy and effort invested produces less and less benefit to skill development. If practicing musicians are not sensitive to this and instead decide to "push through," they may even end up doing damage to their skills.

Accordingly, musicians who wish to maximize the benefits of their practice are best served distributing their practice time over several shorter sessions, instead of cramming a whole day's work into one sitting. Time is needed for the mental representations of learning experiences to be transformed into long-term memory (Roesler & McGaugh, 2010). Mental rest and particularly sleep facilitate this neural process of *memory consolidation*. University music majors may contend that last-minute practicing right before the weekly lesson with their performance professor can work, that they can fool their professor into thinking that they did some productive practicing over the previous week. Be that as it may, any short-term gain accomplished through a single session of massed practice will likely *not* become permanent learning that can be further built upon going forward. From one day to the next, musicians can lose newly acquired skill without the memory consolidation that happens with adequate rest and sleep (Duke & Davis, 2006; Simmons, 2012).

Component Cognitive Skills of Music Performance

A number of researchers in music psychology have advanced a three-component model of the mental representations used in music performance that are built through practice (Ericsson & Harwell, 2019; Lehmann & Davidson, 2006; Miksza, 2005; Woody, 2003; Woody & Lehmann, 2010).

This model suggests that musicians must be able to generate (1) performance goal representations, (2) motor production representations, and (3) representation of current (ongoing) performance. Because generating these representations reflects abilities that are developed over time, they can also be thought of as the three component cognitive skills of goal imaging, motor production, and self-monitoring as shown in Figure 4.3.

Goal imaging is the ability to mentally represent what a piece of music should sound like. For nonmusicians, a goal representation of music is what allows them to recognize a song they hear or to judge that the output of a poor singer "doesn't sound right." For performing musicians, much more precise goal imaging is required to function as a plan for their desired performance of a piece of music. A wealth of experience listening to music (live and recordings) contributes greatly to musicians' ability to carry out detailed and robust goal imaging. This cognitive skill accounts for the proficiency of expert sight-readers, who use the notation of a printed score as cues to access musical knowledge in long-term memory to quickly construct a goal representation of what the unfamiliar music should sound like (Fine et al., 2006; Kopiez & Lee, 2008).

Mental representations for *motor production* are largely what separate musicians from nonmusicians. Goal imaging leads to music performance only if it is realized by executing the physical actions needed to produce musical sound with one's instrument or voice. If goal imaging represents musicians' "intention" for performance, then motor production represents their "action plan" (Pfordresher, 2019, p. 5). As explained previously, well-practiced physical performance skills progress from being very thought intensive (cognitive stage) to having more of a "feel" to them (associative stage) to eventually becoming automatically executed without thinking

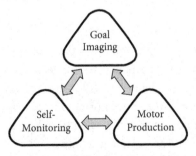

Figure 4.3 Component cognitive skills of music performance.

(autonomous stage). Musicians provide evidence for the existence of a motor production representation every time a performance skill, which once could only be done consciously and methodically, has become more automatically produced.

Coordination between goal imaging and motor production is especially important in playing by ear and improvising. Instrumentalists who are especially adept in these subskills of music performance possess this expertise "not due to better goal images but because of a greater ability to execute them" (Woody & Lehmann, 2010, p. 112). A link between goal imaging and motor production is also critical in reading music notation properly (i.e., understanding the symbols to represent musical sounds). This is why many music pedagogues throughout history have advocated a "sound before sign" approach in the learning activities of beginning instrumentalists (McPherson & Gabrielsson, 2002; Woody, 2012).

Self-monitoring is the ability to mentally represent the sound of one's own performed music. To judge whether their own performance is matching their goal, musicians must be able to objectively hear their music making. This can be especially difficult for musicians who have not yet attained any automaticity in their performing; if all of their attentional resources are spent on goal imaging and motor production, they will likely be unable to accurately hear the results of their efforts. Self-monitoring is critical for practice sessions to be productive. Developing musicians must be able to bear in mind both the sound of their desired goal and the sound of their produced attempts at it. Only with a comparison between these two representations can they "make the differences targets for generating a new and better attempt" (Ericsson & Harwell, 2019, p. 4). The importance of self-monitoring is also seen in research showing that musicians' motor skill learning is significantly impaired when performance conditions prevent them from hearing their own performance (Brown & Palmer, 2012).

Note that in Figure 4.3, there are two-way arrows between all three components. This emphasizes that it is the interaction of the three that supports skilled music performance and its learning throughout practice. This three-component model accounts for the aspirations and goal setting of musicians, their continuous monitoring of concurrent performance, and the error detection and correction needed to reduce discrepancies between desired performance and actual musical output.

Mental Practice: Valuable Supplement
in Some Circumstances

Given the importance of mental representations in music performance, musicians may wonder if purely mental practice can offer an advantage. One may call to mind stories of basketball players, struggling with free-throw shooting, being coached to skip going to the gym altogether (lest poor shooting there further demoralizes them) and instead spend time imagining lots of made free-throws *in their mind*.

In mental practice, a musician thinks through a performance task in absence of any overt physical movement. Research suggests that as a learning strategy, mental practice (1) is better than no practice, (2) can enhance physical practice, but (3) by itself is rarely as effective as physical practice alone (Miksza, Watson, & Calhoun, 2018). It is interesting to consider how mental practice can serve to supplement physical practice. It may be especially useful in moments when a musician's body is tired but mind is sharp. As alluded to earlier, when skilled musicians think through music (in terms of its sound), the movement areas of the brain can be coactivated. Although research on the topic is complex, mental practice does seem to work, especially with a musician who is mentally fresh, who has strong technical proficiency, and who can vividly imagine the sounds and feelings of the music being practiced (Holmes, 2005; Loimusalo et al., 2019). Mental practice is in itself a skill that must be learned to be effective (Connolly & Williamon, 2004).

Silent score reading is a specific kind of mental practice that is used by Western classical musicians who perform repertoire from memory (Loimusalo & Huovinen, 2018). This approach is considered an important part of the memorization process and is especially facilitated by strong aural skills—so musicians can mentally "listen" to the music while looking at the score; aural imagery is especially useful in learning melodic material in tonal music. More conceptual memorization strategies can be aided by the ability to carry out traditional musical structural analysis, for example, "harmonic progressions, thematic connections, melodic or rhythmic patterns, bass lines, etc." (p. 227).

Further supporting the idea that mental practice can work is research showing that among musicians, the brain seems to process imagined music similarly to how it perceives music that is audibly present. This is particularly true among more advanced musicians (Seung et al., 2005) and with

music material that is familiar (Herholz et al., 2012). Thus, a sensible conclusion about mental practice is that it should not be considered as a substitute for physical practice but can be effectively used as a supplement. Also,
it is a strategy best suited to advanced musicians with very robust mental
representations of the music they are learning and of the physical skills
needed. Also, because precise mental representations are needed, mental
practice is likely not effective with unfamiliar music material or new skills.
Finally, sessions of mental practice should be kept short because mental fatigue can disrupt the focus and concentration needed.

Productivity and Efficiency in Quality Practice

Despite their best intentions, sometimes young musicians do not practice effectively. In a practice session, their goals for being there may escape
them or they may lack strategies to correct problems, or they are simply too
tired to muster up the necessary attention. Also, as conditions become less
favorable—for example, when musicians are hungry or have tired of using
the same strategies—then practice as a whole can become a waste of time.
For many developing musicians, the *quality* of their practice (i.e., its structure and strategy use) is a better determinant of progress than quantity of
practice. Consequently, a musician's apparent lack of progress in spite of
reported adequate amounts of practice might actually be related to suboptimal conditions before, during, and after practice (Duke et al., 2009; Valera
et al., 2016).

Because novices differ from higher-achieving musicians in their observable practice (Miksza, 2011; Valera et al., 2016), it appears that quality
practicing is learned behavior. Beginners, especially children, are not capable of generating the necessary mental representations and structuring
their practice time accordingly. Recall the three component skills presented
in Figure 4.3. Until beginning musicians have acquired these cognitive skills
for themselves, they rely on the input and feedback of others to support their
practicing. Poor goal imaging can be bolstered by hearing performance
models provided by music teachers and more proficient musical peers.
Motor production representations can be supported through a teacher's
written instructions, or even verbal reminders provided by parents who
sat in on their child's last music lesson. Inadequate self-monitoring can be
compensated for through the use of computer and smartphone applications

that can audio record performed music and even assess its pitch and rhythm accuracy.

As musicians become more cognitively self-sufficient, they can better regulate their own practice. The concept of *self-regulation* is used to describe learners' overseeing and managing their own learning. Self-regulation is important because deliberate practice often takes place while learners work in isolation. Practice and self-regulation go hand in hand for musicians as they become active participants in their own learning process (McPherson & Zimmerman, 2011). In situations in which musicians' accumulated practice hours do not add up to produce the expected skill acquisition, the addition of self-regulation seems to improve the equation (Bonneville-Roussy & Bouffard, 2015).

Research on self-regulated learning has described a three-phase cyclical model that consists of (1) preparing for, (2) executing, and (3) reflecting on practice. Most of the research has used terminology originally offered in the context of educational problem-solving and, as such, labeled the three phases Forethought, Performance, and Self-Reflection (Zimmerman, 1998). To avoid confusion in this application to a musical context, the term *execution of practice* is used instead of *performance*.

Forethought Before Practicing

Deciding where to practice is often the first step in a young musician's practice planning. Whether they do so in their bedroom, a woodshed (as the old idiom goes), or designated "practice rooms" that conservatories and university music programs offer, musicians can boost the quality of their practicing simply by thinking about it before stepping into the space where they start a practice session. Adding a phase of forethought is a key element in making practice become a part of true self-regulated learning (Hatfield et al., 2017).

Musicians who practice from sheet music—repertoire or etudes/exercises—can add forethought simply by looking over the music before practicing to identify spots that will likely challenge their current skills; this advance planning strategy can help musicians avoid a practice approach of merely " 'passing the time' by playing a piece 'over and over' " (Austin & Berg, 2006, p. 547).

A particularly powerful part of the forethought phase is the hierarchical planning that amounts to identifying long-term goals for practice and, for each of those, selecting shorter-term goals and strategies for organizing sessions (Hatfield et al., 2017). The ability to carry out this higher-level planning seems to depend on musicians' self-efficacy, that is, a self-assessment of their ability to approach and accomplish goals. Keeping a practice diary is a practical technique that can help musicians improve their planning and productivity by explicitly stating (in writing) performance learning goals and ideas for what they need to practice to approach the goals (McPherson, 2005; Osborne et al., 2020).

Coming to believe in the value of practice is an important point that many young people reach in their musical development. Fewer, however, come to understand the value of thoughtful practice planning. Nonetheless, the research is clear: the strategic planning, self-assessment, and goal setting that define the forethought phase position musicians to succeed in the next phases of executing practice and reflecting afterward (Hatfield, 2016; Hatfield et al., 2017; Nielsen, 2015).

Execution of Practice

Sometimes referred to as the phase of "volitional control" (Zimmerman, 1998, p. 2), this second phase of self-regulation involves learners in monitoring themselves and focusing attention on the tasks of practicing. Their effectiveness in executing practice depends in part on how they use the resources they have available to them (e.g., books, recordings, technology tools, the expertise of others) and how they choose strategies for making improvements (McPherson et al., 2019). Because deliberate practice is designed to approach a new level of skill not yet attained, musicians must devote special attention to error detection and correction. This is not to say, however, that they are merely waiting for mistakes to happen. Rather, since this execution of practice has followed the forethought phase, they are able to anticipate problems or weaknesses and have already begun trying to diagnose them to best choose corrective strategies (Miksza et al., 2018).

The strategies that have been shown to be effective during musical practice include the following (Miksza, 2015):

1. Whole-part-whole repetition. With a reasonably sized chunk of music containing a performance problem, the practicer works on a smaller isolated section or a specific objective within it and then recontextualizes the practice by repeating the original entire chunk again.

2. Chaining. When identifying a specific moment in the music that is particularly difficult, the practicer repeats a few notes that make up that
   spot and gradually lengthens the amount repeated by adding notes before or after.
3. Slowing. With a passage that cannot be performed well due to the
   tempo, the practicer performs it at a tempo slow enough to ensure accurate execution, and then, using a metronome to keep the pulse steady
   and preserve rhythmic precision, the practicer gradually increases the
   tempo to the target.

When practicing music from notation, a practical technique that can help is
for musicians to write on the sheet music (e.g., "marking the score") to offer
themselves reminders of the performance goal for that part of the music or of
the technique required to achieve it.

Perhaps the most critical element in the execution of practice is for
musicians to be proactive versus reactive. Proactive practicing highlights the
connection between the forethought and execution phase: when musicians
begin a practice session, they are already aware of what is likely to need
special attention or extra work, so those moments do not become sources
of surprise or disappointment. On the contrary, musicians who take a reactive approach to practicing—that is, choosing corrective strategies only in
the moment when problems are encountered—are more likely to experience
frustration and procrastinate in practicing (Hatfield, 2016).

Proactivity can be critical. When practicing a particular piece of music,
reactive learners tend to start at the beginning of the piece, stop only as difficulties are encountered, and exclusively repeat the trouble spot. Proactive
learners, instead, use a greater variety of corrective strategies, such as starting
at different parts of a piece (not just the beginning), which may aid in
building a more precise and multifaceted mental representation of the music
being learned (Rohwer & Polk, 2006).

Reflection After Practicing

In addition to identifying goals in advance of a practice session and monitoring themselves while practicing, self-regulating musicians engage in
postpractice reflection regarding the extent to which they achieved the
goals they set. As with the previous phases of self-regulatory practice, the

self-evaluation done during reflection occurs at multiple short- and long-term levels. Musicians can reflect on a practice session's completeness (did they get to everything they planned to?), effort level (were they able to stay focused throughout?), and productivity (did they experience progress being made?).

Finally, having a disposition for *coping* can be an important part of self-reflection (Hatfield et al., 2017). Musicians benefit from an orientation to deal productively with negative experiences, to use them to gain insight and to adapt going forward. How they explain relative successes and failures in their practicing can be very consequential. Because the phases of self-regulation are cyclical, it is also important to note that effective self-reflection informs the forethought phase of future practice efforts, perhaps leading musicians to adjust long-term goals or choose new goals for the short term.

After expending mental effort in the forethought phase and execution of practice, some musicians may feel themselves without the energy to engage in any intensive reflecting. This phase, however, should not be neglected. Making reflection a part of practice contributes to musicians' motivation in two important ways. In the short term, it can aid in the ease and effectiveness of goal setting for the next practice session. More generally, reflection can be a powerful contributor to musical self-efficacy.

As alluded to earlier, effective self-regulation is cyclical. Musicians constantly choose, modify, and evaluate the strategies that guide their performance attempts in practice and use the self-evaluated feedback thereby gained to inform subsequent strategy use and performance attempts. This summary description may portray the processes of self-regulation as particularly effortful or even painstaking. To be sure, musical self-regulation is *multidimensional* (McPherson et al., 2012; Miksza et al., 2018). It involves musicians' thoughts and feelings, and it deals with the *why* and *how* of practicing (i.e., goals and strategies). Although self-regulation does not need to be unpleasant, it does take time for developing musicians to adopt this approach to practice. They will likely only do so if their learning environment encourages this (Valera et al., 2016). Their music performance instructors and peer-mentors can do much to help, as can parents for younger learners.

The elements of high-quality practice appear to become more important as a musician's skill level increases. That is, beginners can improve from any kind of practice, provided they put in enough time. But this is not the case for advanced musicians. More skilled music performers may be able to refine their skills with less overall time invested, but only if they carry out efficient and productive practice that features goal setting, focused attention, and deliberate strategy (Bonneville-Roussy & Bouffard, 2015).

In the preceding pages, this chapter has emphasized the value of practice and explained what is accomplished when musicians do it well. Adopting practice into a musical lifestyle is largely a matter of motivation (see Chapter 3, especially the section "Internalizing Extrinsic Motivation"). There are, however, actions that musicians can take and attitudes they can adopt outside of practice sessions that can help make their practice more productive.

Musicians do well to remember that the overriding goal of practice is not just to log time. Being realistic about the demanding nature of practice should compel many to expect better results if they focus less on quantity and more on quality. It can be counterproductive when parents or teachers push beginners into logging practice time without first equipping them with the support and strategies needed to make it worthwhile to them; these youngsters may never come to experience the truth that practicing improves skills, which makes music making more personally rewarding. More experienced musicians may be able to better advance their musicianship by putting in more modest amounts of practice time and supporting it with other musical activities. Making time to listen to music can get squeezed out of a life in which logging practice time is paramount. Music listening, though, can be an invaluable contributor to goal-imaging ability. Developing musicians can also gain much by attending live performances of other musicians or watching video recordings of these. (Note, there is no support from psychology for the superstition-like fear that taking in the music of others will somehow hinder music learners' capacity for original and personal music making of their own.) At the very least, taking in the performances of others provides insight into the audience perspective, which can be a useful perspective for one's own performance preparations. And finally, providing instruction and mentoring to younger music students can be beneficial to advanced musicians themselves. This level of learning can inform their own practicing. Many experts have expressed that they never truly understood their craft until they tried to teach it to others.

Because practicing is so effortful and can be so powerful in musical skill acquisition, developing musicians who are especially committed may find themselves becoming serious students of and advocates for the very process of practice. They apply self-regulation to their practicing at a macro level. They constantly do "big picture" evaluation of their practicing approaches and results. Put more practically:

Perhaps in the best-case scenario, musicians become so engaged that they become fascinated with the phenomenon of practice itself. It becomes a time to experiment with new strategies and test theories about oneself. . . . Musicians who do this with their practicing can come to think of themselves as private investigators of the performance process or musical explorers. Beyond just capturing a great performance at the end of the process, practicing is about the "thrill of the hunt." (Woody, 2019, p. 46)

Taking the Stage: Keep a Practice Journal

Since all musicians are susceptible to mental fatigue, it behooves them to find ways to lighten the load during practice. A good way to do this is by keeping a practice journal; this written record can facilitate productive goal setting before practicing starts and self-reflection afterward. Journal entries can be organized around individual practice sessions or around each day of practicing (it is better to distribute daily practice across multiple sessions, rather than in a single extended one). However musicians decide to organize individual entries, they should also goal-set and plan in longer periods (perhaps weeks or months) that are structured around general skill goals. For example, a university music major decides to use a particular semester of trombone study to approach the goal of improving her slide technique. In a practice journal, therefore, for each daily entry, she includes a category heading of "Slide Technique." Before beginning practice the first week of the semester, she reviews what she has learned about trombone generally and about herself as a trombonist more specifically to diagnose what is most lacking in her current slide technique skill level. Based on feedback from trombone teachers, she decides that a good way to approach her goal is to practice music material she is already familiar with (in terms of notes and rhythms) so when she plays through it, she can focus intently on getting her slide precisely in the correct position and moving between positions very quickly. For this purpose she decides to use major scales and exercises from a method book she often used during her senior year of high school. So for Week 1 in her practice journal, under the "Slide Technique" heading of each daily entry, she indicates her plan to practice the chosen musical material for 10 minutes and leaves space on the page to add comments after practicing for reflection on how well it went and any adjustments to try with her approach.

Leading Learning: Teach and Reward Practice Process

Music teachers commonly face difficulty getting young musicians to practice. No matter how much they preach the value of practicing, it seems a continuous struggle to motivate their students to carry out the practicing needed to produce results. In an effort to keep students accountable, many music teachers require their students to keep a record of their practicing. Weekly practice logs typically ask music students to put in writing the amount of time spent practicing daily and have parents sign off to validate that the amounts have been recorded honestly and accurately. In evaluating the effectiveness of this typical approach, though, music teachers should consider what it is they *most* want for their students to learn about practice. They do not likely want their students to put in time *regardless of results*. Music teachers may want to consider how English and math teachers assign homework. They do not simply ask students to spend a certain amount of time reading or doing mathematical things; rather, they assign specific material to read or a collection of math problems to solve. Also, good math teachers would never assign students a set of problems as homework without first providing them instruction on *how* to solve them and giving them an opportunity to first try under teacher supervision. Rather than asking music students to just spend time practicing, instructors should provide the guidance young musicians need to know *what* and *how* to practice. Thus, instead of students completing a weekly practice log on which they merely report time spent, they can give an indication of the *process* that they used in their practice, including strategy use and postpractice reflection.

Chapter 4 Discussion Questions

1. Think back to when you first started practicing as a young musician. Do you remember why you were practicing? If, in the future, you find yourself working with young musicians as a parent or teacher, how will you support them in their early practice efforts?
2. In your experience, what are the biggest barriers or distractions that interfere with the attention and concentration needed to make practice effective?
3. Of the phases of self-regulation that fall outside the actual execution of practice (i.e., forethought and self-reflection), which is harder to add as part of your practice routine? What could you do to more readily incorporate it into your practice?

PART II

MUSICAL SKILLS

5

Learning and Remembering Musical Works

Beginning the book's Part II on musical skills, this chapter considers the very common goal of learning pre-existing pieces of music. It is equally common in vernacular music—for example, young hip-hop fans may aspire to learn a rap recorded by their favorite artist—as it is in formal music education, in which young performers are often assigned to learn a piece from published sheet music provided by a teacher. Whether learning to a piece by ear or from notation, the processes of memory involved are very similar.

The learning of musical works can also be understood as an important precursor to additional kinds of music making and performance skills. As described in Chapter 2, receptive skills precede productive skills in musical development. Young people are able to perceive and imitate familiar music before being able to produce original musical ideas. Typically, in formal music education, teachers expect their students to have learned the "notes and rhythms" of a piece before devoting much attention to the expressive qualities of its performance. In addition, most learners are taught to read music by working with the notation of *familiar music* before taking on the challenge of *sight-reading*. For its part, making music by ear is a well-accepted precursor to improvisation and, in fact, appears to be a foundational musical skill that contributes to all others (as will be shown later in the chapter).

This chapter explains the following points about learning and remembering pieces of music:

1. Learning music means encoding it into memory, and doing so efficiently relies on identifying the meaningfulness of the material to be learned.
2. Reading the symbolic representations of music notation is a reconstructive process that depends on musicians' previous knowledge as much as on the notated music.

Psychology for Musicians. Robert H. Woody, Oxford University Press. © Oxford University Press 2022.
DOI: 10.1093/oso/9780197546598.003.0005

3. Making music by ear is a learned skill that is foundational to other skills of music performance.
4. The ability to learn and remember musical works is domain specific and can be improved through experience and deliberate practice.

Core Mechanisms of Remembering Music

A solid understanding of human memory can be very beneficial to musicians. Memory within the human mind is the means by which musicians build the internal repertoire of pieces of music that they "know" and keep a knowledge base of information and principles that facilitate high-level music making. It is also the location of the "muscle memory" that executes the physical actions of skilled music performance.

For these reasons, memory may even be more important for skilled musicians than for people involved in other domains (Talamini et al., 2017). One definite exception to this would have to be the domain of chess, which has been a favorite of cognitive psychologists to study because of the memory-intensive nature of the game (e.g., Gobet & Simon, 1998; Lane & Chang, 2018). Like musicians, chess masters accumulate many hours of practice, in which they study transcripts of past world-class match competitions and commit to memory situational circumstances and the tactics that are most advantageous. The study of aspiring chess experts is similar to the description of deliberate practice (explained in the previous chapter). That is, the aspiring chess master devotes focused attention to published chess matches of masters and at various points tries to predict the next move, then checking the prediction against the actual move of the master. Identifying discrepancies from a master's moves constitutes error detection. Consequently, error correction is attained through understanding why the master's move is better than the learner's choice.

The performance of experts in music, chess, and other domains is facilitated by great knowledge bases of domain-related information and skill. Experts are not born with larger memory capacity; rather, they become proficient remembering what they learn from their experience and practice. They build their internal repertoires of knowledge and skill not through rote memorization or memory tricks, but by finding meaning in the material and experiences from which they can learn.

Chunking and *pattern recognition* are important psychological concepts related to how humans process information. Rather than processing information bit by bit, humans tend to search for patterns that allow processing of several units of information at the same time. For this, perceptual input is grouped into meaningful units or chunks. Knowledge, speech, and physical movements are organized into memory in chunks.

The size of chunks that people can mentally handle is variable and depends on their level of expertise. This is partly why a professional orchestra of advanced musicians can work up a concert-ready performance of a new piece of music with much less rehearsal time than a student ensemble would need. The ability to group and make sense out of information depends on previous knowledge, be it procedural (performance skills) or declarative (generalizable music principles and concepts). Similar to spoken language, musical meaning also depends on regular and predictive structure. Knowing the probability of certain events and qualities—gained through experience, study, and practice—helps experts establish meaning; for instance, experienced musicians are advantaged knowing that in tonal music a dominant seventh chord often resolves to the tonic, that many melodies occur in four- and eight-bar lengths, and that musical "runs" are composed of known scales patterns. Chunking is a memory mechanism that links perception to previously stored knowledge.

Human memory is very dependent upon the meaningfulness established at the point of perception. This is seen in the superiority of memory with domain-specific familiar material, as compared to that with unfamiliar or structurally incoherent material. Many advanced musicians would attest to the difficulty of sight-reading or memorizing atonal or 12-tone serial music. Typical chunking mechanisms do not apply, and instead of coding larger meaningful units (tonal melodies and harmonies), they have to group individual notes or intervals.

Research in a variety of domains has found that with meaningful content, experts do far better than novices on memory tasks, but this is not the case when the content is random or lacks the kind of structure that is typically present in the domain. Figure 5.1 offers some examples of the importance of the meaningfulness of material in learning and remembering in the domains of written text, music, and chess. It is much easier to remember the material as it is presented in the column headed "Meaningful in Real Context" because prior domain knowledge can be used. The letters of the word *fortissimo* are more readily committed to memory as a single item (the word) than as a

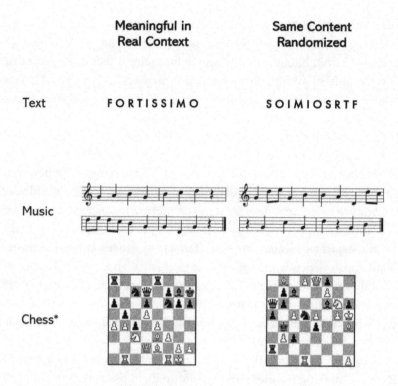

*Chess board configurations taken from Gobet, 1998

Figure 5.1 Meaningful versus randomized content.

random sequence of the individual letters contained therein (especially by classically trained musicians who use the word *fortissimo* regularly in their music activities). And the 16 notes of notated music in Figure 5.1 are more easily remembered when they are recognized as the four phrases of the folk song "Frère Jacques," rather than as a random sequence of the same notes. Although the chessboard configurations in Figure 5.1 may not appear all that different to some readers, they are plainly different in memorability to chess experts, who can almost instantly memorize an arrangement of pieces that can occur in a real game but whose memory is quite faulty with a random configuration. Incidentally, the research that has elucidated expert performer memory has exposed so-called photographic memory as extremely rare and not at all useful, if it exists at all.

Information Processing Model of Memory

Based on thousands of experiments, psychologists have developed sophisticated models of how information is perceived, processed, and stored. The information processing model indicates three types of memory: sensory memory, working memory, and long-term memory (LTM; Figure 5.2). *Sensory memory* lasts only fractions of a second. If the stimuli are not attended to at this stage, they are lost forever. Even though sensory memory is so fleeting, it is still important in music perception; because music occurs across time, only a fraction of a musical work is ever physically present at any point in time. For musical tones to be perceived as a sequence of sounds—let alone understood as a meaningful melody—sensory memory is required.

Cognitive scientists agree that deployment of attention is tantamount to learning (and recall) of information. When stimulus information is attended to, a representation of it enters short-term memory (STM), where it can reside for varying amounts of time. STM is also called working memory because it contains currently relevant information for usage and manipulation. Working memory can be thought of as mental workspace in which items are held and operated on; it compares to random access memory (RAM) in computers that loses its content when the computer is turned off. Information in working memory can be newly perceived stimuli that only recently passed through sensory memory, or it can be information that had been learned more permanently—that is, stored in LTM—and has been retrieved back into STM for further processing.

Information in working memory that is meaningful can be transferred to LTM. As the name suggests, stored information in LTM can be retrieved even after a very long time. Transferring information from STM into LTM—called encoding in the information processing model—is what constitutes "learning." For example, if students in a music class are taught to build

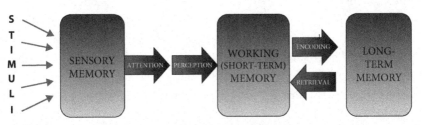

Figure 5.2 Information processing model of memory.

seventh chords in jazz harmony but they cannot remember how to do it a few days after the lesson, they did not actually learn it.

Because encoding information into LTM is so important, additional detail into the process is warranted here. Cognitive psychology has identified a number of ways that new information is encoded into LTM. The following are presented here roughly in order of increasing efficiency and meaningfulness:

1. Rehearsal. Not to be confused with the common musical meaning of "rehearsal," psychology uses this word to label rote repetition of information in its original form.
2. Organization. Relationships within new material are identified via grouping and categorization strategies.
3. Elaboration. Prior knowledge is applied to the new material, creating new associations with what is already known.
4. Imagery. Information originally perceived in one sensory mode is "cross-coded" into another; for example, music originally heard is visually imagined as notation.
5. Activity. New information is used meaningfully by personally responding to it, experimenting and creating with it, and otherwise using it in ways valued by learners.

Expertise Facilitated by Knowledge Base of Long-Term Memory

The achievements of expert performers, including in music, can be a challenge to explain with the information processing model of human memory. This is because expert performers seem to command immediate access to large amounts of learned material. Highly skilled expert memory is explained through the *long-term working memory theory* (Ericsson & Moxley, 2013). Through their skilled activity experiences, including deliberate practice, experts develop a privileged access to information stored in LTM. In skilled performance, all the relevant information need not be retrieved from LTM back into STM; rather, information stored in LTM is kept directly accessible by means of retrieval cues. Essentially, these cues are pointers to relevant knowledge in LTM and are built to suit the tasks that experts persistently engage in.

Acquiring musical expertise is about building a knowledge base of performance skills and conceptual knowledge. Both are important. Skills help conceptual knowledge become useful in a practical sense. And conceptual knowledge allows new skills to be experienced and practiced with deeper understanding. Both approaches help new material become meaningful, which makes it more likely to be encoded into LTM, thus making it permanent learning.

In this way the growth process that leads to expert musicianship is exponential in nature. The more meaningful knowledge musicians have in LTM, the easier it becomes for them to learn new information and move it into LTM. Also, a memory-based understanding of learning highlights the importance of retrieval cues in expert performance. Acquiring musical expertise is not just a matter of storing knowledge and skill in LTM but also using it persistently enough to build the retrieval structures that make that knowledge and skill readily accessible. This is why deliberate practice and performance experience are so critical in the development of musical proficiency.

Performing Music by Ear

Inasmuch as sound is the artistic material of music and hearing is the sense by which humans process sound, it would seem that the most natural way to learn a piece of music is by ear. As mentioned briefly in Chapter 2, hearing and imitating familiar music are hallmarks of typical development in childhood. Moreover, a survey of human musicality around the world and throughout history shows that learning music by ear is the norm, even though it may be somewhat of an exception among formally educated musicians in society.

Indeed, the values of Western classical music prioritize the performance of published "masterworks" written by noteworthy composers. This value system is plainly evident in formal music teaching and learning practices. It might, therefore, surprise modern-day classical performers to know that at the time when many historically significant composers penned their works, it was common for student musicians to learn them by ear. This practice only began to change with the advent of printing machines and the mass production of musical scores (McPherson & Gabrielsson, 2002). Even since then, however, many prominent music educators, researchers, and pedagogues— some of them noteworthy composers themselves—have strongly advocated that music learners not be exposed to the symbol system of music notation until they possess an ear-based fluency in their musicianship (Woody, 2012).

Skilled ear musicians do not require cues from notation (or any other source) to know what notes to sing or play on their instrument. Rather, their performance is guided by an internal model of what they want their music to sound like. And as the phrase "by ear" suggests, this guiding internal model was built by hearing music and remembering it. Making music by ear involves two skills: (1) learning a piece of music so well that it is encoded precisely in memory and (2) being able to realize this music on one's instrument (or voice).

Explaining Ear Playing by the Component Cognitive Skills

Chapter 4 presented the three component cognitive skills of goal imaging, motor production, and self-monitoring (see Figure 4.3). Making music by ear requires a link between goal imaging and motor production. This can be thought of as an "auro-motor coordination" (Baily, 1985; see also, Woody, 2001; Woody & Lehmann, 2010). If motor production is well coordinated with an aural image of the music, then simply having a precise goal image (i.e., having learned the music) allows a musician to produce it on an instrument. That is, the production of known musical sounds has become automatized. Skilled ear musicians do not need to consciously identify the musical pitches (e.g., by note name) of the music and cognitively instruct themselves about how to produce them on their instrument. Rather, the sound-to-action process exists in the autonomous stage of skill acquisition.

Developing musicians seem to acquire this automatized skill through ample opportunity to make music without notation. Many music students gain such experience only through vernacular music making done outside of the context of school music or formal lessons (Woody & Lehmann, 2010). Instrumentalists without these experiences may never gain the sound-to-action skill required to perform even simple music material by ear. Composer and pedagogue Zoltán Kodály decried the poor musicianship of brilliant pianists who "play only with their fingers" and not their ears and musical minds. "They are not musicians," he asserted, "but machine operators" (Kodály, 1974, p. 196).

Note that Kodály did acknowledge that some concert musicians can attain a level of competence—even brilliance!—without developing their ear-playing ability. Indeed, many musicians who learn to play an instrument without learning to play it by ear may be inclined to attribute the ability to a special giftedness. There is, of course, a more scientifically based explanation. A study by Woody and Lehmann (2010) compared the ear-playing abilities of two groups of advanced music students: (1) those whose past music learning experiences had occurred exclusively in formal instructional settings and (2) a similar group who had additionally participated in vernacular music making in their past music development. One of the main purposes of the research was to identify whether superior ear-playing ability is more attributable to better goal imaging or motor production. In the study, the musicians learned two melodies by ear; in each learning session, a musician would listen to the target melody and then attempt to perform it themselves, and the researchers tracked how many trials through this listen-then-perform cycle the musician needed to reach accurate performance (in pitch and rhythm). With one melody, the musicians learned it in order to sing it back; this served as a measure of their goal-imaging ability. With the other melody, they learned it to perform on their primary instrument; this indicated their motor production ability. The research participants also verbally reported the thought they had while carrying out the musical learning tasks.

Not surprisingly, the results showed that musicians with vernacular experience were significantly better at playing by ear, and that their motor production was superior. A more unexpected finding, however, was that those with vernacular experience also demonstrated significantly better goal imaging—that is, they were able to commit music to memory more quickly. Data analysis indicated that their superior ability was facilitated by "a more sophisticated knowledge base" applied while listening to the target melodies (Woody & Lehmann, 2010, p, 101). Musicians with vernacular experience more often employed a harmonic approach to learning melodies (e.g., using underlying chord progressions to chunk melody notes), whereas those in the "formal musicians" group tended to use less efficient interval-based or note-by-note approaches.

These findings were reinforced by more recent research that demonstrated that playing by ear can be improved by directing the attention of developing players' cognition to the underlying harmonic properties of a melody they are learning (Woody, 2020a). For some musicians, this move toward more advanced cognition can be accomplished by providing the implied chord changes of melodies being committed to memory:

> When the presence of the printed chord changes led to superior ear-based performance, cognitively speaking, the difference for the better was largely accomplished through faster encoding of the melody into memory. Not only was a goal image more quickly generated, it also seemed to support more facile instrumental performance (i.e., it aided musicians in being able to find the right notes on their instruments). (Woody, 2020a, p. 689)

The results of the Woody and Lehmann (2010) study indicated that the aural imaging cognitive component skill of musical memory is not exclusively sound oriented. That is, it does not function merely as a "tape recorder in the head" (p. 112). Rather, there is a conceptual aspect to it, for which musicians' prior knowledge—stored in LTM—is applied. This corroborates earlier research showing that when performing music informed by an aural model, musicians' explicit identification of features in the model produces better performance (Woody, 1999, 2003, 2006a).

Ear Musicianship as a Foundation for Other Performance Skills

It should be noted that the musicians with vernacular experience in the Woody and Lehmann (2010) study were not true vernacular musicians. They were music majors at a university. They had all the requisite "formal musician" performance skills required to be admitted into advanced study of music in higher education; they additionally had vernacular music-making experience. Musicians such as these are among those who populate university bands and orchestras. Although such ensembles do not require the skill of playing by ear per se, still university musicians with past vernacular experience bring to these groups' rehearsals and performances a musicianship that features strong aural skills and efficient goal-imaging ability. Applying ear musicianship research to traditional school ensembles in the United States, Musco (2010), affirmed, "We would do well to value playing by ear in the band and orchestra curriculum" (p. 60).

This discussion points to a conclusion reached by many music researchers and pedagogues over the years: music making by ear in no way detracts from the ability to read music. In fact, playing by ear is a key contributor to other instrumental performance skills, including sight-reading and performing rehearsed music from notation. Based on a thorough review of research literature, extensive field testing, and original research conducted with high school instrumentalists, McPherson et al. (1997) offered a theoretical model of the interrelation of musical skills. This model, shown in Figure 5.3, features playing by ear as the only one of the five music performance skills that contributes to all others. The theory that ear musicianship contributes to other performance skills has since been supported by additional research (Bernhard, 2004; Kopiez & Lee, 2008; Lee, 2006; Musco, 2009; 2010; Woody, 2020a; Woody & Lehmann, 2010). In their review of research literature related to the teaching and learning of music notation, McPherson and Gabrielsson (2002) concluded that emphasizing notation separate from opportunities to make music by ear "restricts overall musicianship and the types of skills needed for a musician to succeed long-term" (p. 113).

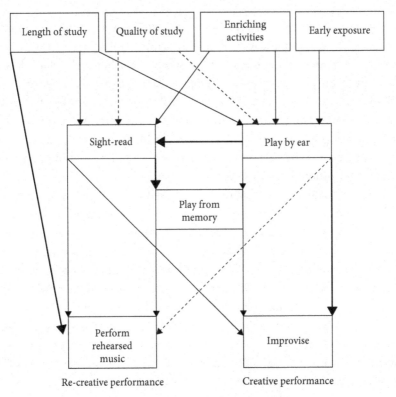

Figure 5.3 McPherson model of interrelated musical skills.

From McPherson, G. E., & Gabrielsson, A. (2002). From sound to sign. In R. Parncutt & G. E. McPherson (Eds.), *The science and psychology of music performance: Creative strategies for teaching and learning* (pp. 99–115). New York, NY: Oxford University Press. Reproduced with permission of the Oxford University Press through PLSclear.

Reading Music

The ability to read music notation—or attaining what some consider musical literacy—requires instrumental musicians to establish a link between the eye and the hand that is mediated by the ear. Without the ear in this process, young instrumentalists can become mere "button pushers," for whom "notation indicates only what fingers to push down" (Mills & McPherson, 2016, p. 181). The proportional contributions of the eye, ear, and hand seem to vary greatly across musicians, likely according to instrument (or voice), performance genre, and learning background.

Musical Symbol Systems

The system of notation that uses a five-line staff is very common in many traditions of Western music making. The symbol system used today, which evolved over time before the advent of sound recording technology, has as its primary purpose to archive sounded music so it would not be forgotten (Rankin, 2018). This system, which classical musicians consider "standard" or traditional staff music notation, represents pitch and rhythm (in Western tonal music) precisely, but not much else. For this reason, it can be quite effectual when used by skilled performers who are well versed in the performance conventions of the style of music notated.

There are other music symbol systems used in the Western world to archive music and to allow others to learn to play it. Tablature or TAB notation is used by many players of fretted instruments, most popularly guitar (Waldron, 2009). Guitar TAB uses a six-line staff, on which each line corresponds to a guitar string. While traditional staff notation is intended to represent musical sound, TAB represents how to perform the music on the instrument. Most learning musicians who use TAB today use it in conjunction with audio recordings to know what the music is supposed to sound like; the TAB functions more like technical instruction, which meets the needs of the musicians it serves. Other music systems do the same, including the Nashville numbers system, used by pop/rock and country musicians to indicate chord progressions in songs (Johnson, 2009).

Traditional five-line staff notation, although commonplace in music education, is not particularly intuitive to learners. For example, in terms of symbol size, a whole note is spatially smaller than a quarter note, even though the sound duration of a whole note lasts four times as long as a quarter note. Learning to read traditional staff notation can be "slow and tortuous for children" and other novice musicians who are asked to use the symbols of notation without first being familiar with what they represent (Mills & McPherson, 2016, p. 184). When researchers have asked children to notate familiar songs, their drawings tend to consist of iconic representations that may include scribbles, body parts (hand, foot, mouth), and instruments. Typically, it is only after children have started receiving music lessons that their created notations include some of the attributes of standard notation (e.g., letter names for pitches; shapes and visual spacing relationships to represent timing, duration, and rhythm; Upitis, 2018).

If nothing else, children's invented representations of music serve as a reminder that symbols of notation are intended to represent sound. This is why an automatized sound-to-action coordination mentioned previously in the context of playing by ear is also important in performing music from notation. This can be especially important in teaching beginners to play a musical instrument. When most children begin music study, the symbol system that they are already familiar with is that used to represent their native language; that is, they have either already learned to read the language proficiently or are well into that learning process. The experience of learning that symbol system can serve as an example for learning to read music notation, but only if music teachers consider it carefully. As outlined in the "Music and Language" section of Chapter 1, children can best learn a symbol system if they have first gained a level of aural fluency through hearing and imitating the sounds represented by its symbols. Sloboda (2005f) encouraged music teachers to re-examine their methods for helping learners acquire sight-reading proficiency, noting that no one would consider teaching children to read text when still at a very early stage of learning the spoken language. "Yet it seems the norm," he wrote, "to start children off on reading at the very first instrumental lesson without establishing the level of musical awareness already present" (p. 20). It need not be that way, of course. For many years, music educators have drawn upon research to advocate for a developmentally natural progression of "sound to symbol" when providing learning experiences to beginning music students (e.g., Clauhs, 2018; Gordon, 1999, 2003; Mainwaring, 1941, 1951; McPherson & Gabrielsson, 2002; Suzuki, 1966; Woody, 2012).

Explaining Music Reading by the Component Cognitive Skills

Highly skilled music reading uses the same sound-to-action coordination that is developed through experiences playing by ear. With this skill in place, musicians use the notation they are reading for cues to build a goal image of what the music is supposed to sound like. It is that mental representation that informs what they perform. With ample experience making music by ear—for example, as gained through vernacular music-making activities—the process of turning a goal image into motor production can be an automatized response.

Of course, not all instrumental musicians learn to "think in sound" like this (McPherson & Gabrielsson, 2002, p. 103). There are those who learn to use music notation like the "button pushers" mentioned earlier and the "machine operators" that Kodály criticized. Instead of using symbols to mentally represent a goal sound that can be fluently realized through sound-to-action motor production, they instead use a symbol-to-action process. The symbols of music notation are not understood as representing musical sounds as intended; rather, they act as direct cues to carry out actions on an instrument. Although musicians can become quite skilled at this—especially on instruments for which there is a unique key, fingering, or action for each producible note—it is not optimal sight-reading. Eliminating musician-imagined sound from music making is a humanly unnatural way of performing, and it ultimately limits the musicianship of learners.

Sight-Reading

The ability to sight-read music notation has captivated people for about as long as it has existed. Lowell Mason, considered the father of public school music in the United States, emphasized learning to read music and sing from a score. This was well valued and likely contributed to the Boston school board's allowing him to bring music into the curriculum in 1838 to improve hymn singing in the church (Scanlon, 1942; Volk, 1993). One of the first sight-reading researchers, Bean (1938, p. 3), stated that "efficient reading seems to involve a trick of which neither teacher nor pupil is conscious." Fortunately, research since then has revealed some of the psychological processes that make up the "trick" of sight-reading.

To value sight-reading and the cognitive tasks associated with it, it is helpful to understand how the eye works. It surprises many people to learn that human sight does not work like a snapshot camera in which the entire picture is photographed; rather, it captures only one small area at a time. It operates more like a camera that can only zoom in on small portions of a picture, and to capture an entire picture, it must take many successive snapshots.

At a typical reading distance from a book, the area in focus is about two words (10 letters) long. The focal area of human vision cannot be enlarged by training, although expert readers can learn to use partially perceived information in the periphery of the area. To view a larger scene, the focus of vision must jump from one point to another about three to six times per second, while the mind constructs an image of what is experienced as a coherent whole. These small jumps are called *saccades*, and the pauses in between these movements are called *fixations*. Researchers can record fixations and saccades with eye-tracking equipment to study how people deploy attention when taking in visual stimuli.

Research has shown that sight-reading musicians look forward and backward in the process of gathering information from notation. Put differently, they look ahead, as well as back to the point of execution, because the eye is always a little ahead of the body (producing the music on an instrument or voice). The rate of saccades and duration of fixations depend on a sight-reader's pre-existing knowledge and ability to apply it with the music being read. That application takes the form of expectations about the music represented by the notation. Based on a meta-analysis of sight-reading research spanning eight decades, Mishra (2014) concluded that "deeper musical understanding and the development of expectations appear to be the most effective in improving sightreading skills" (p. 19).

The exact locations of eye fixations are dependent on the sight-reader's experience (Goolsby, 1994). Goolsby studied the eye movements of musicians (skilled and less skilled sight-readers) while they were sight-singing unfamiliar music. More skilled readers peeked around, searching for information, backtracking to places they did not identify at first, whereas less skilled musicians looked at every consecutive note (and still made mistakes). Unlike the less skilled musicians, the skilled ones also scanned expressive/dynamic markings.

In sight-reading, the eyes do not simply move about but actively extract meaningful information. The distance between the current point of performance and the point ahead where the eye is looking is called perceptual span.

Better sight-readers have a larger perceptual span (roughly seven notes) than poorer readers (roughly four notes). That superior performers have larger spans suggests that information is being stored in more or larger chunks. Chunks are constructed internally based on information taken in with several fixations. Being able to construct larger chunks faster during the time-constrained activity of sight-reading gives performers an advantage as they must also access motor programs to produce the music.

Eye movement and perceptual span are affected by the structure of the music being read—recall the preceding explanation of Figure 5.1—which points to the intricate interplay between vision, knowledge, expectation, and performance in sight-reading. Pieces of music are not random arrangements of notes but rather coherent works originating from the minds of musicians, usually created in a certain style, and containing a fair amount of redundancy (e.g., recurrence of thematic material). These qualities allow musicians to build up expectations about the music, which aids in identifying patterns and abstracting chunks of music. For example, if sight-reading musicians see a run of notes that could be a scale and identify the first few notes as the start of the expected scale, they will not bother to visually inspect each of the notes in the notated run, but rather just perform the scale that they know. This is where expert readers can take advantage of blurry information in peripheral areas of vision as a basis for inferences or guesses of what is there.

Language reading research shows that readers do not actually read all the words and letters of printed text but essentially overlook short and common words such as *a* and *the*. They also focus more on word boundaries than on the center of words. A similar process has also been shown in music. When classical musicians work from a score with notational errors in it—either misprints of a publisher or mistakes deliberately planted by a researcher—the results can be interesting. Accomplished sight-readers are likely to play the music not as notated, but the way it should be (i.e., they correct the errors); lesser musicians, especially if given time to work with the score, may end up playing it as written (Sloboda, 2005f).

As already alluded to, skilled sight-reading relies on quick pattern recognition and the application of pre-existing musical understanding. Experts so equipped require fewer eye fixations to gather information from notation—likely constructing larger mental chunks—and decide what to perform. This process of inference or knowledgeable guessing is very important to the best sight-reading musicians, such as pianists who make a living accompanying other performers. It is probably the closest thing to a "trick"—to use Bean's

(1938) terminology—that exists for expert sight-readers. Although rapid pattern recognition facilitates reading music very efficiently, it also makes musicians susceptible to so-called proof-readers errors. This is why atonal or 12-tone serial music compositions can challenge even the best sight-readers, because much of their musical knowledge and expectations are rendered useless.

This discussion suggests that a sight-reader is not merely engaged in a mechanical process of translating visual input automatically into motor programs (see the Chapter 4 section on automaticity). Rather, skilled readers reconstruct in their heads what the music should sound like based on the perceptual information, no matter how scarce it may be due to the time constraints. In the process, expectations and knowledge are integrated. What eventually feels for the performer like "intuition" and allows for quick and accurate guessing is really access to knowledge of style, performance practice, and music theory.

Memorizing Music From Notation

Musical memorization comes in two variations: one that happens incidentally as a by-product of repetition and one that requires great deliberation and effort to establish. When a musician repeatedly performs a piece of music and does so exclusively start to finish, the mental representation of the music will take the form of chunks connected sequentially (i.e., forward chaining). In this case, each chunk functions as a cue to the next; therefore, when performance goes as expected, performing one chunk will trigger the memory to perform the next one. This is what many call rote memory. The disadvantage of this kind of memory is evident when something in performance does *not* go as expected, such as when anxiety deteriorates performance skills. In such situations, the connection between two sequential chunks can break down; if one chunk cannot be performed as typically done, then the next chunk may not be performable at all.

Many expert performers take a different route to musical memorization. These musicians work to establish a very precise mental representation of the piece to be performed. That representation may include tactile-kinesthetic cues, but it is not entirely dependent on them. The representation of the piece may include sound and visual images too. Memorization strategies include writing down parts of the piece, analyzing it away from the instrument, starting performance in different places, or singing parts (that are normally played on an instrument) to test one's memory (Ginsborg, 2004). This work leads to meaningful units (chunks) being stored more robustly, such that they can be retrieved more readily regardless of circumstantial elements. The Chaffin et al. (2005) case study of a professional pianist learning the Presto movement in Bach's *Italian Concerto* has provided an example of how expert classical musicians memorize. Although initially some rote memorization may take place as a by-product of practicing interpretive and technical aspects of the piece, musicians may essentially restart learning a piece by deliberately identifying places in the score where they plan to give specific technical or expressive attention during performance, for example, "this is the sunrise part here," "make sure the crescendo comes to a sudden *pianissimo*," "watch that jump now." Performers can create cues that produce a hierarchical memory that allows them to conceive of a piece from higher overall artistic goals down to detailed thoughts about individual keystrokes in their performance. For performers who memorize a piece like this, the practical advantage is that they can jump at will from one point in the piece to the next meaningful point in case of a problem. This type of approach also facilitates longer storage and retrieval of memorized music, such that the piece can be accurately recalled even years after initial memorization (Chaffin et al., 2005).

Musicians and master teachers often give advice about how to commit music to memory that encompasses musical meaning and instrumental demands alike (Hughes, 2010). Their best advice often endorses a multiple coding system in which tactile-kinesthetic considerations, musical analysis, and emotional imagery/metaphorical associations work together to build a rich mental representation of the piece. Singers are often advised to memorize music and words together, giving them two possible modes of retrieval (Ginsborg, 2004). Eventually, consecutive chunks and sections are interconnected on different levels, and when one level fails during performance, another one can take its place. Although highly experienced artists may put their performance on "autopilot," their robust memorization allows them to retake command if desired.

Psychological research on musical memory indicates that performing pieces of music is a reconstructive process. The mind's ear does not function like an audio recorder and the mind's eye does not photograph music notation. Sources of input, whether by sound or by sight, result in performers' mentally constructing a goal image of the music being learned, and *this*—not a model recording and not sheet music—is the representation that guides their performance of the work.

In this music learning process, prior knowledge—gained from performing experience and deliberate practice and study—is critical. How efficiently musicians can learn a piece of music depends on their understanding of relevant musical concepts (e.g., harmonic structure) and instrument-specific performance techniques. Such understanding allows performers to more readily recognize the *musically meaningful* elements of a work, which aids in creating a performance-ready mental representation of it, whether that learning is accomplished by ear, by reading notation, or through a combination of both.

Research has revealed similarities in how musicians make music by ear and by notation. With both performance skills, experts use a pre-existing knowledge base to conceptualize musical works in more sophisticated ways. Novices tend to use less efficient memory encoding strategies. One example is how experts try to learn melodies according to the underlying harmonic structure, whereas novices may try to commit the music to memory note by note. The expert approach facilitates larger, more meaningful chunking, and the novice approach is much more mentally cumbersome. Because expert memory mechanisms (involving access to LTM) are domain specific, musicians wishing to improve their learning and remembering of music material need not turn to any mnemonic devices or memory "tricks." Rather, they can rest assured that sharpened memory for music results from increased engagement in the domain of music, in terms of both increased time and increased deliberateness and use of learning strategy.

Taking the Stage: Build a Better Knowledge Base

Whether by ear or by notation, learning and remembering music are enhanced by the ability to apply pre-existing knowledge to new musical works encountered. This allows musicians to quickly recognize the most musically meaningful parts of unfamiliar material and mentally process them for immediate performance. The more experienced and knowledgeable about music people are, the more efficiently they can learn new material and move that learning into long-term memory. There are multiple ways to improve one's ability to find musical meaning in new music experiences. Although using multiple strategies is always helpful, certainly individual musicians can factor in their musical tastes and preferred learning styles when choosing for themselves. Strategies they can select from include analytically listening to recordings, talking in depth to experienced performers, reading about music and musicians, and formal study in music theory and analysis. All of these—and other strategies not listed here—can aid in building a better musical knowledge base. Of course, musicians also can accomplish much by upgrading their deliberate practice through increased self-regulation (see Chapter 4). This strategy points to the fact that all potential learning will only make it into long-term memory if it is successfully encoded through meaningful and persistent use. Musicians must remember that human memory is not exactly like computer storage; human beings cannot "save" information indefinitely in long-term storage and expect it to be readily accessible far into the future after a long period of nonuse. Just as deliberateness is a key in learning new knowledge and skills to the point of getting them into long-term memory, persistent use is the key in building the retrieval structures that make the knowledge and skills available to musicians when they need them.

Leading Learning: Give Vernacular Music-Making Experiences

Playing music by ear is not a skill best left to "jazzers" and rock guitar soloists. Psychological research and pedagogical study have confirmed it as a foundational ability for virtually all kinds of musicianship. Engaging learners in making music by ear can pay major dividends for aspiring instrumentalists. This experience may provide necessary learning variety, especially to students who have come to believe that music education is all about taking the printed music they are given and decoding the notation into keypresses or fingerings that produce a sound on their instruments. In such cases, young learners may need to be given "make music by ear" assignments. Teachers can issue their students a "Ten Tune Challenge" (or whatever number teachers like), with which learners must show that they have learned to play by ear music of their choice from whatever sources are readily available to them, including popular music, television commercials and show themes, and music from videogames or online sources. For some music learners who are already entrenched in notation-dependent performance, making music by ear may be a scary prospect. Their apprehension can be eased by using a portion of instructional time to give students experiences with the elements of authentic vernacular music making and its informal, peer-collaborative, and exploratory nature.

Chapter 5 Discussion Questions

1. Which do you think would be more of a challenge: teaching an instrumental musician who plays only by ear to read notation or teaching a notation-dependent instrumentalist to play by ear?
2. In your experience, what are the strengths and weaknesses of standard staff music notation as a symbol system?
3. Are any of the three performance skills covered in this chapter—playing by ear, performing rehearsed music from notation, and performing memorized music—neglected among the musicians you know? Why do you think this is the case?

6

Expressing and Interpreting

Victor Hugo, author and poet of the Romantic era, eloquently stated: "Music expresses that which cannot be said and on which it is impossible to be silent." The sentiment was echoed by prolific storyteller Hans Christian Andersen, who wrote of music: "Where words fail, sounds can often speak." Maria Von Trapp, the real person immortalized by the historically popular musical *The Sound of Music*, wrote, "Music acts like a magic key, to which the most tightly closed heart opens."

It is striking that writers—masters of expressive language—have extolled the power of music, perhaps even with some envy. Indeed, such sentiments about the emotional power of music are etched deep into artistic culture. During great performances, both listeners and performers can experience a sense of awe at the emotional power of the moment. The emotions of the music seem to flow directly from the hearts of performers. Listeners are not, of course, privy to the hours of work and shaping that performers can devote in preparation.

Artistry is at the crux of expressive performance. It is the craft of the artist to design, shape, and produce works with great intention and skill. Because sound is the medium of musical artists, their work requires an "ear for detail." Artistically expressive musicians craft the details of sound parameters—timing, loudness, timbre, pitch—to make their music sound alive and human. The fine distinctions of these parameters are important in every musical genre, such as the swing rhythms of jazz and the wide dynamic range of Romantic orchestral music. Because nuance and feeling are so involved in emotional expression, musicians may struggle to find the words to describe their performance process.

For this reason, some performers may be uneasy when psychological science attempts to capture and analyze musical expression. It can seem to them as though researchers are encroaching on the unknowable and personal core of their artistic being. The fear is, perhaps, that if science identifies a "formula" for musical expression, then the unique contributions of human musicians will be devalued. A balanced assessment of the research renders

Psychology for Musicians. Robert H. Woody, Oxford University Press. © Oxford University Press 2022.
DOI: 10.1093/oso/9780197546598.003.0006

such fear groundless. Recall the music psychologist's perspective offered in Chapter 1 that the processes of music need not remain shrouded in mystery for its power to be remarkable. In fact, the insights afforded by psychological research on musical expression can directly assist performing musicians. If anything, scientific discovery adds layers of new richness to the appreciation of human artistic expression.

This chapter summarizes the findings of research that lead to the following conclusions about expression and interpretation in music performance:

1. It is primarily through variations in tempo, dynamics, and articulation that musicians add emotional expression to the pitches and rhythms they perform.
2. The expressive features applied by musicians in performance originate from several basic sources related to the structural characteristics of the music they are performing and to their own humanness.
3. Interpretation, which is the selection and combination of expressive ideas applied across an entire piece, remains at its core an artistic enterprise. Although effective interpretations may share some general characteristics, the specifics of an artist's interpretation always depend on the individual's skill level, motivations, and expressive intentions.
4. Musical *communication* occurs only if listening audience members experience the emotion or feeling that performing musicians intended to express. Musical expression is more reliably communicated when performers engage in explicit planning and artistic decision-making.

Expression

Expression refers to the small-scale variations in the sound properties of music that performers insert at specific points in a performance. An expressive gesture can often be completely contained within a sequence of a few notes. *Interpretation* refers to the way in which many expressive moments are chosen and combined across an entire piece of music to produce a coherent and aesthetically satisfying experience. Expressive performance gestures are thus the basic building blocks of the larger design of interpretation.

One of the most important features of human musical performance is the fact that it is not, and can never be, free from note-to-note variation. This is what makes any human performance instantly distinguishable from machine-generated music in which each note plays at exactly its notated duration and at the same loudness level; for this reason, more recent computer music applications have their "playback" functions programmed to simulate human variability. The variations found in human musical expression are of several types, and performance research has identified multiple sources of variation. These can be organized under the three categories of random/unintended variation, meaningful sources of expression, and idiosyncratic style.

Expressive performance has long whetted the curiosity of music scholars, who have used the technology available to them at the time to study its processes. Nineteenth-century music theorist Mathis Lussy listened intently to live performances of then-current virtuosos, such as Hans von Bülow and Anton Rubinstein; while doing so, he annotated the printed scores of the works to document the details of their timing and dynamics. This study led him to define musical expressiveness: "the behavioral manifestation in sound of the performer's affective response to the tonal are rhythmic features of the music" (Lussy, 1874, 1883, as cited in Doğantan-Dack, 2014, p. 3). American psychologist Carl Seashore later used early audio recording technology to examine acoustical data to identify that "expression of feeling in music consists in aesthetic deviation from the regular—from pure tone, true pitch, even dynamics, metronomic time, rigid rhythms, etc." (Seashore, 1967, p. 9).

The notion of *deviation from the regular* has endured. More recent researchers have examined the variations in sound properties that musicians put into their performances and to which listeners emotionally respond. Of particular psychological interest is determining what variations are intentionally used by performers, and for those that are not, what their origin is.

The Human Factor: Random and Unintended Variations

Random variation in performance properties comes about because of the limitations of the human body's timing and motor control systems. Even the most highly trained performers are incapable of playing a sequence of notes that have exactly the same sound properties from note to note. Research on simple repetitive motor tasks, such as tapping, suggests that this variation is partly dependent on the speed of movement—for example, the slower the tempo, the more variable—and also on experience: not surprisingly, repeated practice at a motor task can reduce the level of random variation (Repp, 2005).

It must be noted, of course, that music performance is a much more complex motor task than repetitive tapping. As such, not all unintentional variations are necessarily random. When researchers have asked musicians to perform in a deadpan manner—that is, lacking any variability in the expressive sound properties—they are unable to do it (Woody, 2002b). Their attempts retain instances of expression at a reduced level. Large exposure to certain idiomatic performance features likely results in musicians' building such features into their expectations for music to the point that they may not be able to identify the features in music they hear; in other words, they automatically include the features in their own performance (Woody, 2003).

Meaningful Sources of Expression

The performance of idiomatic expressive features leads to the conclusion that much performer expression, even if produced unconsciously, is meaningful in a musical context. The musical expression used by musicians, especially those in classical music, can be very consistent from performance to performance (Chaffin et al., 2007; Noice et al., 2008). This indicates that expressive performances result from mental representations that can be quite stable. Consistency in expressive performance is not confined to classical music; an analysis of Paul McCartney's vocal expression showed remarkable stability in his singing of "Yesterday" across a span of decades (Ashley, 2004).

Such consistency in expression and interpretation raises some interesting questions. How can a performer remember the thousands of subtle performance variations that allow almost exact reproduction from performance to performance? Why isn't the memory of the performer overwhelmed?

Recent research shows that a great deal of performance variation can be accounted for by certain heuristics or principles of expressive performance. In general psychology, heuristics refer to mental shortcut strategies that allow human beings to make judgments quickly by lightening the cognitive load that is required by deliberate rational decision-making (imagine having to think through the "pros and cons" of each of the many choices made in everyday life). In understanding the psychology of expressive music performance, heuristics can be thought of as quickly adopted principles or "rules." Although there are many individual examples of these, they fall into three major groups: generative principles, emotional coding, and motional patterns.

Generative principles stem from the structure of the music and help to make that structure clearer to a listener. For instance, *accenting* (i.e., increasing the loudness of a note's onset) is commonly used to direct listeners' attention to the most structurally important parts within a musical line. Research has shown that performers play the same music differently if the rhythmic notation is shifted from metrically regular to syncopated, in relation to the note sequence. Compare the two melodies in Figure 6.1. Purely from a pitch and duration standpoint, the two melodies—at least the first 24 notes of them—are identical; if each note is played with the exact same loudness and tempo, they would be indistinguishable. Because of the notational difference, however, human musicians perform them differently. The notes considered most metrically important would tend to be stressed by musicians by performing them relatively longer, louder, or with a longer attack time (Moelants, 2012). This is one simple example of a generative principle.

Another example of a generative principle relates to *phrasing*, which is the timing-related segmentation of musical structure. The *grouping* of notes, through performers' variations in expressive sound properties, helps listeners to understand which elements in a piece "go together" and are separated structurally from what precedes and follows them. For instance, a common development of a musical phrase involves building melodic tension to a peak, then lessening to the phrase's end, called "tapering the phrase." Thus, performers tend to use expressive variation to bring focus to phrase boundaries (i.e., the ending of one musical idea and the start of the next). Specifically, the tempo and dynamic trajectories of the phrase tend to be arch-like; that is, it begins more slowly and softly, increases in tempo and dynamic level in the middle, and then slows and softens again at the end (Bisesi

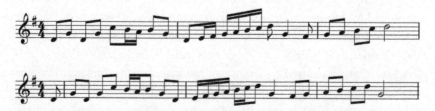

Figure 6.1 Metrical versus syncopated notation of the same melody.
Based on Sloboda, J. A. (1983). The communication of musical metre in piano performance. *Quarterly Journal of Experimental Psychology, 35*, 377–396.

& Windsor, 2016). Because the notes at phrase boundaries are performed significantly more slowly and softly than the others, it creates a perceptual gap between phrases, which in effect segments the music; elements on one side of the gap appear to be grouped together, in distinction from elements on the other side.

It deserves reiterating that some generative principles are so ingrained in music culture that they are often not deliberately executed by musicians and not explicitly noticed by listeners. Nevertheless, these generative features are extremely meaningful and important to the perception of music as "human" and expressive. Although performers and listeners may not explicitly identify idiomatic expressive features, they would surely notice if the features were not present (Woody, 2002b). In other words, mental representations for expected musical expression may lie below consciousness, but they quickly rise to the surface when the expectations are not met.

Emotional coding is defined by performers' intentions to convey emotions to listeners. This is perhaps the heart of artistry for performing musicians. As such, the common term *emotional expression* can be misleading in the context of music performance:

> It is only occasionally that performers are truly expressing their own emotions during the performance—perhaps because optimal performance requires a certain state (e.g., relaxed concentration; see Williamon, 2004) that is incompatible with experiencing certain emotions. Usually what the performer presents in a music performance is not the emotion itself but rather its "expressive form." (Juslin & Lindström, 2016, p. 598)

This is why "coding" is the correct descriptor for explaining how musical emotion is conveyed to listeners. Performers' emotional intentions must be converted to a material format that may be imparted to others.

The musical expression of certain basic emotions can be accomplished based on human emotional experiences. Basic emotions such as happiness, sadness, and anger are considered universally expressed and understood. Facial expression, vocal sounds, and other behavioral indicators of these are generally recognizable across all human cultures. The most basic human emotions can be defined by two dimensions: valence (positive or negative) and activity level (low or high) (Eerola & Vuoskoski, 2011; Posner et al., 2005). The combinations of these produce the four emotions labeling the quadrants of Figure 6.2. The emotional coding of these are

Positive Valence

	TENDERNESS	HAPPINESS	
	slow tempo, moderate tempo variability, medium-soft dynamic level, small dynamic level variability, legato articulation, small articulation variability, medium-fast vibrato rate, small vibrato extent	fast tempo, small tempo variability, medium-loud dynamic level, small dynamic level variability, staccato articulation, large articulation variability, medium-fast vibrato rate, medium vibrato extent	
Low Activity	SADNESS	ANGER	*High Activity*
	slow tempo, large tempo variability, soft dynamic level, moderate dynamic level variability, legato articulation, small articulation variability, slow vibrato rate, small vibrato extent	fast tempo, small tempo variability, loud dynamic level, small dynamic level variability, staccato articulation, moderate articulation variability, medium-fast vibrato rate, large vibrato extent	

Negative Valence

Adapted from Juslin & Lindström (2016) and Juslin & Timmers (2010)

Figure 6.2 Summary of Western musicians' coding of basic emotions.
Based on Juslin, P. N., & Lindström, E. (2016). Emotion in music performance. In S. Hallam, I. Cross, & M. Thaut (Eds.), *The Oxford handbook of music psychology* (2nd ed., pp. 597–614). Oxford, UK: Oxford University Press.

largely learned though typical human emotional life, especially human vocal expression (Juslin & Laukka, 2003; Juslin & Scherer, 2005). Because music borrows from pre-existing coding used in emotional speech and behavior, experience with these may be all that is required for people to understand musical coding, such as that "angry music," like an angry voice, tends to be loud, and "peaceful music," like a peaceful day, tends to proceed slowly.

The musical expression of more complex emotions, however, requires more deliberate coding on the part of performers. This kind of expression also is more culturally constrained. People unfamiliar with classical music often struggle to recognize emotional expression in it, instead dismissing it as alienating or "boring" (Dobson, 2010). In the same way, many Westerners would fail to understand the emotional communication contained in Japanese traditional music, due to lack of exposure to the genre (Laukka et al., 2013).

The leading researcher of musical emotion is Swedish psychologist Patrik Juslin (2019). The work of Juslin and collaborators over recent years has provided much insight into how emotions are coded for communication through music performance (Juslin, 2013; Juslin & Laukka, 2003; Juslin & Lindström, 2016; Juslin & Sloboda, 2010; Juslin & Timmers 2010; Juslin & Västfjäll, 2008). Figure 6.2 summarizes research findings about the coding Western performers use to communicate basic emotions through music. This line of research has also shown that performing musicians can improve the effectiveness of their emotional communication through feedback based on the coding usage (e.g., Juslin & Laukka, 2000; Juslin et al., 2006).

Motional patterns are expressive features in musical sound that resemble natural human movement or biological motion (Juslin & Lindström, 2016; Juslin & Timmers 2010). Indeed, movement has long been a focus of attention among people in the larger field of music (performers, scholars, philosophers, pedagogues, and psychologists among them). One team of researchers explained how musical expression can be viewed as a coupling of perception and action:

> It is assumed that the human body is the natural mediator between experience and physical reality. Music-driven movements of the listener are seen as corporeal articulations that reveal a mirroring (in movement) of the perceived sonic moving forms. Through this mirroring, it is assumed that musical expression can be captured more fully, experienced, and understood. (Leman et al., 2008, p. 264)

Music and movement are often described as a "natural" coupling, likely because both phenomena exist across time (as does human speech and other vocalizations).

Regarding time, concepts related to tempo and rhythm (duration) appear to be especially transferrable between musical expression and human movement. This may be due to biological rhythms of the human body, such as heartbeat and gait. One theory suggests that the same mirror system regions of the brain activate when perceiving and performing action (Sievers et al., 2013). In a particularly interesting example of the motional patterns of musical expression, research has shown that the rate of slowing that classical musicians use in a ritardando can be remarkably similar to the pattern of deceleration that runners naturally take in coming to a stop (Kleinsmith et al., 2016).

Idiosyncratic Style

Some musicians reading this chapter may be inclined to prefer the notion of idiosyncratic or personal style over the aforementioned sources described as principles, heuristics, or "rules." Real expressive performance, however, is created from all the sources already covered in this chapter. Musicians cannot choose to use only idiosyncratic style (at the exclusion of the other sources) in an effort to be maximally unique and personal in their expressive performing. All of the sources are important and even when maximally employed still leave much room for individuality in musical expression. In fact, explicitly knowing and understanding the other sources of expression likely offer musicians the best possible position for personal creative and expressive performance.

The combination of the aforementioned sources accounts for much expressiveness in most musicians' performances. Even so, emotional expression can be quite dissimilar from one performer to another. Musicians tend to differ in how they employ the sources and focus on certain types of expressive variation. For example, one performer may place more emphasis on tempo changes, another on variations in dynamics. Alternatively, one musician's emphasis on score study may bring generative principles to the fore, while another musician's penchant for detailed advanced planning may result in emotional coding being very prominent. The emphasis on some expressive sources over others is one example by which expressive performance is idiosyncratic or personal to individual musicians.

With understanding of how expressive performance tends to be done in a certain cultural context, performers may choose to deliberately flout common expressive conventions. Advanced musicians seem to do this carefully though. In a review of some seminal research on how professional concert pianists show individuality, Margulis (2014) concluded that the pianists who were studied showed similar "expressive patterns over the larger scale— slowing down at phrase and section endings, for example—but tended to show different patterns of expressive lengthening at the very smallest, note-to-note and chord-to-chord levels" (p. 1220). Stylistic unexpectedness can convey added emotional tension and surprise to listeners. Too much idiosyncrasy, however, can "all too easily spill over into eccentricity and incomprehensibility," which is why greater idiosyncratic expressiveness may be more characteristic of prestigious musical performers:

The recorded performances of the pianist Glenn Gould, for example, provide a case. Gould was (according to some commentators) famously idiosyncratic — and some of his recordings seem to bear out this reputation.
His recording of the opening movement of the Mozart piano sonata in
A major (K. 331) is taken at about half the speed (20 dotted crotchet beats
per minute) of almost any other recording, and with a strangely deliberate
style of articulation. (Clarke, 2005, pp. 162–163)

Other aspects of idiosyncratic style may be less volitional and more
constrained by a performer's physical traits. For example, a pianist with
small hands may need to arpeggiate or "roll" chords that other players do
not (Deahl & Wristen, 2017). Also, vocal track size is a largely biologically
determined trait that contributes to vocal timbre, a sound property that
makes some singers so easily identifiable; the singing voices of performers
are often given expressive descriptors such as breathy, growly, or even dark
and sobbing (Heidemann, 2016). Such physical traits either are unchangeable or affect performance in a manner that is outside the conscious control
of musicians, so they develop distinctive performance styles that reflect their
physical constraints.

Interpretation

Musician individuality is especially salient at the larger level of interpretation.
How musicians interpret works they are performing is seen in the aggregate
of their expressive moments across entire works. Inasmuch as artistry is defined by the skillful execution of ideas from a creative mind, interpretation is
a paramount ability for musical artists.

Outside of the specific context of music, interpretation is defined as the
action of explaining the meaning of something. An interpreter is someone
who converts one language to another so people can understand what a foreign language speaker is saying. Similarly, when musicians perform an interpretation of a musical work, they are expected to convey the meaning of the
work by artistically converting it to the sound properties of music so listeners
can understand it. This idea of *conversion* may be extremely critical in understanding artistry and the nature of emotional communication through
music. In fact, some art philosophers have suggested that the artist's role is

not the expression of emotion, but rather the *interpretation* of it through a chosen artistic medium, such as music (Dilworth, 2004).

From a practical perspective, a performer's interpretation is essentially that musician's coherent set of choices about expression applied over an entire piece. For this reason, interpretational goals can be quite unique to a specific performer, a specific piece, and a specific time. That said, research findings support at least two quite firm conclusions about the nature of effective interpretations, namely that (1) musicians' interpretations reflect patterning and structure that are perceptible and evident upon analysis and (2) they happen on a large-scale as well as a small-scale basis.

In classical music solo performance, interpretation is manifested in a strong relationship between compositional structure and variations in expressive sound properties, including dynamics. This relationship can exist at multiple levels, including on a large scale, suggesting that variations in dynamics (and other properties) are important not only for expressive moments at specific points of a piece but also in musicians' broader interpretative purposes. One example of this is the "arch" structure, characterized by a gradual increase in loudness followed by a symmetrical decrease (Langner et al., 2000; Sundberg et al., 2003). Expert performers can employ hierarchically organized arches at both note-to-note and phrase-to-phrase levels (Cheng & Chew, 2008). It is relatively easy for a musician to perform arch dynamic variation over a single phrase of four measures. It requires far more skill to do this while simultaneously constructing and controlling an arch that spans an entire piece lasting many minutes. Expert performers can manage a hierarchy of separate, multiple arches embedded within the same piece, such that 8-bar phrases containing dynamic arches could occur within a 64-bar "meta-arch," in which the average dynamic of each phrase also rises then falls in a controlled manner. The same kind of hierarchical use of arches can be applied in expressive timing and duration (Ohriner, 2012). Advanced performers' use of arches indicates that experts bring to their interpretations a deep structural understanding.

This knowledge assists musicians in identifying the key structural locations within a piece, so as to choose which expressive tactics to employ. Advanced musicians have been shown to be cognizant of specific locations in the music where particular expressive outcomes are intended, in addition to knowing where those local points fit within the piece's global context (Sloboda & Lehmann, 2001). At such "target points," performers' expressive intentions generally result in objective differences in performance properties, and these points coincide with "changes in perceived/experienced emotionality" on the part of listeners (Sloboda & Lehmann, 2001, p. 107).

The importance of compositional structure in interpretation is hardly surprising, given how musicians are expected to "explain" the meaning of a musical work through their performance of it. This is seen in the *Werktreue* concept, which refers to a responsibility to be true to a piece of music and its composer's intentions (Crispin & Östersjö, 2017). Some musicologists have suggested that the musical concept of interpretation, as now understood, only appeared in the 19th century as the roles of composer and performer diverged (Goehr, 2007), and performance was demoted to "a position as mere vessel for the musical work" and performers were expected to "play as if from the soul of the composer" (Hunter, 2005, p. 357). Relegation to a "mere vessel" is hyperbole as performers surely show individuality in the variety of interpretive approaches they take. Strategies for developing an interpretation of a piece include gaining expansive knowledge about the work and its composer through reading biographies and other writings about the historical-cultural time period (Silverman, 2008). Performers make myriad expressive decisions when preparing a piece for performance, and although they are generally expected to be true to the piece and its composer, they are also expected to contribute their own sensibilities related to emotional expression. Balancing individual expression with faithfulness to the score is viewed by some to be among the "ethical issues" faced by performers (Silverman, 2008, p. 266).

Key interpretational decisions are made early in the learning history of a particular piece and guide the practice process. Learning a new piece of repertoire is, for most performers, a lengthy process that can require many hours of practice spread over weeks or months. A prevalent belief among music learners is that technical and expressive practicing are separate processes that can be accomplished in sequence, first one, then the other (Nielsen, 2001). Some talk of "learning the notes" as a process that must be completed, or at least that has significantly progressed, before interpretation is added, as if it were a final coat of paint.

Research on the process of more advanced performers has shown a different story. These musicians are likely to consider interpretation before working on technique (Chaffin et al., 2009). It appears to be something of an expert strategy to begin performance preparation with a "big picture" idea of the overall musical shape of a piece. Musicians can use such an overall interpretive plan to guide technical work (e.g., knowing what tempo a section of music needs to be worked up to) and avoid having to relearn motor production skills that might change if interpretation decisions are put off until later. Unlike expert performers, novices "tend to focus on superficial characteristics, plunging into the details without developing a clear idea of the big picture" (Chaffin et al., 2003). Early ideas about interpretation are often informed by listening to many performances of the piece, which would include different interpretations (Lisboa et al., 2005; Philippe et al., 2020). Musicians can engage in this concentrated listening focused on the emotion of the work and supplement it with score study to gain greater structural familiarity, all the while devoting practice time primarily to technical performance aspects (i.e., note security and fluency). Later in their performance preparations, their practicing may begin to focus more on expressive aspects, and interpretation is refined through the feedback of others (for whom they give practice performances) and through self-feedback by making recordings of themselves (Philippe et al., 2020).

Drawing from the extensive study by Chaffin et al. (2005) of a professional concert pianist preparing a Bach concerto for performance, a number of researchers have advanced a multiple-phase model of how a performer's interpretation of a piece is built into a mental representation that guides preparation and practice (Héroux, 2016, 2018; Lehmann et al., 2018; Miksza, 2011; Wise et al., 2017). In the first phase, *scouting it out*, the musician reads through the piece and analyzes its structure to gain a clear understanding of the piece as a whole. In the second *section-by-section* phase, the musician practices to gain the technical skills required to produce the desired performance of the piece. In the third phase, called the *gray stage*, the piece progresses from being deliberately and consciously performed to being more automatically executed; the gray stage can involve complete run-throughs during solitary practice, giving practice performances for small informal audiences, and doing dress rehearsals in concert attire and in the actual performance venue (if available). The final *maintenance* phase occurs after the musician considers the piece fully learned and when efforts for additional refinement have begun to yield diminishing returns; at this point the big picture interpretative goals return to the forefront of the musician's attention.

While corroborating the four phases offered by Chaffin and colleagues, the research of Héroux (2016, 2018) has suggested an additional stage of "artistic appropriation," an individualized and creative process during which a musician develops an artistic image or message to convey through performance of the piece. Artistic appropriation can occur at different points in the larger process of interpretation development, depending on the individual performer and that person's conception of musical expression. One performer's process may consist of experimenting with sound properties to convey a perceived internal meaning of the composed work, while another performer's artistic appropriation may center on conveying a personal message aided by "extramusical elements" such as the performer's biographical memories or even a fictional dramatic narrative (Héroux, 2018, p. 3). As the term *appropriation* suggests, in this process, performers take a musical work—though originally composed by someone else—and make it their own.

Communication of Meaning in Performance

Interpretation in the sense described previously—as musicians' planned shaping of a piece according to their ideas—highlights the understanding that interpretation is a cognitive undertaking that involves planning and use of ideas. This may lead some to surmise that musical interpretation is different from musical expression: even if interpretation is cognitive in nature, might expression be more emotional? Musicians may speak of learning to "feel the music" or "use your soul" so as not to merely "simulate" emotional expression (Woody, 2000). Even if musicians' production of expressive performance is *experienced* as simply inducing felt emotion within themselves, there is surely higher-level cognition mediating it. Research has indicated that moments of expressive music performance and the broader context of interpretation are part of a highly cognitive enterprise.

Musical expression is also like musical interpretation with regard to the element of conversion, as emotional ideas are transformed into the material of an artwork (i.e., sound, in the case of music). Like all cognitive skill development, what begins as a highly conscious and effortful process can ultimately become an ability that is automatically performed below consciousness. Along these lines, music performance research suggests that expressive musical communication is often best accomplished when it is begun with deliberateness and explicit planning.

Approaches to Learning and Performing Musical Expression

This chapter began with a quote about how music can express that which cannot be said. From this perspective it is not surprising that some musicians may purposefully avoid talking about emotional expression in music and instead, when addressing it with other musicians or teaching students, rely primarily on demonstration. Teacher *aural modeling* (with student imitation) is a traditional and still widely used instructional approach to musical expression. As shown in Chapter 5, making music by ear is a foundational skill and the means by which music is exclusively learned in many cultures. For music learners of all ability levels, hearing expressive exemplars can always be beneficial. When live demonstration is not possible, many music learners turn to audio recordings. Some classically trained musicians, however, may harbor a fear that listening to other people's performances will "contaminate" their ability to perform authentic expressive performances of their own. This fear of contamination seems very specific to the classical conservatory culture. Wider cross-cultural evidence suggests that musical masters in virtually all genres study other people's performances, sometimes very intensively. In the development of popular and jazz musicians, exact imitation appears to be a universal primary stage in the learning process. In some musical cultures, it is only after apprentice musicians typically perfect their imitative skills that they earn the right to deviate from the master with original artistry. Ultimately, there is no evidence that avoiding the performances of others is a beneficial strategy for performing musicians, and it is certainly not appropriate for those who are not yet established as professionals.

An approach of aural modeling and imitation is not without limitations, however. Musicians and music teachers do well to remember (from Chapter 5) that human musical memory is not an audio recorder in the head, such that listening students can imitate a teacher model with some kind of mental playback function. When provided a model performance, what students hear, process, and encode into memory depends on how readily they recognize the meaningful elements of the model. This, of course, is affected by students' pre-existing musical knowledge, expectations, and preferences. Research has shown that listening musicians' expectations can prevent them from identifying expressive features in an aural model, and without the features explicitly built into a plan for performance, their imitative efforts are unlikely to be accurate (Woody, 2002b, 2003, 2006b).

Those who believe musical expression is all about nuanced mood, feeling, and gesture may prefer an approach featuring *verbalization of emotional imagery and descriptive metaphor.* Many music teachers endorse this approach and routinely offer instruction to students in this form (e.g., Karlsson & Juslin, 2008; Lindström et al, 2003; Woody, 2000). Schippers (2006) reflected on the appeal and breadth of this approach:

> It appears to be a matter of degree: although the emphasis lies on relatively unambiguous, physical instruction, it extends to imaginative use of language, evocative of the right attitude needed to play the right technique. From there it moves to references to the interpersonal and abstractly aesthetic. Many master musicians across the world are aware of these aspects and often have found creative ways of communicating to specific students what they consider important mechanisms to achieve expression. It is not uncommon to encounter in biographies or anecdotes specific mention of a teacher's expertise in creative use of metaphor. (Schippers, 2006, pp. 212–213)

Advanced music students come to understand that imagery and metaphor are likely to be heard among musicians. As such, they are able to accommodate this type of instruction (Sheldon, 2004; Woody, 2006a, 2006b). It can prove ineffective, however, if imagery/metaphor examples are vague or unfamiliar (Karlsson & Juslin, 2008; Woody & McPherson, 2010).

As pointed out earlier in this chapter, the creative material of the musical artist is sound, and as such, some music performers and teachers prefer to address the musical sound properties directly through *verbalizations about concrete musical properties.* In explaining how they make their music expressive—or how student musicians should do it—they may describe the variations in tempo, dynamics, and articulation employed in performance, perhaps even linking certain variations to emotions to be expressed (as in Figure 6.2). When researchers have used such an approach with student musicians, it has been shown to be effective in improving emotional communication through their music (Johnson, 2000; Juslin & Laukka, 2000).

Explicit Planning and Cognitive Engagement

There is some indication from research that when each of these approaches is used in music teaching, the instruction must eventually take the form of concrete musical properties in the minds of students to be effective. As explained in previous chapters, music performance is precipitated by underlying mental representations, including a goal image of what the music is supposed to sound like. More expert performance, including with respect to emotional expression, is facilitated as performers engage in deliberate practice and carry out detailed listening to music, thereby building more precise and robust goal imaging for their own expressive performing.

A research study that compared equivalent instruction in three different approaches to teaching musical expression—aural modeling, verbalization of imagery/metaphor, and verbalization about concrete properties—found that university pianists were able to use all three types of instruction to improve their expressive performance of melodies (Woody, 2006b). In this study, performance data were supplemented by the musicians' verbal reports of their thoughts while considering the instruction and practicing in light of it. Their verbal reports suggested that the imagery/metaphor instruction "effected greater performance change when it was used to build an explicit performance plan addressing the properties of loudness, tempo, and articulation" (p. 34).

This finding offered provisional support for a theory that musicians use a cognitive translation process with certain kinds of expressive instruction. This theory was corroborated by subsequent research that specifically examined how university musicians use imagery-based instruction to create their own expressive performances (Woody, 2006a). Data collected in this study indicated that musicians do use a translation process whereby they convert imagery and metaphors into more explicit plans for the expressive properties of performance. The translation process was especially evident among musicians in the middle range of expertise (as measured by cumulated years of private lessons received). The musicians with the least and most expertise (private lesson–wise) tended to use a more emotion-based strategy to process imagery-based instruction, suggesting that (1) the least experienced musicians' failure to translate imagery reflected a lack of appreciation for audience members' reliance upon sound properties to perceive emotional expression, and (2) among the most experienced musicians, the translation process had become an automatized skill.

In cases when an advanced musician can automatically transform imagery or metaphor into expressive sound properties of performance, it would appear that they use extramusical ideas (related to emotion) to encode and retrieve expressive performance devices in long-term memory. Recall from Chapter 5 that a defining feature of expert memory is privileged access to information stored in long-term memory by means of efficient retrieval cues. Instead of having to retrieve a vast amount of detailed information to perform a properly nuanced crescendo or ritardando, for example, the memory processes are made more manageable for expert musicians by abstracting the expressive information into a single emotional image or motional metaphor (Sloboda, 2014; Wolfe, 2019; Woody, 2000, 2002a).

This process can account for why many advanced musicians may endorse a felt-emotion approach to expressive performance, with which they may encourage developing musicians not to "overthink it" but to simply feel the emotion they want to express and trust that it will happen naturally. Research suggests that this may be bad advice in some cases, because the complex process that works for expert performers often is not available to less skilled musicians. The cognitive translation of emotion to expression has been proposed as "a 'bridge' between the naïve use of felt emotion (which may or may not result in perceptible expressivity) and the most advanced musicians' use of the approach" (Woody & McPherson, 2010, p. 414).

Before they have acquired the expert skill of automatic processing of emotional ideas, musicians are advantaged by applying explicit attention to their expressive performance efforts. As mentioned earlier, aural modeling works best in teaching expressive performance when listening students identify sound properties (in the model) to be explicitly built into their goal image for imitative performance (Woody, 2002b, 2003, 2006b). Similarly, emotional imagery/metaphor examples will likely only effect change in student musician performance if they convert the extramusical ideas into an explicit plan for expressive sound properties.

Seeking Feedback and Acquiring Expertise

Developing musicians likely learn the artistic conversion process through music listening, deliberate practice, and other cognitively engaged experiences in the domain, including formal music instruction. From the aforementioned research study that compared the approaches of aural modeling, verbalization of imagery/metaphor, and verbalization about concrete properties (Woody, 2006b), one practical implication that emerged was that using multiple approaches in conjunction with each other "may in fact be the key to success" (p. 34). Teachers who demonstrate expressive performance and accompany their aural model by pointing out the features therein can ensure that student musicians truly learn from the demonstration. Similarly, by combining aural modeling with imagery-based instruction, music students can better understand what emotional and motional ideas actually *mean* in the context of musical sound. Wolfe (2019) called the connecting of extramusical associations to musical sound "cross-domain mappings," offering as an illustration: "the image of a flock of birds taking to the sky, for example, may encapsulate a change in dynamics and tempo in a particular passage" (p. 282).

Of course, teachers talking about their own performance is not the only verbalization that promotes expressive performance learning among student musicians. Having students state what expressive features they hear in an instructor model is a good strategy to ensure they appreciate the importance of converting emotional ideas into expressive sound properties. A music teacher can also challenge students to explain how they intend to make their sounded music reflect the emotional or extramusical ideas that they are using to guide their performances. This prompt by a teacher can elicit a rather direct indicator of whether students are using the explicit planning that is so important in producing reliably perceptible musical expression.

Music learners also benefit greatly from teacher feedback offered about their expressive performing. Such interactions with music teachers and other musicians make it much more likely that developing musicians will make explicit what is behind their expressive and interpretive impulses. It is likely commonplace for musicians in a chamber group rehearsal to ask each other questions such as "What exactly are you doing in measure 10?" or "At what tempo do you want to start the second movement?"

In public performance, rather few opportunities exist for performers to obtain detailed feedback from audiences concerning the reception of their expressive intentions. Applause, enthusiastic or otherwise, is not very informative. It does not tell a performer whether the audience was able to hear, for example, a carefully planned transition from tension to peacefulness that a musician wanted to communicate. Contrast this plight of musicians with performers in competitive sports. They often get immediate and unavoidable feedback—they either win or lose—and can adapt their future preparations in light of it.

Although feedback to expressive performance may be difficult for musicians to obtain, it is nonetheless critical in their development. Musicians can help themselves in this respect if they are perceptive of the "structure-emotion link" whereby certain musical properties produce certain emotional affects (Sloboda, 2005e). Musicians can take this understanding into their own music making and use an experimental approach to discover which expressive devices elicit responses from listeners—including themselves—that match their emotional intent (Woody, 2002a).

Expression and interpretation are at the heart of musicians' artistry. Although music making is a natural human activity in a broad sense, musical artistry is not a natural outgrowth of human development. Just as sculptors must learn to work the stone with mallets and chisels, musicians must learn to craft their sound with their available performance tools.

Taking the Stage: Become an Expressive Improviser

According to the standard definition of musical interpretation—and corroborated by research with expert musicians—interpretation necessarily involves advanced planning and careful preparation. It requires deliberately designed and creative decision-making and usually involves revision and refining throughout the preparation process. In this way, interpretation is the "composition" of performer communication. Within this context, the "improvisation" of the process consists of more specific expressive moments within a performance. Classical musicians and other performers who never learned to improvise (in the most common sense of the term) may enjoy testing the waters of improvisation through the expressive variations they include in their performing. That is, instead of making final decisions in advance about precisely when and how they will precisely execute, say, crescendos, ritardandos, and special articulations, they can instead decide that more spontaneously in the moments of performance. As shown in the following chapter's coverage of improvisation, improvisatory performance takes more, not less, preparation on the part of performers. For example, instead of repetitively practicing and polishing the *one* way they *will* execute a particular crescendo in a piece being performed, performers can practice a variety of crescendo styles at that location in the music. With sufficient practicing, instead of automatizing the very specific skill of performing a single crescendo in a single musical context, they can automatize the transferable skill of choosing the right expressive feature for the moment during performance. This can be very rewarding for performers and can help them to be more mindful of their surroundings during performance (e.g., audience responsiveness, coperformers' music making, etc.). By approaching expressive performance in an improvisatory way, their practicing not only helps add a new piece of music to their repertoire but also contributes to their overall musicianship.

Leading Learning: Use Peer Evaluation

Because music students' expressive skills are best developed through conscious attention and explicit performance planning, music teachers should consider adding more verbalization to their instruction. Teacher talk is seldom a scarcity in music teaching (see Chapter 10), so the added benefit comes in having student musicians verbalize more, specifically about their thought processes around expressive performing. In group instructional settings, this can take the form of peer evaluation. One student (or a small subgroup) can be asked to perform an excerpt of music expressively, while the remaining students, charged with listening carefully, afterward describe the sound properties they heard that contributed to emotional expression. This activity can pay dividends to all students involved. The students who perform can gain insight into which aspects of their music are most communicative to a listening audience, or perhaps discover that their emotional intentions are not being realized as perceptible sound properties. Listening students can make the same discoveries vicariously. They additionally are likely to be motivated to soon apply what they have learned in their own performing. This learning strategy can be especially beneficial when a teacher's expressive instruction consists primarily of imagery and metaphor or aural modeling. In effect, this instruction promotes the cognitive translation process, whereby students convert instruction into a goal image for their own expressive performance. Verbalization about sound properties can also help in one-on-one instruction when peer evaluation is not possible. If a teacher provides an aural model for a student whose performance is lacking expressivity, it is a good idea to have the student verbally report the features heard before attempting imitation of the model. If the student has not explicitly identified expressive features (so as to build them into a mental representation of the music), there is little reason to expect that his or her imitative performance will include any added expressiveness.

Chapter 6 Discussion Questions

1. How have you sought feedback about the effectiveness of your emotional communication in performance? Has that feedback prompted you to alter the approaches you take to being expressive?
2. What are some ways that musicians can familiarize themselves with a composition they will be performing, in order to maximize their generative expression?
3. How important do you think it is for performers to accept the "ethical" responsibility of balancing their personal expressive goals with the intentions of a work's composer?

7

Composing and Improvising

Creativity is often associated with great musicians of the past and less frequently used by today's performers to describe their own everyday musical
activities. Historically significant composers have been imbued with a "creative mystique," foremost among them Mozart, who has been regarded by
many as a "genius endowed with superhuman powers, as if his music mi-
raculously fell from the heavens to fete the world with his divinely inspired
masterpieces" (Lucey, 2013).

Studying composition and improvisation from a psychological standpoint must begin by defining creativity not by divine inspiration but rather
as a *generative* process, that is, the act of generating new musical material
or new renderings of pre-existing music. Musical generativity is best understood as a component of basic musicianship rather than part of a specialized
skill set. Many composers of the past were also performers and improvisers.
Many musicians of today also enjoy similar breadth as composers and
performers, as seen in the common descriptor "singer-songwriter." Indeed,
today's specialized classical performer who plays exclusively pieces composed by others (and without improvised material) is a recent phenomenon,
historically speaking. Up to the late 19th century, many musicians—though
not necessarily orchestral musicians—were composer-performers mainly
playing their own works. Clara Schumann, for instance, was one of the first
performers who played pieces composed by others, specifically promoting
her husband Robert's works. Modern musicians still play pieces by Liszt and
Paganini, touring virtuosi who improvised a great deal and often played variations of then popular melodies. Additionally, there are well-known works in
music history that are said to have emerged from improvisational practices
of a given historical time, such as baroque fantasias or classical variations.
J. S. Bach's *The Musical Offering* (*Das Musikalische Opfer*, BWV 1079) is said
to have been derived from an improvised fugue on a musical theme given to
him by Frederick the Great.

Improvisational practices remained active in classical music well into the
20th century, as famous concert performers often changed the score at will to

Psychology for Musicians. Robert H. Woody, Oxford University Press. © Oxford University Press 2022.
DOI: 10.1093/oso/9780197546598.003.0007

suit their artistic goals. Thus, musical creativity need not be viewed as a specialized activity engaged in by only the artistic crème de la crème. Virtually all musicians engage in generative activity. As explained in the previous chapter, even musicians who exclusively perform the music of others are expected to create personally unique interpretations of composers' works, and they often make improvisatory decisions about musical expression during the moments of performances.

Studying creative processes in the arts can be challenging. Despite creativity being of great interest to scholars for a very long time, it eluded scientific study until fairly recently. Of all topics within music, creativity may be the one with which musical traditionalists resist the relevance of psychological insight. After all, one might surmise, imagination, like intuition, exists outside of the realm of conscious thought and human intellect. Swanwick (2003) characterized an attitude of resistance to science's attempts to study the almost magical power of music: "Are we trying to weigh a moonbeam or measure a thought? Can the clanking apparatus of the social sciences really throw light on intuitive knowledge?" (p. 66). Even the most committed music researchers must acknowledge that psychological study of musical creativity can be challenging. One reason is that artists often have difficulty verbalizing their creative processes, and secondly, their creative products do not always reveal the steps of production. Another reason is that works of art can elicit vastly different opinions about creative quality. Such subjectivity is off-putting to many would-be researchers. A final challenge in studying creativity is that some artists may not want to explain their creative process lest it destroy some of the mystique associated with musical creativity. Psychologists call this impression management, and it is quite common.

Challenges notwithstanding, the psychological study of creativity has borne some useful insights for musicians. This chapter explains the following points about the musical processes of composition and improvisation:

1. Many principles of human creativity, revealed by research across many domains, are applicable to creative activity in music.
2. Composing music involves a combination of nonconscious processing—perhaps experienced as inspiration or intuition—and effortful deliberate working out of ideas.
3. Although improvised performance is spontaneously executed, it is in no way a product of chance. Becoming a fluent improviser requires

substantial investment on the part of musicians to build a musical expertise that supports the automatized skill of improvisation.

4. Musical creativity is best built by nurturing the naturally creative behaviors of childhood and facilitating young musicians' adopting a creative mindset to explore composing and improvising as a basic part of their musicianship.

The Psychology of Creativity

The field of psychology has offered multiple theories to explain human creativity. Although there is much variation across these offerings, there is general agreement about one aspect of defining creativity. For an idea to be truly creative, it must be *both* new and useful (Cropley & Cropley, 2010). Eminent creativity researcher Dean Keith Simonton described the "most favored definition" of creativity this way:

> It must produce an idea that is both (a) original, novel, or surprising and (b) adaptive or functional. So Einstein's general theory of relativity is highly creative because it was highly original (i.e., constituting a substantial break with Newtonian physics) as well as highly functional (e.g., it solved a problem in Mercury's orbit that hitherto lacked any workable solution). (Simonton, 2010, p. 179)

Gardner (2011) stated the dual definition of creativity as being "initially considered novel" and that it "ultimately becomes accepted in a particular cultural setting" (p. 33).

The two-dimensional nature of creativity is also congruent with the well-accepted concepts of *divergent* and *convergent thinking*. Divergent thinking involves the ability to generate multiple solutions to a problem, or a variety of ideas within certain parameters. This kind of thinking is expansive in nature and what is commonly referred to as "brainstorming." Convergent thinking, on the other hand, involves considering multiple ideas and determining the best one. It is selective in nature and results in a creative product ultimately becoming useful, functional, or culturally accepted. These two ways of thinking are quite different, and it would seem that being truly creative necessitates engagement in both. Accordingly, psychologists have described these contrasting types of thinking as two broad types of creative thought: (1)

generation, in which divergent thinking is used to produce ideas that are original, and (2) selection or exploration, in which convergent thinking is used to identify and refine the best ideas to be most functional (Kaufman & Gregoire, 2015). Recognition of these two broad processes has led to the so-called geneplore (*gene*rate + ex*plore*) model of creativity (Kozbelt et al., 2010; Sternberg, 2005).

Another popular approach to considering creativity within psychology is a framework of the "Four Ps of creativity" (Gruszka & Tang, 2017; Kozbelt et al., 2010). Traditionally, these aspects refer to the person, process, product, and place. Research focused on the creative *person* has examined the lives of people widely recognized as highly creative and sought to identify the character traits that distinguish them from the general population. Psychological investigations of the creative *process* have yielded theories to explain the mental mechanisms engaged in during creative thinking and activity. The most well-known theory of the creative process, the Wallas four-stage theory, is covered in detail in this chapter's forthcoming section on composition. Research focusing on creative *products* has often taken the form of studies that measure and analyze the artifacts produced by artists, inventors, and creative thinkers. Finally, research on *places* has examined how contextual setting, cultural climate, and environmental factors can affect creativity.

The four Ps framework was prevalent in mid- to late 20th-century psychology before being expanded to six Ps. The addition of *persuasion* refers to the impact creativity has on others; the addition of *potential* embraces consideration of everyday creativity and the creative capabilities of children (Runco, 2008; Simonton, 1995). Glăveanu (2013) proposed a similar model using the letter A rather than P, and emphasized the interdependence of the components, which was not often done with the older P model (the components were often studied separately); the five As in the model are the actor, action, artifact, audience, and affordances of creativity.

Also common in the psychological study of creativity is the so-called *Big-C/little-c* dichotomy. Big-C creativity refers to breakthrough ideas of historically eminent artists, inventors, and creative geniuses. Musical examples might include the symphonies of Beethoven, which ushered classical music into the Romantic era; the work of Stravinsky, whose *Le sacre du printemps* famously caused an audience uproar at its Paris premiere (but later was widely praised as one of the most influential works of the 20th century); and the "visionary music" of jazz saxophonist John Coltrane (Burniston, 2011, p. 204).

Little-c creativity is often described as "everyday creativity" and would include the work routinely done by musicians, artists, and creative thinkers whose works do not garner widespread acclaim. Although the Big-C/little-c dichotomy has been referenced for decades, it has also been recognized as inadequate for categorizing real-world creativity, as illustrated in this musical example:

> Highly accomplished (but not yet eminent) forms of creative expression are (mis)categorized into the little-c (or even Big-C) category. For instance, the accomplished jazz musician who makes a living playing jazz (but clearly is no John Coltrane) might be put into the same category as the high school jazz student who plays (passable) jazz in school concerts and the occasional birthday party, wedding, or family gathering. (Kaufman & Beghetto, 2009, p. 2)

Learning From the Exceptionally Creative

Although there is some debate as to whether Big-C creativity and little-c creativity should be treated as similar or different psychological constructs, a general fascination with the Big-C has resulted in a great deal of research attention being paid to the creativity of eminent artists, inventors, and innovative thinkers (Merrotsy, 2013). Some creative works are of such magnitude that their effects are felt for centuries (or more), they are hailed as breakthroughs, and they earn their creators immortal fame, as is reflected in the names Michaelangelo, Newton, and Beethoven (among others). While the folklore surrounding such "geniuses" may not offer reliable information about the true nature of creativity, psychological study of the real lives of such individuals has proved insightful. Simonton's (2010) study of creative geniuses concluded that eminently creative individuals tend to be prolific in output. Not only do they tend to start being productive unusually young, but also they maintain a high rate of productivity throughout life until they are advanced in years. Creativity as a regular way of life was also a conclusion drawn by Gardner (2011), who examined the lives of historically innovative individuals, including Pablo Picasso, Igor Stravinsky, and Martha Graham. His research offered these principles, which are pertinent to musical creativity (see also Gardner & Weinstein, 2018):

- *Domain specificity*—Rather than being a multidisciplinary personality trait, creativity is exhibited in specific domains (e.g., science, music, painting).
- *Mastering the domain*—Exceptionally creative people are first experts in their fields. They do not become innovators by ignoring what has already been done in a domain but by comprehensively understanding and wanting to add to it, in effect deciding to change the domain as a whole.
- *Success and failure*—Creative individuals accept that they will experience both successes and failures in their work; failure is understood as part of the process, not a reason to quit.
- *Alone and others*—Balancing the need for isolation (to focus on their work) and the need for the support and reassurance of others, highly creative people can have strained personal relationships in their lives.

Creativity as an Extension of Expertise

Not everyone in psychology has endorsed domain specificity as an absolute characteristic of creativity. It is possible to identify aspects of creative thinking that apply across disparate domains (Lothwesen, 2020; Lubart & Guignard, 2004). The case for domain generality begins with the argument that creativity is an attitude toward life or a style of intellectual inquiry (Sternberg, 2018; Zhang & Sternberg, 2009). Still, creativity cannot "be entirely free-floating and abstract, but must touch down and embrace some content" in a particular domain (Baer & Kaufman, 2005). The whimsically titled amusement park theoretical model of creativity attempts to bridge the gap between domain-specific and domain-general notions of creativity. Using the metaphor of an amusement park, this model acknowledges that the park is made up of multiple thematic areas or domains; thus, fields like music, science, and writing are analogous to water park, animal exhibit, and thrill ride sections of an amusement park. There are, however, certain initial general requirements that apply; just as a general admission ticket and interpark transportation pass is required no matter what section of the park visitors will focus on, general traits such as intelligence and motivation are thought to support creativity across domains. The amusement park model also identifies micro-domains; a person's affinity for rollercoasters might compare to a creative musician's specialization in jazz improvisation.

As mentioned earlier, Gardner (2011) emphasized the domain specificity of creativity, and additionally concluded that a certain level of domain mastery is attained before meaningful creative contributions are made (see also Baer, 2018). This view seems to validate the common practice—among formally trained and vernacular musicians alike—of familiarizing themselves with the work of those who have come before them. There can, however, exist a superstitious fear among some that spending too much time listening to and studying others' past creative works can impede their own creative musicianship; that is, becoming too familiar with pre-existing music can limit their own imagination and potential for originality. This perspective is not supported by psychological research, nor is it corroborated by musicological study.

Composers, for example, are known to have studied the old masters by literally copying, paraphrasing, and imitating them; such exercises can provide greater understanding of counterpoint techniques and orchestration. For their part, many popular musicians typically start off covering the songs of past artists before attempting to create original music (Green, 2002; Maruyama & Hosokawa, 2006; Negus et al., 2017). Also, jazz musicians, whose performance is expected to include much improvisation, do a great deal of listening to other musicians' recordings and often try to duplicate (or "transcribe") the improvised solos of past jazz greats. The mastery of existing musical accomplishments seems to be a prerequisite for inventing new material.

Listening to music is a central activity that fosters generative abilities through the formation of aural skills. Before the advent of recording technology, musicians had to physically attend performances to hear music. For instance, Leopold Mozart traveled with his son Wolfgang to Italy to familiarize the young composer with Italian opera (Sadie, 2006). Similarly, as a teenager, early jazz great Louis Armstrong peeked into dance halls and snuck into honky-tonk clubs where jazz music was played (Brothers, 2007). On the other side of the globe, in the *guru-shishya* tradition of musical apprenticeship in India, students are expected to "live the music" of their master teacher and "imbibe" the artform thoroughly (Grimmer, 2011, pp. 91–92). Since modern music learners now have great access to recorded music, they can readily familiarize themselves with the creative works of experts in the field.

By listening to and studying master works analytically and finding out how past great composers produced certain musical effects or structures, aspiring composers develop the ability to mentally represent and ideate similar structures. This background study and listening support the aural imagery that many composers mention in their writings as being rather vivid and crucial in their creative process.

A musician who has acquired all the necessary knowledge and skills has a chance to produce something new—maybe even outstanding. As mentioned earlier, by first mastering the domain, creative individuals are positioned to become so innovative that they essentially change the domain (Gardner, 2011). Thus, it is clear that having knowledge of what has been done in a field facilitates—and does not impede—personal creativity (see also Hao, 2010). Put another way, ignorance is not promotive of creativity.

It must be noted, however, that highly creative individuals are not "merely extreme experts in their chosen domains" (Simonton, 2000, p. 284). Exceptionally creative individuals tend to show a number of character traits that distinguish them from high-achieving domain experts. These traits include independence, openness to experience, nonconformity, and risk-taking (Kaufman, 2013; Kaufman & Gregoire, 2015; Simonton, 2000, 2009; Zhang & Sternberg, 2009).

The importance of prior knowledge is a quite prominent element of the "remix" model of creativity. Although some may associate the word *remix* with the relatively simple practice of modifying sound recordings to produce different versions of pre-existing musical material, the term can also describe a more complex process of generating work that is perceived as original (Hill & Monroy-Hernández, 2012; Knobel & Lankshear, 2008). The remix model of innovation identifies the three phases of the creative process as copy, transform, and combine. A study by Flath et al. (2017), done in the field of 3D printing design, offered empirical support for the remix model and led the researchers to conclude that remixing relies on both convergent and divergent thinking and that "recombinations of distant and diverse knowledge" can produce "breakthrough innovations."

Explaining how new ideas emerge from pre-existing knowledge is one of the goals of *spreading activation theory,* which comes from cognitive science. This theory asserts that prior knowledge is mentally stored as small, discrete "nodes" of information, which are interconnected in a vast network of the mind. The links between nodes reflect a person's associations between the concepts or ideas stored at the nodes. For example, a classical musician might have a node for the key of E-flat major, which, among its many connections, links to its relative key of C minor, which is connected to known works in C minor, including a node representing the second movement Marcia funebre of Beethoven's Symphony No. 3, and subsequently nodes representing the musical concept of a funeral march and other ideas related to funerals, death, and expressions of mourning. When engaged in creative thinking, as a node is activated (i.e., brought into consciousness), further activation may spread through the network, making it more likely that the ideas or concepts stored at associated adjacent nodes will come into consciousness. Creativity, then, happens as node activation spreads to form new pathways.

It follows, then, that the more knowledgeable creative artists are, the greater potential they have for a "rich fabric of interconnected nodes" with which to discover new pathways toward creative products, ideas, and solutions to problems (Schubert, 2012, p. 127). The knowledge that builds a creative thinker's mental network can come from formal study as well as mere exposure to one's environment and culture (enculturation). Even with similar education, experience, and exposures, individuals' mental networks surely differ because (due to individual differences of attention and prior knowledge during the perception of said education, experience, and exposure) there are myriad possibilities for how nodes and links are mentally structured. Conventional thinking, and not creativity, occurs when typically paired nodes are connected (e.g., a funeral march with another expression of mourning, to use the example offered in the previous paragraph). More imaginative thinking, however, results as node activation through an extensively linked pathway produces a distant relationship between previously unconnected nodes (Schubert, 2012). In the well-constructed mental network of a domain expert, spreading activation can happen without conscious attention, and thus be experienced as intuition or a "flash of insight" (Topolinski & Strack, 2008; Weisberg, 2006).

The remix model of creativity and spreading activation theory fit well together, and both speak of the importance of having an expert knowledge base and enriching background experiences to draw upon. South African jazz musician Jason Reolon described his own valuing of such factors this way:

> The artist that you are is about what you've absorbed through your life, in terms of what you've taken in listening-wise, but also what you've absorbed in terms of life experience. So creating is not necessarily about inventing something that wasn't there before. It's about taking all these things, mishing them together, and coming up with something that nobody else will, because your combination of influences is unique—because you're unique in your own experiences in all the different genres that you've absorbed, all the

melodies you've grown up with. That's what sets my creativity apart from somebody else's is that they have a different set of what they've gathered in their creative tool box. (Hill, 2018, pp. 7–8)

Impediments and Facilitators to Creativity

Of the many models of creativity, most share some broad commonalities. They suggest that (1) some preparation or readiness is required before engaging in creativity; (2) creativity typically begins with "insight," that is, the generation of original ideas; and (3) a working out of ideas takes place through conscious reflection or refinement.

The creative process can be hindered at any one of these broad phases. At the earliest phase, individuals can lack the readiness to be creative if they have not acquired the requisite knowledge and experience in the domain in which they aspire to be creative. After that, however, a more likely hindrance can occur when they generate original ideas and too quickly reflect critically on them. To do so is to attempt to engage in divergent and convergent thinking simultaneously; this often produces the phenomenon known as "writer's block."

Because generating original ideas (brainstorming) requires a noncritical and uninhibited mindset, some musicians have speculated that *altered mental states* can facilitate creativity. Certain naturally occurring states of consciousness may facilitate the generative part of creativity. Imaginativeness and openness to ideas may be greater in trance, hypnagogic states (semiconsciousness before sleep), and hypnopompic states (transition from sleep to wakefulness); this may be why a number of composers have reported musical ideas coming to them in dreams (Fachner, 2006). Also, a deep state of absorption or heightened state of mental awareness, which can be induced by certain types of meditation, has been linked to the experience of creative insight, that is, the movement of an idea into consciousness (Horan, 2009).

Some musicians have turned to alcohol, drugs, and other psychogenic substances in hopes of increasing creativity (West, 2004). More often than not, however, any short-term progress experienced as the result of chemically induced altered states does not develop into outstanding creative output. Although certain substances can surely reduce inhibition, increase activity level, or otherwise affect mood, they also can severely impede the processes of reflecting on and refining one's creative work. In fact, the same effect that can cause musicians to feel more productive may also result in their overrating the quality of their production.

Similarly, some theorists have speculated whether certain pathological conditions may actually facilitate creativity; this notion has posited a possible link between "genius and madness" (Simonton, 2005). Between historically perpetuated anecdotes about tormented artists and sensationalized headlines in modern mass media, there is much reinforcement of the idea that creativity is "closely entwined with mental illness" (Roberts, 2012). Although certain pathological conditions can affect a creative individual's mood, activity level, and productivity—most notably periods of mania within bipolar disorder—the preponderance of psychological evidence indicates that "mad genius" is a myth (Dietrich, 2014; Schlesinger, 2009; Simonton, 2014).

Composition

Clear understanding of the processes of musical composition remained mysterious for a very long time, in part because of the awe and admiration shown to great composers. A sense of wonderment toward composers has been reinforced both by music aficionados and within communities of composers themselves. In the past, when scholars did have the opportunity to probe the minds of great composers, the musicians' descriptions of the creative process—as they experienced it—usually provided little psychological insight. For example, in a conversation about creativity between composers' Johannes Brahms and Joseph Joachim, Brahms asserted that obtaining inspiration does not happen through the conscious mind (Abell, 2016/1955). Citing Mozart's creative process as a "vivid dream," Brahms described his own composing experience this way:

> I immediately feel vibrations that thrill my whole being. These are the Spirit illuminating the soul-power within, and in this exalted state I see clearly what is obscure in my ordinary moods; then I feel capable of drawing inspiration from above, as Beethoven did. (Abell, 2016/1955, Chapter 1, "How Brahms Contacted God" section, para. 4)

More recent psychological understanding of creativity has suggested that musicians' descriptions of a vague or mystical composing experience is the result of the complex and sometimes conflicting processes that underlie creativity. Divergent thinking and convergent thinking are, by definition, opposite processes. Both, however, are required for great creative works to be produced. In this way, it is understandable why composers might experience at least some aspects of creativity as originating outside of themselves.

Creative Process Stage Theory

Among researchers of creativity, an oft-cited model of the creative process is that offered by early psychologist Graham Wallas in his book *The Art of Thought* (Wallas, 1926). He originally theorized that the creative process consisted of four stages: preparation, incubation, illumination, and verification. These stages have endured over the last century and have continued to be embraced by researchers studying the processes of music composition (e.g., Burnard & Younker, 2002; Chen, 2012; Collins, 2005; Katz, 2009). The Wallas stage theory has also been revised by a number of researchers, including Csikszentmihalyi and Sawyer (2014), who called the illumination stage "insight" and subdivided the final stage of verification into "evaluation" and "elaboration." An amended stage model like the one summarized and explicated to follow has been advanced by a number of researchers, including Bogunović (2019), Csikszentmihalyi and Sawyer (2014), Hansen et al. (2011), and Lumpkin et al. (2004):

1. Preparation. Creative individuals such as composers must have acquired enough musical knowledge, skills, and perceptiveness to be fully functional in the domain. If a proposed composition seeks to be expressive of a particular emotion, situation, or life event, the composer must know how to apply said extramusical referents to their music (Konečni, 2012). This first stage of creativity consists of both lifelong preparation for the activity of composing in general and the "project planning" that musicians do for a particular composition. It may include making initial decisions about the parameters of the composition, for example, for what instrumentation the piece will be written and whether the piece will take on an established musical form (e.g., concerto, 12-bar blues, love song).

2. Incubation. This stage may not yield much observable behavior on the part of composers. After preliminary decisions about the parameters of a composition are made in the preparation stage, composers may

intentionally take some time away from the work, during which they devote little conscious attention to their composition, as if they are waiting for ideas to present themselves. Although incubation in the original Wallas (1926) theory likely reflected early psychology's general fascination with the "unconscious mind" à la Sigmund Freud and Carl Jung, a more modern understanding simply acknowledges that creative solutions can be facilitated by taking a break from conscious problem-solving efforts. As for *why* incubation is beneficial, it may be that it offers relief from mental fatigue or functional fixedness (i.e., a cognitive bias to consider materials only for their conventional uses). It appears that the nonconscious processes of incubation work best when creative individuals enter into the stage intending to later return to their work consciously (Gallate et al., 2012).

3. Insight. Originally labeled "illumination" by Wallas (1926), the point of insight refers to the "Eureka! moment" or "A-ha! experience" when creators suddenly think of creative ideas or solutions to problems. Anecdotes of insight moments are the stuff of legends, such as Archimedes discovering the principle of buoyancy while in the bath, and Isaac Newton creating his theory of gravity when hit on the head by an apple falling from a tree. Similarly fantastic accounts have been shared by composers. This includes Richard Wagner, who reported that the orchestral prelude of Das Rheingold came to him in a daydream (Carafoli, 2017), and popular musician Paul McCartney, who woke up one morning with the melody of "Yesterday" in his head (Kaufman & Gregoire, 2015). Illuminative insight marks the point in the creative process at which a composer's work returns to consciousness.

4. Evaluation. Originally part of the final "verification" stage of Wallas (1926), evaluation is the stage when creative individuals decide whether the ideas that have come to them are good ones and worthy of development. Evaluation can include much self-reflection on the part of creative individuals themselves or also involve "bouncing ideas off others" (Hansen et al., 2011). Upon coming up with the tune for "Yesterday," Paul McCartney is said to have gone around for weeks "asking friends whether they had heard the melody before. It took him a month to become convinced that he had not plagiarized anybody" (Carafoli, 2017, p. 461).

5. Elaboration. This was also originally part of the "verification" stage of Wallas (1926). Eminent inventor Thomas Edison famously defined creative genius as "1% inspiration and 99% perspiration." Csikszentmihalyi

(1996) asserted that elaboration is the stage in which the 99% is situated, being the most time-consuming and requiring the hardest work within the creative process. For composers, the stage of elaboration can involve the trial-and-error work of revising, extending, transforming, and refining germinal ideas (Collins, 2005; Collins & Dunn, 2011; Pohjannoro, 2014).

These stages occur more recursively than linearly. That is, the latter stages of elaboration and evaluation can see the emergence of new creative problems requiring their own incubation, insight, etc. Thus, a composer may proceed through "several cycles of creation" before producing a final version of a work (Bogunović, 2019, p. 96).

Types of Composers

Some researchers of music creativity have categorized composers as either "working types" or "inspirational types" (Bogunović, 2019; Holtz, 2009). These categories differ in how composers find and solve musical problems, what methods they employ when working, and how they assess their products. The inspirational types appear to be less conscious about their work, and they experience the source of their ideas as somewhat mystical and coming from outside of themselves. Working types, in contrast, labor systematically and experience their creative products as directly resulting from such efforts. The inspirational type may be seen in famous composers such as Schubert, Tchaikovsky, and Berlioz, and the working type may be represented by musical greats such as Bach, Beethoven, and Stravinsky.

Because of how they experience creativity, inspirational-type composers may struggle to verbalize much about their process. They may speak of a muse, spirit, or the universe imparting creative ideas to them. From a psychological perspective, what is likely happening is that composers put themselves into a mental state that facilitates divergent thinking and unfettered spreading activation across their mental network of musical knowledge. Celebrated modern composer Ellen Taaffe Zwilich described what she called "informed intuition" this way:

I want to inform myself as much as possible about everything concerning the piece that's going to be, and then I want to trust my instincts. If I have a plan for a piece, and then as I'm writing, the piece wants to do something different, I will *always* go with the piece and throw away the plan. But it's never just total inspiration, or total reliance on inspiration, it's a question of trusting yourself to make judgments that are beyond your emotional or intellectual grasp. (Raines, 2015, p. 9)

There is also ample evidence that the working-type and inspirational-type approaches to musical composition are not mutually exclusive. In the same conversation with Brahms, mentioned earlier, in which he spoke of the Spirit illuminating him while composing, he also acknowledged that composers must *work* to acquire technical mastery of theory, harmony, counterpoint, instrumentation, and orchestration (Abell, 2016/1955). Additionally, despite the widely propagated lore that W. A. Mozart's music came to him fully formed (i.e., without need for any conscious revision or development), it is now known that the composer did in fact work on and refine his compositions through multiple sketches and even explicitly stated his penchant for "experimenting—studying—reflecting" (Konrad, 2006, p. 102). More recently, Pulitzer Prize- and Grammy Award–winning contemporary classical composer Jennifer Higdon described a blending of inspiration and working approaches as she shared advice on composition: "Students often ask me, 'Should I wait until I am inspired?' No, you should be sitting there writing every day to get the inspiration in the first place" (Raines, 2015, p. 124).

Review of the psychological research on musical composition suggests that all composers use a creative process similar to the amended Wallas stage theory detailed in the preceding section of this chapter. The real difference between inspirational-type and working-type composers likely depends on which stages of the process are most evident to them. With the inspirational type, the composer may be most attuned to their experience of incubation and insight, that is, the stages involving the least amount of consciousness. Also, their preparation preceding the incubation stage likely consists not of specific planning for a piece, but of the cumulation of more general musical knowledge and lived experience. In contrast, working-type composers are likely to be most aware of their evaluation and elaboration—the most effortful stages of the process; their initial preparation stage probably includes much careful planning for the specific composition project about to be undertaken. Thus, it is reasonable to conclude that across all musicians, composing involves a combination of intuitive and deeply cogitative mental processes.

Katz and Gardner (2012) offered an alternative way of understanding how different types of composers may use the same stages of the creative process. Those who use a "Within-Domain" approach focus on the musical elements and musical materials of their compositions. In the preparation and incubation stages, they imagine the musical sounds they wish to create and supplement mental exploration with hands-on experimentation through vocal or instrumental improvisation. In subsequent stages, Within-Domain composers use sketching to fill in the details to get the written composition to match what they have imagined in their mind's ear. In contrast, the "Beyond-Domain" approach begins with extramusical ideas or human experiences to be expressed artistically. The initial stages of preparation and incubation involve consideration of such larger themes, sometimes for very extended periods of time. True to the original notion of incubation, Beyond-Domain composers are content to not concentrate but instead let ideas "marinate." The latter stages of their creative process include the effortful translating of ideas into artistic decisions about broader musical parameters and then specific musical elements, work that can be very tedious and time-consuming (see also Giesbrecht & Andrews, 2015). Table 7.1 shows how Katz and Gardner integrated Within-Domain and Beyond Domain processes with the original Wallas stages of creativity.

Composing as Dialogue

A recent study by an international team of music researchers has advanced the idea that musical creativity can be conceived of as interactive dialogue (Schiavio, Moran, et al., 2020). In their study of active professional composers of contemporary classical music, their results suggested that their creative outcomes emerge as composers explore, interact with, and constantly adapt to their environment. Much of this formative interaction consists of sociocultural relationships with people, including other musicians (those who perform their compositions, members of a composer's community). Engagement with these musical people allows composers to receive feedback on their work, shape their musical identities, and even dialogue with dead composers (by learning about them from more experienced musicians). Accordingly, one of the best ways that music teachers can support student composers is to provide them with an environment with useful resources and a community of musical peers (Wiggins & Medvinsky, 2013).

Table 7.1 Within-Domain and Beyond-Domain Process Mapped Onto Stage Theory

	Stage 1 Preparation	Stage 2 Incubation	Stage 3 Illumination	Stage 4 Verification
Stage Theory	Creator becomes acquainted with and evaluates a problem	Creator is distanced from a problem; conscious work is put on the back burner	Creator has a "flash of insight" when there are signs that the solution is imminent	Composer refines and develops the basic model
Within Domain	Experimentation with musical materials (e.g., sound, instrument) in a hands-on fashion		Bits of music gel into a more cohesive work	Details of piece are worked out and notated
Beyond Domain	Attachment into a conceptual model from outside of the music domain		Major characteristics of the conceptual model defined and mapped onto piece	Fleshes out models with smaller ideas and associations connected to the larger framework

From Katz, S. L., & Gardner, H. (2012). Musical materials or metaphorical models? A psychological investigation of what inspires composers. In D. J. Hargreaves, D. E. Miell, & R. A. R. MacDonald (Eds.), Musical imaginations: Multidisciplinary perspectives on creativity, performance, and perception (pp. 107–123). Oxford, UK: Oxford University Press, p. 111.

The *audience* is another important human element of a composer's environment. While some may outwardly insist that they do not care how their work is received, most express an understanding that they have a kind of relationship with the audience, even seeing themselves as "the audience's representative" while doing revision work in the compositional process, such as asking, "Is it interesting enough?" (Zembylas & Niederauer, 2018, p. 22). Beethoven may be considered an exemplar for composers acknowledging the important role of the audience; said one professional composer, "He was clearly trying to knock people out of their seats, trying to knock their socks off; that's what Beethoven was trying to do. I think it's what we're all trying to do" (Raines, 2015, p. 150).

Composers can also have relationships with musical instruments and technologies that that they use (Schiavio, Moran et al., 2020). Although these may be seen simply as tools for inspiring or realizing creative ideas, a psychological perspective recognizes musical instruments as enactive factors in a composer's conceptual space that can present creative limitations or affordances. Composition can be understood as a form of situated cognition, meaning the creative process is inextricable from its sociocultural context and the artifacts and practices contained therein (Folkestad, 2012; Roels, 2016).

The benefit of dialogue and interaction underscores the importance of composers being receptive to learning from the musical people and material with which they interface. *Openness to experience* is one of the character traits most often associated with creativity (Kaufman, 2013). In a creative context, openness to experience includes both emotional engagement and aesthetic engagement (i.e., appreciative involvement with the arts). Especially among contemporary composers, such openness may take the form of exploration and adaptation of a variety of musical genres. Obviously, this element connects to the remix model of creativity. Some composers have benefited by having experiences with both serious art music and more popular styles (e.g., Waldron, 2018). When asked in an interview about becoming a composer, musical artist Pamela Z recalled her experiences as a rock musician while also formally studying music in college:

> I felt inspired to try to expand what I was doing and became more interested in experimental music. My work was coming from a performance-art sensibility, and I realized that I could combine these two worlds in my own work, so I begin practicing other styles of singing and making vocal sounds. I started playing with electronics, processors, and multi-track tape recorders to compose music. I think that's when I first started calling myself a composer. People who come from the popular music world would write songs and sing and perform their music, but usually don't refer to themselves as composers. (Raines, 2015, pp. 308–309).

Speaking to the same interviewer, composer Kevin Puts acknowledged that his symphonic composing had been influenced by blues, jazz, and rock, including "certain harmonies . . . which might be attributed to '90s soft rock" (Raines, 2015, p. 158). It is likely no coincidence that jazz, which places a premium on originality, improvisation, and innovation, has also historically shown openness to a very diverse array of cultural influences. Examples of cross-genre creativity include Duke Ellington's recording Tchaikovsky's Nutcracker Suite, Miles Davis's *Sketches of Spain* album, and Charlie Parker performing with chamber orchestra musicians (Montuori, 2020).

Improvisation

Because composition is so clearly a generative process with multiple stages, improvisation is sometimes viewed as a different creative activity altogether. The research, however, confirms that composition and improvisation are more similar than different. In fact, improvisation could quite rightly be called "instant composition" (Johansson, 2012). Performers draw on previously acquired musical knowledge and past experiences as they seek to create new musical products "in the moment," and their creative activity combines both reproductive and innovative aspects. Like the compositional process, skilled improvisation requires preparation, as well as the ability to generate musical ideas and refine them, albeit in a manner different from composing.

Especially among formally educated musicians in the "classical" realm, the most apparent difference between improvising and composing may be that compositions are written down. More careful consideration, though, shows that this is not always the case. Most composers want to preserve their musical creations, but not all of them do it through written music notation. Some "archive" their work by making audio recordings of it, and others ensure its preservation simply by performing it repeatedly. This brings to mind the scenario of a loving parent who sings a made-up song to a child every night at bath time or bedtime. It is also likely that such a personally composed song began as an improvisation but over time became a more finished and consistently performed composition.

In fact, the characteristics of improvisation that most distinguish it from composition have to do with the element of *time*. Although improvising is often talked about as spontaneous or even "instantaneous," in reality, musicians devote a great deal of time to the skill of improvisation. Because the musical decision-making *during* improvisation must happen so quickly and automatically, it demands of a skilled improviser great investment both before and after the performance activity itself.

Processes Underlying Improvisation

The *constraint of time* dictates the processes of improvisation and distinguishes it from composition. In the many musical settings in which improvisers must coordinate their performance with coperformers, improvisers cannot alter the timing of their performance to accommodate deliberate thinking and musical decision-making. The creativity of improvisation must happen *in real time*. Time, however, is not the only defining constraint. As Ashley (2016) has pointed out in his review of research literature on musical improvisation, a performer's extant knowledge is another significant constraint. Improvising musicians can only act on what they know.

In different musical styles and performance settings, improvisation can vary greatly in the amount of musical freedom afforded to performers. Even within the specific genre of jazz, it ranges from traditional styles, in which improvised solos are expected to communicate the underlying harmonic progression of the pieces performed, to free jazz, in which performed music usually does not even indicate a tonal center. In this way, improvisation can be conceived of as a continuum on which one end is structure and the other is freedom.

Especially when improvising in a highly structured context, musicians' acquired knowledge and experience are important. This point is especially relevant to note selection in improvisation. Skilled improvisers do not just pick notes out of thin air. Rather, their pitch selection is meaningful and reflects an assimilated understanding of musical qualities such as tonality. Within jazz, for example, improvised solos—such as those of saxophone great Charlie Parker—have been shown to more prominently feature scale degrees that indicate the tonality of the composition within which the solo is being created (Ashley, 2016). This kind of performance fluency reveals skill that has moved well beyond the cognitive stage (at which deliberate thought and decision-making take place) and has advanced into a state of automaticity. As explained in Chapter 4 of this book, performance skills only reach automaticity with much purposeful practicing and performance experience.

Therefore, practically speaking, some of the most important processes that facilitate improvisation are those that have taken place well before the moments of real-time performance. Berkowitz (2010) has provided a detailed and cogent explanation of how performers acquire the knowledge base that facilitates expert improvisation. The process is like the acquisition of a language knowledge base that allows people to express themselves in spontaneous conversation. Just as a language knowledge base includes phonology (i.e., the sounds used to make words) and syntax (i.e., how to combine words into understandable phrases and sentences), a music knowledge base includes familiarity with musical sound material and an understanding of how to transform and recombine components into performed music that is meaningful to listeners (see also Berkowitz & Ansari, 2008). The building of an improvisation-supportive knowledge base includes the preparation for improvising, that is, the initial stage of creativity. In jazz, for example, the necessary preparation is accomplished by gaining a broad familiarity with the style to be improvised in and prelearning music material, such as "licks," patterns, and chord progressions. This preparation is accomplished mostly via listening (Berliner, 2009/1994). In his algorithmic explanation of how jazz musicians improvise, Johnson-Laird (2002) described how performers' ability is facilitated by both (1) consciously known ideas about the musical context within which they are improvising and (2) assimilated principles governing musical elements of melody, harmony, meter, and rhythm. Although the latter procedural knowledge is nonconscious, it is nevertheless "acquired at the cost of considerable work" (p. 439).

Through practicing and other experiences in the domain, musicians build the acuity of their musical "ear" and gain a functional understanding of what musical material is expressive in their chosen genres of performance. Pressing (2001) explained:

> By the time advanced or expert stages have been reached, the performer has become highly attuned to subtle perceptual information and has available a vast array of finely timed and tuneable motor programmes. This results in the qualities of efficiency, fluency, flexibility, and expressiveness. All motor organization functions can be handled automatically (without conscious attention) and the performer attends almost exclusively to a higher level of emergent expressive control parameters. (p. 139)

Perceptual competence can be passively acquired through enculturation. Prior to gaining improvisation expertise, however, the enculturation experiences must be supplemented with deliberate learning of productive skills.

Once automatized improvising skill has been acquired, accessing and executing it in the moments of performance require a mindful "letting go" on the part of improvisers (Berkowitz, 2010, p. 125). The psychological state of flow (Csikszentmihalyi, 1990), previously mentioned in Chapter 3, appears to be a correlate of skilled improvisation (Biasutti, 2017; Biasutti & Frezza, 2009; Forbes, 2020a). The "letting go" of flow and improvisation is *not* accomplished by disengaging mentally. On the contrary, it is more of a "complete absorption" (Berkowitz, 2010, p. 127) or "full immersion" in the moment (Ford et al., 2020, p. 141).

Brain scans of musicians engaged in improvisation indicate that the "letting go" consists of suspending self-assessment and allowing automatized music-making processes to happen (Berkowitz, 2016; Limb & Braun, 2008; Pinho et al., 2014). This point addresses the question of whether improvisation is under the deliberate control of the performer. This question remains debated among some musicians and researchers even, but one thing is clear: the performance created by an expert improviser is not a product of chance. Although all aspects of improvised performance do not result from performers' conscious decision-making and executive control (the constraint of real-time spontaneous performance prevents it), improvisation is still the product of the musicians' expertise, which has been deliberately acquired. Among expert improvisers, a strong connectivity between automatized motor processes and executive control function amount to a "greater neural efficiency" (Beaty, 2015, p. 114).

Although improvisation is clearly facilitated by the suspension of self-assessment *during* performance, it is not to be eliminated altogether. In fact, attending to feedback about one's own improvised performance can be a critical contributor to the acquisition of improvising skill. In improvisation, the "working out" of ideas—that is, the latter stages of creativity, evaluation, and elaboration—does not occur the same as in composition, but revising ideas is still important in the development of the skill. When composers try out a musical idea, perhaps sketching it in pencil on paper, they may decide against using it and then erase it from the sketchpad. Obviously, improvisers cannot erase from a past moment in time a musical idea they tried, but they do use feedback received in that moment to inform their improvising going forward. Internal feedback consists of their own feelings and self-appraisals. External feedback can come from two sources, coperformers and the listening audience, as explained by Biasutti and Frezza (2009):

On the first level, the external feedback could be visual (while improvising, musicians look to each other), gestural (musicians state some conventional signs to define the order of improvisation), verbal, and musical feedback (musicians can settle a priori a certain sequence of notes that indicates, for instance, the passage from a harmonic progression to another). On the second level, external feedback might be listeners' positive or negative reactions to improvisation. (p. 238)

Improvisational choices receiving positive feedback will likely be repeated or explored further in the future, whereas ideas that elicited negative feedback will be modified in subsequent practicing or performing.

The research of Biasutti and Frezza (2009) found supporting evidence for a theoretical model of five dimensions of improvisation, as shown in Figure 7.1. This model nicely encapsulates the component processes of improvisation identified by the research and reviewed in the preceding paragraphs here. Flow and feedback appear verbatim in the model, their "use of repertoire" refers to prelearned "licks" and other material, and their dimension of "anticipation" also reflects acquired knowledge. Assimilated musical understanding allows anticipation in multiple ways, including for planning an improvised solo to form a meaningful unified whole, and accurately knowing what to expect of coperformers. Acquired musical knowledge is also important in their final dimension of "emotive communication." As explained in Chapter 6, it is through music listening and performance experience that musicians learn emotional coding, that is, how certain musical sound properties are expressive of emotion.

Interestingly, because improvisation is understood to be an expression of one's personality and feeling, it has been used as a "clinical tool" in music therapy (Wigram, 2006, p. 223). It has been used for a variety of therapeutic purposes, including in work with children with autism, individuals with

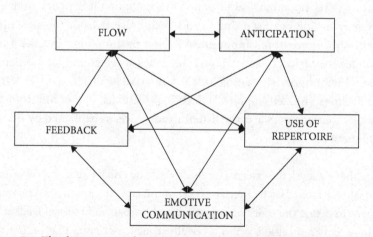

Figure 7.1 The dimensions of musical improvisation by Biasutti and Frezza (2009).

From Biasutti, M. (2015). Pedagogical applications of cognitive research on musical improvisation. *Frontiers in Psychology,* 6, article 614. https://doi.org/10.3389/fpsyg.2015.00614

learning disabilities and psychotic disorders, and older adults with dementia. In such clinical settings, the music therapist employs flexibility in leading improvisational activities and encouraging expressive and imaginative play from clients.

Social Interaction as a Defining Element

Much performed improvisation is done in a group setting. This became so common in certain musical traditions that it brought about the word *jamming*. Jam sessions are defined by musicians gathering together socially and making music together extemporaneously, that is, without any specific preparation.

Just as the psychological state of flow is conducive to individual improvisation, the concept of *group flow* refers to an ensemble performance situation in which all members seem to be mentally and emotionally "in sync" and "things are clicking" (Sawyer, 2003, p. 43). Also called *shared* flow, it is often presented in psychology with the example of the jam session of a musical group (Nakamura & Csikszentmihalyi, 2014). A sense of group flow emerges when performers feel connected to one another and their performance is especially well coordinated. While performing in group flow, musicians are very receptive and responsive to their coperformers.

As explained by Sawyer (2003), the parallel processing of group flow—that is, performing while simultaneously attending to the music made by other musicians—is facilitated by the mindful and immersive consciousness of the flow state. An "open communicative channel among performers" is experienced through nonverbal communication, primarily eye contact and bodily gesture (Sawyer, 2003, p. 44; see also Duby, 2020; Walton et al., 2015). Coperformers also communicate with each other through musical cues. For example, members of a jazz combo may only know when an improviser will end a solo by listening to the music within the solo itself (Seddon, 2005).

It deserves emphasis that group creativity with improvisation is more than just exceptionally precise coordination of performance. Through their improvisatory music making, well-attuned group members can communicate their individual intentions and ultimately *construct shared intentions* in the musical context of the moment (Bishop, 2018). The musical result can be collectively borne ideas, the creativity of which is greater than that which any one person could generate, a psychological phenomenon known as *emergence*. These types of performance experiences are so artistically and personally rewarding to musicians that they describe them in terms such as "special, cherished moments," "ecstasy," "divine experiences," and feeling "telepathically" connected to coperformers (Berliner, 2009/1994, pp. 389–390).

Becoming Musically Creative

People typically show plenty of creativity in their everyday lives. They routinely compose email messages and engage in spontaneous conversations with others in a real-time improvisatory way. Thus, it is somewhat surprising that so many consider composing and improvising to be specialty skills that relatively few musicians will acquire. As pointed out earlier in the chapter, it is a relatively new phenomenon in classical music to have musicians who specialize in reproductive performance, that is, exclusively performing music created by someone else. With this point in mind, perhaps instead of wondering how people become musically creative, a better question is why so many developing musicians lose their natural human creativity. Pablo Picasso is widely quoted as having said, "Every child is an artist. The problem is how to remain an artist once he grows up" (Time Magazine, 1976).

Experimental composer-songwriter Tom Waits has also pointed to children to illustrate the mindset of openness that artists need. "Children make up the best songs," he once told an interviewer. "Better than grown-ups. Kids are always working on songs and throwing them away, like little origami things or paper airplanes. They don't care if they lose it; they'll just make another one" (Gilbert, 2002, p. 255).

Research into the musical creativity of children has long been an important source of insight into child development, as well as the nature of human creativity. The Swanwick and Tillman spiral model of musical development, featured in Chapter 2 of this book (see Figure 2.1), was based primarily on research done in the late 20th century in which the creative music making of children age 3 to 11 was tape recorded and analyzed by researchers. The children's "compositions" ranged from spontaneous utterances to more carefully constructed and rehearsed performances. The model reflects well-established psychological concepts known to be a part of creativity, including mastery, imitation, and imaginative play.

Subsequent research has revealed that music composition is carried out in a great variety of ways among children. Constrained by their background and available resources (e.g., whether they play an instrument or have access to technology for mixing/looping), children's musical creations can range from quick made-up pieces to more "proper pieces" that indicate a stepwise process of generating ideas followed by working with, fixing, and finalizing them (Burnard, 2006, p. 121). If a single theme permeates the development of musical creativity, it may be that it is a *source of meaning making* for young people. Creating original music, whether in individual or group settings, allows children to explore and gain insight into themselves and the world around them. It can be a particularly meaningful vehicle for children to grow musically, as well as in socioemotional ways.

In this vein, the specific compositional activity of *songwriting* has shown particular promise for nurturing the creativity of young people (Adams, in press; Draves, 2008; Hess, 2018; Hill, 2019; McGillen & McMillan, 2005). Songwriting allows young musicians to choose the styles of music they will work in, which allows the activity to align with their lived cultural experiences. Situated in familiar musical contexts, songwriting promotes personal expression, identity formation, and a greater sense of self. It also can facilitate social development through membership in a songwriters' community. The Chapter 7 sidebar box offers specific recommendations to music educators about how to incorporate songwriting into the learning activities they lead.

Similar musical and personal benefits have been identified for young people from engaging in improvisation. In the recent past, improvising has mainly been incorporated into music education through jazz pedagogy. The primary focus has been on the creative *products* of improvisation (e.g., spontaneously performed solos) and accordingly has operated through a music theory–based approach emphasizing chords, scales, arpeggios, patterns, and harmonic progressions (Biasutti, 2015). As previously mentioned, improvisation can be conceived of as a continuum on which one end is structure and the other is freedom. The theory-based approach clearly favors structure. Hickey (2009) adopted the continuum concept in explaining how traditional approaches to improvisation in school music begin by instructing student performers to embellish known melodies and utilize patterns. Hickey has argued that students who start at the structure end of the continuum seldom progress across the continuum to experience greater freedom in their improvising; in fact, as time passes in this approach, students may venture less and less away from already-known material (see top panel of Figure 7.2). Calling the traditional approach didactic and teacher directed, she has proposed a more learner-directed approach, in which students are first guided to develop an "improvisatory disposition" through *free improvisation*, in which creative process is emphasized over product (Hickey, 2009, p. 292). Instead of being concerned whether students' improvised solos sound like jazz should, emphasis is placed on exploring the processes of musical choice, listening, and expression. This alternative model, illustrated in the lower panel of Figure 7.2, indicates that over time, young musicians will learn to do musical problem-solving individually and eventually be able to add stylistically expected structure to their improvisations.

For many musicians, childhood playful and exploratory creative experiences are much more than passing fancy. The experiences and insights gained form a foundation for a lifetime of creative musicianship. As previously explained in the context of composing, both inspiration and hard work are part of the creative process. This is also true at a life-span level, especially for musicians who go on to distinguished careers as composers. Research on the creative productivity of great composers has produced some interesting theories. For example, based on extensive research on the careers of classical composers, Simonton (2000) reported that the most productive and acclaimed composers required relatively fewer years of training before beginning serious composition and before making their first lasting contribution to the repertoire. This suggests that they required less time to attain the necessary level of musical mastery and that perhaps composing became a career goal for them early in life. More recently, Kozbelt (2008, 2012) offered support for a theory that past classical composers' career peak—that is, when their creative output was at its best quantitatively and qualitatively—could be explained by their creative process and whether they evaluated their own work based on raw originality of creative concepts or on the perceptual effect of their artistic creations. Composers whose process was rapid, was ideation focused, and used conceptual evaluation criteria tended to peak earlier in their careers. In contrast, those whose process involved greater elaboration and perceptual evaluation criteria tended to have long-term productivity, even later in life. Additionally, composers who could be classified as "one-hit wonders" (i.e., they produced only one outstanding contribution to classical music), as compared to those who enjoyed more sustained productivity, were

Traditional Approaches to Improvisation in School Music

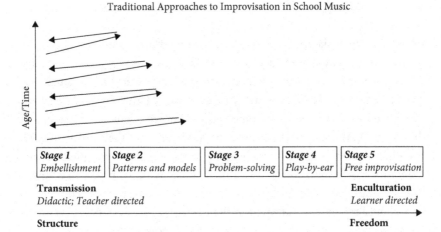

Proposed Approaches to Improvisation in School Music

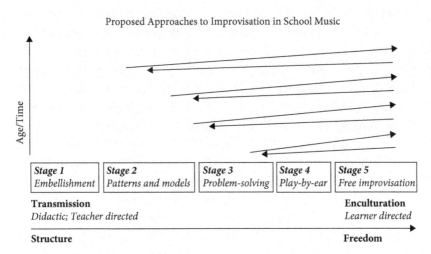

Figure 7.2 Traditional versus Hickey's proposed approaches to improvisation on a structure-freedom continuum.

From Hickey, M. (2009). Can improvisation be "taught"?: A call for free improvisation in our schools. *International Journal of Music Education, 27*(4), 285–299.

more likely to write "mainstream, even conservative, small-scale works" (Kozbelt, 2008, p. 190). Multihit composers more often produced large-scale works consisting of numerous well-elaborated musical ideas and as such were more likely to be seen as innovators who altered the course of music history.

Taking the Stage: Give an Inspirational Recital

Musicians can make the activity of performing more creative by employing the character trait that is most often linked to creativity across domains. Openness to new experience reflects an innovative mindset, adaptable expertise, and flexibility in one's artistic endeavors. Many of the most innovative musicians not only point to their musical knowledge as a creative tool but draw also upon their life experiences for inspiration in their music making. Even the hardest-working "working type" composers have sought to express aspects of the human condition in their music (case in point: Beethoven's Eroica Symphony). As performers have new and interesting life experiences, they should try to connect them to their music, even if connections do not obviously present themselves or it takes a heavy amount of artistic interpretation to make a musical application. For example, when young musicians fall in love for the first time, it would be a shame for this once-in-a-lifetime experience to occur without it impacting their performing. Even if they are not moved to compose and perform original music for the object of their affection, they could still program a recital of selected works around the unifying theme of love (there is plenty of existing repertoire from which to choose!). The new experiences that spark creativity can also be less emotionally charged. Musicians who identify more with certain issues of social justice can find ways to feature those causes in their performing activities. Also, when musicians gain exposure to and enjoy a style of music that is different from the ones they typically perform, they need not relegate that new style to the status of a "guilty pleasure." Rather, they could try borrowing from the new style. For example, György Ligeti, the great composer of contemporary classical music, upon hearing a recording of Michael Jackson's "Billie Jean," remarked, "This drum machine is very interesting. I think you could compose fascinating polyrhythmic music with this new technology" (Raines, 2015, p. 169). Musicians can explore musical genre crossover, even if it is a relatively superficial aspect such as costuming or stage behavior. In whatever way musicians apply new experiences to their performing, they should also consider informing their audiences about their intentions, be it through personally written program notes or spoken remarks from the stage between pieces performed. Most audience members cherish opportunities to go "behind the music" and get a glimpse inside an artist's mind, especially as it relates to how personal experience interacts with creative work.

Leading Learning: Give Students
Songwriting Opportunities

Songwriting is a great way for young people to demonstrate their current level of musicianship and make music study more personally meaningful to themselves. Much of the guidance shared here is based on Adams (in press), who has drawn on research and his own experiences as a singer-songwriter and music educator to offer many practical suggestions for teachers interested in adding this music-making activity to their instruction. Because creating original music requires a certain level of musical expertise as preparation for creativity, students should be encouraged to explore songwriting in the musical genre with which they are most familiar. For many of today's students, these genres will be pop, rap, hip-hop, or country music. Even if teachers are not well versed in these musical styles themselves, they should nonetheless allow their students be creative in them. Teachers should trust that their own musicianship is robust enough to provide the musical guidance students need to grow as songwriters. Teacher-led songwriting instruction can take the form of mini-lessons on common song forms or chord progression options. They can also lead students in "analytical" listening of professionally recorded songs and guide students in identifying the most salient song properties and musical elements that students can borrow to use in their own song creation. Teachers should also make a concerted effort to educate their students about the mindsets that facilitate creativity, particularly the openness needed to experiment with music, to persist through failed ideas, and to be receptive to feedback and revision. Perhaps the most important contribution teachers can make is to arrange for students to be a part of a community of songwriters. This can be accomplished in a music classroom context by facilitating "songwriting circles," within which a group of aspiring songwriters gather to share their works in progress and offer each other encouragement and helpful ideas for revision efforts.

Chapter 7 Discussion Questions

1. As you reflect on your own musicianship and that of the other musicians you know, to what extent are composing and improvising part of regular music activities? What developmental experiences likely

account for composition and improvisation either being a part of or being missing from different people's musicianship?

2. What anecdotal evidence can you point to in support of domain specificity or domain generality of creativity? In your experience, are the most creative musicians also creative in other domains, such as visual art or real-life problem-solving?

3. Recall your most rewarding music performance experience in which you performed music composed by someone else and compare it to your most rewarding experience performing original music you created yourself. What made each so rewarding? Are the reasons mostly the same or different?

8

Managing Performance Anxiety

Most people choose to be musicians based on a love of music and a desire to share it with others. If the reality of music performance were always this simple, then all musicians would enthusiastically welcome opportunities to perform for an audience. Of course, the issue of performance is more complicated. Instead of sensing excitement to share their music with an audience, musicians sometimes feel apprehensive and anxious. This anxiety, commonly called "stage fright," can be a serious and debilitating problem.

Unfortunately, the problem can start early in the lives of musicians. Although parents and teachers usually provide students with the encouragement and assistance they need to develop musically, they can also place such an emphasis on achievement that their young musicians feel pressured (Osborne & Kenny, 2005; Papageorgi, 2020; Patston, 2014). Although very young children seldom experience performance anxiety (they simply enjoy making music), it appears to manifest in the course of development as children become aware of how performance flaws can elicit critical feedback and feelings of embarrassment in themselves (Kenny & Osborne, 2006). Research has shown that adolescent musicians share similar experiences of performance anxiety as older performers (Papageorgi, 2020; Thomas & Nettelbeck, 2014), and that their emotional attitude toward performance can include tension, lack of confidence, and feelings of fear (Kaleńska-Rodzaj, 2020). Based on a review of the research, Osborne (2016) concluded that up to 75% of student musicians experience some form of performance anxiety.

The problem is also prevalent among adult populations of musicians. Kokotsaki and Davidson (2003) found that 65% of the conservatoire musicians in their study reported feeling anxiety that impaired their performing ability. Other studies of university musicians have reported even higher incidence (Zakaria et al., 2013). In a study of professional classical orchestra members, over half reported experiences with performance anxiety (Cohen & Bodner, 2019). Other research has suggested that this problem is prevalent among musicians in a variety of genres (Papageorgi et al.,

Psychology for Musicians. Robert H. Woody, Oxford University Press. © Oxford University Press 2022.
DOI: 10.1093/oso/9780197546598.003.0008

2011). Noted sufferers include virtuosi Pablo Casals, Arthur Rubinstein, and Vladimir Horowitz, as well as hugely successful popular musicians Barbra Streisand and George Harrison (Kenny, 2011). That even successful musicians struggle with performance anxiety attests to the fact that it is fundamentally unwarranted; that is, it does not stem from being untalented or ill-equipped to perform.

Unfortunately, when young musicians reach out to others for help with performance anxiety, sometimes they receive one-size-fits-all folk wisdom. They may be told that "nervousness just means you're not prepared" or given person-specific advice such as "What works for me is. . . ." Even the most revered good advice, "practice, practice, practice," is not always a valid solution to performance anxiety problems. From a psychological perspective, a proper treatment strategy cannot be prescribed without first diagnosing the source of anxiety. Psychologists attempt to look beyond the physiological symptoms to define performance anxiety by its causes and the conditions that produce it. Researchers of music psychology have grouped sources of performance anxiety into three broad categories of the person, the situation, and the task (Papageorgi, 2020; Valentine, 2002; Wilson, 2002). This chapter consists of four sections that consider the following:

1. *The symptoms.* The physiological responses of performance anxiety are produced when a person feels threatened. The activation of the body's emergency system produces physical and psychological symptoms that can be treated through bodily training and medicinal remedies.
2. *Source 1: The person.* One source of performance anxiety is the performers themselves. Whether the underlying cause is a character trait or unrealistic thinking about performing, musicians can benefit from cognitive treatment approaches.
3. *Source 2: The situation.* Another source to consider is situational stress, which relates to the environment and circumstances of performance. Identifying stress-inducing aspects can lead to incorporating helpful strategies into performance preparations.
4. *Source 3: The task.* The final source of anxiety is the performance task. To perform confidently, musicians must attain a level of mastery of the music to be performed. To avoid anxiety, the performance task must not challenge musicians beyond what they believe their skill level to be.

Understanding the Symptoms

When a human being perceives a threat—whether real or imagined—the body reacts naturally. The physiological reaction has long been called the "fight or flight" response (a phrase coined in the 1920s)—but more recently, a third option, "freeze," has been identified by research (Niermann et al., 2017; Schmidt et al., 2008). The physiological response is a defensive mechanism, in which the brain activates the body's emergency system in the sympathetic branch of the *autonomic nervous system*. The nerves stimulate the adrenal glands in the abdomen to release certain hormones into the bloodstream. These hormones, commonly referred to as adrenaline, affect organs throughout the body in characteristic ways. Table 8.1 shows how the changing functions of the organs result in abnormal feelings within the person.

These *physiological symptoms* constitute the physical state of arousal, which is also marked by increased brain activity. Although musicians more readily identify too much arousal (anxiety) as a problem, *too little arousal* would also make it difficult to perform well. Imagine a person just waking up in the morning, feeling very little energy. Heart rate is slow, breathing is shallow, and the mind is anything but alert. Certainly, in this state of low arousal, a person is in no condition to carry out the physical and mental challenges of performing music. Psychologists who work in areas such as the performing arts and sports point to "optimal arousal" as a condition for

Table 8.1 How the Physical Changes of Arousal Translate Into Physiological Symptoms of Anxiety

Adaptive Bodily Function	Sensation Felt
Heart beats vigorously to increase oxygen supply to muscles	Pounding chest
Glands in the skin secrete perspiration to lower body temperature	Excessive sweating, wet palms
Lungs and bronchial airways open to supply more oxygen	Shortness of breath
Saliva flow decreases	Dry mouth, lump in the throat
Digestive system is inhabited as blood is diverted from stomach to muscles	"Butterflies in the stomach," nausea
Pupils dilate to sharpen distance vision	Blurring and focusing problems
Muscles tense in readiness for increased physical exertion	Tension, shaking hands, muscle tremors

high-quality performance. Athletes and performing artists alike talk about the need to get "psyched up" or "pumped" for an event, in effect drawing on the increased arousal that facilitates better performance—for this reason, optimal arousal is considered *adaptive anxiety* in psychology.

Symptoms' Effect on Performance

Named after two psychologists, the *Yerkes-Dodson Law* describes the relationship between arousal and performance as an inverted U (see top panel of Figure 8.1). As arousal increases from low to moderate levels, performance quality improves. Performance is at its highest when arousal is at a

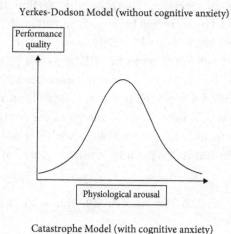

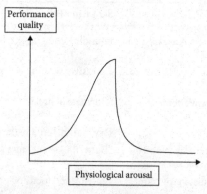

Figure 8.1 Yerkes-Dodson inverted-U model (without cognitive anxiety) and catastrophe model (without cognitive anxiety).

moderate level. Additional arousal amounts to *maladaptive anxiety*, steadily impairing performance quality as anxiety increases past optimal arousal. Practically speaking, what constitutes optimal arousal depends on several factors, including the nature of the task to be performed. For example, greater manifestations of physiological arousal are probably more enabling for a rock-and-roll set drummer than for a flutist in a Baroque chamber ensemble. An accelerated heartbeat and amplified muscle readiness match the physical exertion required to play a drum set, but these symptoms could interfere with carrying out the fine motor skills and breath control required to play the flute. Thus, the same bodily changes of arousal that are facilitative for some performers can be debilitating symptoms for others.

The problem with maladaptive physiological symptoms is that they can lead to deterioration in performance quality. In fact, excessive physiological arousal before and during performance is viewed by many musicians as a primary *cause* (rather than a symptom) of anxiety (Kenny et al., 2014). Visual disturbances caused by the dilation of the pupils can interfere with reading printed music, especially under bright stage lighting. Additional muscle tension can cause twitching or tremors that affect the physical production aspects of performance. The end result might be inaccurate pitch production (e.g., finger placement, arm movement) and rhythmic timing. High arousal often influences the choice of tempo, which tends to become faster in performance than during practice, thus adding technical difficulties. A combination of these physical sensations can make musicians feel so strange that they are unable to concentrate or execute the expressive aspects of the music. The manifestation of symptoms is likely related to the physical demands of different instruments, for example, a greater prevalence of respiratory symptoms in wind players or sweaty palms and finger tension in string players (Studer et al., 2011). It could be, though, that these are just the symptoms that the players notice most often or find most bothersome.

In addition to directly producing performance mistakes and hindering expressive control, these physiological symptoms may cause musicians to change how they normally and properly go about performing. For example, a trumpet player who normally uses strong breath support to produce higher pitches on the horn may suffer from shortness of breath and may therefore try to compensate by using excessive force of the mouthpiece against the lips. The latter method is much less effective and will result in fatigue more quickly. Such undesirable adaptations, as well as the performance mistakes that result, are sometimes referred to as the *behavioral symptoms* of performance anxiety.

Another important factor is the presence of *cognitive symptoms*. When taking the stage, musicians who lack confidence in their performing ability may respond to their increased arousal with fear that the physiological symptoms will ruin their performance. If they become mentally preoccupied with negative thoughts about their performance, they may worry excessively about mistakes and assume a catastrophic performance failure is going to occur (Spahn, 2015). In many ways, such catastrophic thinking becomes more a source of performance anxiety than a symptom, and as such, it is discussed in this context later in this chapter.

In considering symptoms, however, it is important to note that when cognitive anxiety is added to physiological arousal, the result can be even greater damage to performance quality. This outcome also points to the interrelated nature of physiological, behavioral, and cognitive symptoms, which, unfortunately for afflicted musicians, can all occur simultaneously. Borrowing from research in sports performance psychology, Osborne (2016) offered a conceptual model to understand the phenomenon of "choking," that is, failing in a crucial performance situation. This so-called performance-stress model of choking is shown in Figure 8.2. This model illustrates the interactive and cyclical nature of performance anxiety symptoms. For example, musicians' worries (cognitive) going into a performance may cause them to tremble, sweat, and tense up (physiological) onstage, resulting in performance problems and poor technique (behavioral), all of which prevent them from paying attention to what they intended to do (cognitive).

This kind of vicious cycle has led some psychologists to believe that the inverted U is not the best model to illustrate the deterioration in performance that occurs once moderate arousal is surpassed. The *catastrophe model* of anxiety and performance replaces the gradual decline in performance quality (of the inverted U) with a sharp downward plunge, as shown in the bottom panel of Figure 8.1. According to researchers, the key to predicting the course of deterioration is the cognitive components of performance anxiety. With a performer who is suffering only from the physiological responses to stress, the gradual decline of the Yerkes-Dodson model is apt. However, as more cognitive anxiety is introduced into the equation, the more catastrophic the loss in performance quality will be. The catastrophe model has received empirical support mainly in the realm of athletics, but psychologists

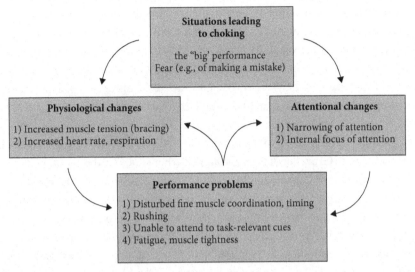

Figure 8.2 Performance stress model of "choking."

From Osborne, M. S. (2016). Building performance confidence. In G. E. McPherson (Ed.), *The child as musician: A handbook of musical development* (2nd ed., pp. 422–440). Oxford, UK: Oxford University Press. Reproduced with permission of the Oxford University Press through PLSclear.

have readily applied it to the realm of music performance as well (Bugos & Lee, 2015; Wilson & Roland, 2002).

Treating the Physiological Symptoms

Sometimes the most expedient course of action is to target the physiological symptoms for treatment. One such approach is the use of *relaxation techniques*. Deep breathing before and during performance may be the most popular relaxation technique (Fernholz et al., 2019; Nagel, 2010). Slow, deep breathing ensures that the body takes in the amount of oxygen it expects in its state of arousal. Another approach directed at physiological symptoms is progressive muscle relaxation training. In these exercises, a person proceeds through areas of the body, alternately contracting and relaxing the muscles one at a time. Often the procedure starts with extremities such as fingers and progresses inward to larger muscles, such as those in the shoulders. Research has shown this training to be effective in reducing several measures of performance anxiety in musicians (Kim, 2008).

In some clinical tests of performance anxiety treatment, relaxation techniques have been supplemented with *biofeedback training*. Using monitoring devices with visual displays, musicians are made aware of the physiological responses their bodies are exhibiting, such as heart rate variability. When they successfully employ relaxation techniques and other coping strategies, they have the benefit of seeing the positive results in physiological measures. Biofeedback assistance has been shown to be an effective tool in decreasing performance anxiety and improving the self-appraised quality of performance (Gruzelier & Egner, 2004; Thurber et al., 2010).

The *Alexander Technique* is a specific method related to relaxation and bodily awareness. Its creator, F. M. Alexander, was a successful Australian actor who went on to develop his system of "psychophysical re-education" in response to performance-related health problems. The technique has a distinctly philosophical component, emphasizing the unity of body and mind, but it also offers solutions to "misuse" of the body through enhanced sensory awareness and physical training. Exercises largely focus on proper bodily posture, position of the head, and use of muscles when moving. The Alexander Technique was not developed with stage fright in mind, but it is widely used by musicians to reduce unnecessary tension that accompanies anxiety. Some research attests to its effectiveness in improving heart rate variance, self-reported anxiety, and positive attitude toward performance (Klein et al., 2014; Valentine, 2004).

Despite the potential help offered by these relaxation approaches, some musicians have turned to medications to deal with the symptoms of performance anxiety. The most common drugs used are *beta blockers*. Surveys of classical musicians suggest that in certain circles, between one-quarter and one-third of performers use beta blockers (Kenny et al., 2014; Matei & Ginsborg, 2017). Beta blockers impede the physiological symptoms that stem from adrenaline being in the bloodstream. Normally, the adrenal hormones in the blood bond to the beta receptors of organs throughout the body, causing them to change their function. When a beta-blocking medication is taken, its chemical agents in the bloodstream also bond to the organs' beta receptors, in effect blocking out the adrenaline. Research has confirmed that beta blockers can reduce physiological symptoms of performance anxiety (Brugués, 2011). Potential benefits, however, are less likely when beta blockers are used without medical supervision (Kenny, 2011). There also is some indication that beta-blocking drugs can have negative side effects in musicians, especially with prolonged use (Packer & Packer, 2005;

Patston & Loughlan, 2014). Another concern raised is that beta blockage also changes the bodily function needed to perform well (Brugués, 2011; Patston & Loughlan, 2014). This includes with respect to expressive aspects of musical performance, as some musicians report a feeling of "detachment" while using beta blockers (Violinist.com, 2017).

Because of the interrelated nature of physiological, behavioral, and cognitive aspects of performance anxiety, treatment targeting physiological symptoms also can have some benefit beyond them. For example, relaxation techniques may help the cognitive processes of musicians by refining performers' powers of attention and concentration. Or perhaps performers feel more at ease simply from knowing that they have done something to address bothersome physical symptoms, and the resulting sense of empowerment allows them to (behaviorally) perform more capably.

Understanding Source 1: The Person

For many musicians, merely treating the physiological symptoms does not completely eliminate the experience of performance anxiety. The brain activates the body's emergency system only when a person perceives some sort of threat. This points to the importance of the cognitive realm. How musicians think—their attitudes, beliefs, judgments, and goals—determines in large part the extent to which they perceive a performance as threatening.

Character Traits

Performers themselves are the first source to be considered in explaining performance anxiety. *Trait anxiety* refers to a disposition to be anxious in all aspects of life. Those with high trait anxiety tend to view the world around them as more threatening than others do and respond anxiously to situations they encounter. Although some view *trait anxiety* as genetic, other research suggests that an anxious personality develops from environmental factors (Lebowitz et al., 2016). Musicians who report high levels of performance anxiety tend to also score high in measures of trait anxiety (Kenny et al., 2004, 2013; Martin-Gagnon & Creech, 2019). There is reason to doubt the folk wisdom that some people are just naturally anxious, especially among musicians. Research with adolescent musicians (Osborne & Kenny,

2008) and undergraduate music students (Robson & Kenny, 2017) has indicated that those who can recall a past worst performance or on-stage breakdown tend to experience high levels of performance anxiety later in life. This finding suggests that some musicians may become unusually sensitized to performance anxiety through a "traumatic conditioning experience" similar to those reported by sufferers of social phobia (Osborne & Kenny, 2008, p. 449; see also Dobos et al., 2019).

Whether character traits are the result of inborn genetics or life experiences (or likely both), they are relevant to musicians' experiences with performance anxiety. Although there is certainly great diversity among the personalities of musicians, research has identified several traits that are common among musicians and often associated with anxiety. One such characteristic is *neuroticism*, or emotional instability (Miranda, 2020). Neuroticism often manifests as a person regularly experiencing a wide array of emotions (mood swings) and showing instability in relationships and interactions with others. Neuroticism appears to also make musicians more susceptible to performance anxiety (Rae & McCambridge, 2004; Thomas & Nettelbeck, 2014).

Musicians also can be well characterized by the passion they apply to their activities. Although two musicians may have a similar level of passion and drive in their professional pursuits, they may differ significantly in their specific motivations. Some musicians' passion may come from an infatuation with the creative and expressive potential of the art. Others' passion may be aligned with their being wholly committed to their success as a professional performer. An emerging line of research has suggested that the *type of passion* that musicians have can determine their susceptibility to performance anxiety, as well as their potential for long-term fulfillment as a musician.

The research of Bonneville-Roussy and colleagues, focusing on advanced classical musicians, has provided evidence for a dualistic model of passion (Bonneville-Roussy & Bouffard, 2015; Bonneville-Roussy et al., 2011; Bonneville-Roussy et al., 2020; Bonneville-Roussy & Vallerand, 2020). *Harmonious passion* is characterized by unpressured choice to engage in an activity, and the experience of positive emotions during and as a result of engaging in it. In contrast, *obsessive passion* manifests as an unmanageable compulsion to carry out an activity, even through negative consequences. Musicians with harmonious passion show a flexible persistence and are able to balance their music activities with other aspects of life. Musicians with obsessive passion are driven to attain the approval of people in their lives or to maintain a self-esteem that is contingent upon success.

Personal Cognition

The practical differences between harmonious passion and obsessive passion demonstrate that characteristics of musicians themselves can greatly influence how they go about their activities and respond to the experiences they have. Personal cognition mediates between personality traits and the behaviors that musicians exhibit in preparation and performance. In other words, how musicians carry out daily activities such as practicing and the resulting experiences onstage are very much impacted by the beliefs they hold and the thought processes in which they engage.

One especially pertinent example is *perfectionism*, which is best understood as a set of thought patterns of unrealistic expectations and a judgmental perspective of performance as categorically good versus bad or correct versus incorrect. A closer examination of the components of perfectionism suggest that striving for excellence is not the problem so much as the negative reaction to imperfection (Kenny, 2011; Stoeber & Eismann, 2007). Among musicians, perfectionism can manifest as a preoccupation with mistakes made in performance (Patston & Osborne, 2016). Although awareness of performance errors—especially in individual practice—is necessary to improve one's skills, an unmitigated perfectionist attitude is irrational. The concept of correctness usually is not applicable among advanced musicians whose ultimate goal is not a "correct" performance, but rather one that is personally expressive and elicits an emotional response in listeners. Minor performance mistakes in and of themselves usually will not ruin the experience for most audiences, but musicians' preoccupation with them can thwart expressive communication. Celebrated pianist Arthur Rubinstein seemed to understand this:

> Never mind if I miss one or two notes. The big line is the thing, and it seems to convey the right thing to the audience. Otherwise I would have been pushed from the concert podiums years ago. The public wouldn't stand for it. I think I am the champion of playing wrong notes, but I don't care. And the public doesn't seem to care much. (Elder, 1982, p. 3)

The general field of psychology has identified perfectionism as a particularly destructive factor; in addition to being a strong correlate to performance anxiety, it has been linked to depression, eating disorders, and self-harm (Flett et al., 2014; Stoeber et al., 2016). A psychologist who drew upon clinical observations from 35 years of psychotherapy practice concluded that "the most successful people in any given field are *less* likely to be perfectionistic, because the anxiety about making mistakes gets in your way" (Dahl, 2014; see also Greenspon, 2014).

As discussed in Chapter 3, musicians' goals for performance can be very consequential. Those with a task-involved goal orientation tend to see performances as opportunities to share music with others. A task-involved goal orientation has been likened to having "mastery goals" because task-involved musicians are more focused on improving their skills than on how others judge them. Musicians with an ego-involved goal orientation, however, see performance as an opportunity for others to judge them and, as such, are more likely to see performance as a potential threat, thus making them more likely to struggle with stage fright. Research has indicated that optimal performance experiences (i.e., not marred by anxiety) are more likely when musicians prioritize expressive communication and their own enjoyment of the experience rather than strive to give a successful performance (Lacaille et al., 2005).

As was mentioned earlier in this chapter, catastrophic thinking about a performance can be particularly deleterious. This type of cognitive distortion, known as *catastrophizing*, is thought to be the best predictor of music performance anxiety (Brugués, 2011; Liston et al., 2003). Catastrophizing occurs prior to performing and often increases in intensity as the performance draws nearer. It consists of inordinately negative thoughts that assume that a performance will go poorly. Often catastrophizing thoughts are vague—they may be experienced more like feelings than thoughts—and as such, it can be very difficult to simply push them out of one's mind. Combined with the trait of perfectionism, catastrophizing can take the form of extremely negative and critical self-statements and feelings of doubt in one's ability to manage the forthcoming performance (Kenny & Osborne, 2006; Mornell & Wulf, 2019; Osborne, 2016).

Self-handicapping is a particularly troubling form of maladaptive behavior that a perfectionistic musician may exhibit as a result of catastrophizing. If convinced they are heading for a performance failure, some musicians may invest more energy in creating an excuse for a poor performance than in preparing their best possible performance. In effect, they believe they can protect their image by having a convincing excuse for failing to attain perfection. Before a performance, musicians might start to complain about feeling sick or publicize reasons for not being able to practice as much as they wanted.

Their desire to have an explanation for a performance failure can escalate to the point of actually sabotaging their performance ability, perhaps by being careless with their physical health or damaging their own instruments. Self-handicapping behaviors are designed "to locate the blame for a bad performance on external factors but to claim extra credit for a good performance, which occurred despite adverse circumstances" (Valentine, 2002, p. 169).

When dealing with performance anxiety, looking outside of oneself is tempting on a larger scale too. This is perhaps why so many musicians and music teachers prescribe "practice, practice, practice" as the ultimate solution to stage fright, rather than doing an honest evaluation of oneself. Even so, the psychological research is clear that musicians' character traits and personal cognitions are highly consequential in their susceptibility to performance anxiety. One final interesting example is that instrumental performers' relationship with their musical instrument is quite telling. Those who feel united or "as one" with their musical instrument (as opposed to something to hide behind or an obstacle to overcome) are significantly less likely to experience performance anxiety (Simoens & Tervaniemi, 2013).

Cognitive Treatment Approaches

Cognitive restructuring is a treatment strategy that targets a person's thought processes. Musicians work to improve self-awareness and identify thinking that is irrationally negative and counterproductive and replace it with thoughts that are realistic and task focused. For example, one team of researchers tested the effectiveness of mental skills training with a group of adult musicians with varied levels of expertise (collegiate, amateur, professional) and various performance areas (pianists, singers, string and wind instrumentalists). The study offered small group training workshops (delivered over a three-week period) in which musicians practiced self-awareness exercises to identify "wasted energy" on uncontrollable factors and dysfunctional "all-or-nothing thinking" and learned how to use self-talk and imagery to eliminate unhelpful thoughts and regain concentration (Hoffman & Hanrahan, 2012, p. 21). Compared to similar musicians in a control group, those who received the mental skills training experienced reduced performance anxiety and improved performance quality. Similar intervention studies have reported similar results (Clark & Williamon, 2011; Osborne et al., 2014). Although not research based, a number of books written by musicians promote the use of self-talk to correct excessively critical thinking, the most popular of which is *The Inner Game of Music* (Green & Gallwey, 2015).

Self-awareness and self-talk can help musicians overcome irrational perfectionistic thinking that promotes performance anxiety. A growing body of research has indicated that musicians can benefit greatly by becoming more mindful and accepting in the moments of performance (Juncos & Markman, 2016; Steyn et al., 2016). Spahn (2015) suggested that catastrophizing can be replaced by realistic thinking when musicians adopt a "meta-level awareness" of performing and work to utilize a full repertoire of coping strategies (p. 133). For many musicians—and all people—it is not easy to change well-established habits, including habits of mind. In such cases, they may want to consider very deliberately addressing the anxiety problem with meditation. Although meditating is done in a great variety of ways, in general, the purpose of meditation is to gain greater awareness and nonjudgmental acceptance of oneself and one's surroundings. As such, meditative practice may hold great promise for reducing performance anxiety among highly perfectionistic musicians (Diaz, 2018; Lin et al., 2007).

Another important quality of productive cognition for performers appears to be directing attention away from the self and focusing it on the performance task at hand (Mornell & Wulf, 2019). This points to the importance of goal setting in musicians' personal cognition. Accordingly, relief for performance anxiety may come for some musicians when they change their goal setting to define performance success by the skills they acquire during preparation, rather than by the performance being free of any mistakes and impressing others (Kenny, 2011; Lacaille et al., 2005). Wilson and Roland (2002) identified goal setting as a cognitive strategy for treating performance anxiety, specifically recommending learning-oriented goals over outcome goals. For performers whose motivation to practice comes primarily from an upcoming performance (Burwell & Shipton, 2011), they would do well to focus on goals that are more intrinsic to music making, such as communicating expressively to listeners and feeling absorbed in the moment while onstage (Kenny, 2011; Lacaille et al., 2007).

As shown in this section, the mental makeup of a performer is a primary source of performance anxiety. Anxiety can manifest itself in troublesome thought patterns such as perfectionism, catastrophizing, and faulty appraisal of other performance aspects. Paraphrasing Wilson (2002), the most effective cognitive strategies are (1) learning to accept physiological arousal and minor errors during performance, (2) appreciating the process of performance rather than dwelling on the audience's evaluation, and (3) using self-talk to supplant overly critical thinking with more realistic and task-oriented thoughts.

Understanding Source 2: The Situation

A second broad source of stage fright is the situation of a performance. Anything in the environment or circumstances surrounding a performance that intensifies a performer's sense of threat will increase the level of anxiety experienced. Perhaps the most significant element of a performance situation is the presence of an audience. The intimidation posed by anonymous faces in a packed concert hall can be surpassed by a smaller audience consisting of more significant listeners—loved ones, music experts, adjudicators.

Context and Consequences

Performing music is not stress inducing per se, but doing so in front of people seems to be. As previously explained, musicians with perfectionistic tendencies or an ego-involved goal orientation may see performances primarily as an opportunity for others to judge them as a failure. This problem of personal cognition may be exacerbated by the presentational style of the Western concert tradition, which is marked by strict observance of performance conventions and a social context of separation between performer and audience (Turino, 2008). The formalities of concert attire and stage behavior can increase the expectations of audience members. Not surprisingly, performance anxiety may afflict classical artists more than jazz and popular musicians, who often perform in informal settings (Kaspersen & Götestam, 2002; Papageorgi et al., 2011). In the presentational-style concert tradition, performers onstage are not just sharing their art but are viewed as specially skilled experts to be considered from afar by the people of an audience, some of whom are adoring fans and others critics. In this context, it is understandable why many musicians might worry about not "measuring up" and struggle with a kind of impostor syndrome (Kenny, 2011; Lazarus & Abramovitz, 2004).

In terms of public performance, anxiety is greater when performance conditions put musicians "on the spot," that is, feeling special scrutiny. Situational stress has been shown to vary according to the characteristics of audience, as well as the onstage performers. Kenny (2011) summarized past research this way:

> Larger audiences whose members are respected by the performer for their status in the field and expert knowledge of their repertoire will elicit more performance anxiety than audiences without these characteristics. Moreover, the size of the performance ensemble influences the level of anxiety, with solo performances eliciting the highest anxiety, followed by small ensembles, orchestras, and teaching settings (p. 63)

Many times for musicians, the size and status of the audience are not as nerve-wracking as the stakes of a performance. This is why auditions, juries, and performances in competitions can be especially stressful. In such evaluative settings, musicians often have very little choice in the conditions around performance, and the lack of control can be debilitating. When musicians cannot control performance conditions and cannot control the consequential results determined by others, they must acknowledge what they *do* control, namely the *preparation* with which they take the stage for an audition or competition performance. This includes the mental preparation done before performance. Though performers do not decide for themselves whether they win the job or prize, they can resolve in advance how consequential they will consider the results to be in terms of their self-esteem and commitment to their musical life.

Managing Situational Stress

Musicians dealing with performance anxiety should appreciate the influence of situational factors, but they should also realize that they often have some decision-making power over the conditions of their performances. Collegiate music students, in particular, are usually in charge of making the arrangements for their recitals. If they have a choice in the venue of their performance, they may choose according to the size of the auditorium and the physical layout of the stage area and audience seating. Also, since the presence of coperformers onstage tends to reduce felt anxiety, musicians may benefit from including duets or small chamber works on their programs instead of performing solo pieces exclusively.

In other words, the first strategy for managing situational stress is for musicians to take control of performance factors that they can in fact control. Some musicians may unthinkingly conform to the typical performance settings and circumstances that they assume are expected of them, or surrender their decision-making power to teachers or others (who might actually prefer that the musicians themselves handle preperformance arrangements). Performers can help prevent stage fright by taking control of situational factors when possible and not acquiescing to uncomfortable conventions or "unwritten rules" for performance.

Related to this, one unconventional way that some musicians have overcome audience-induced anxiety is through improvisation. By experimenting with free improvisation or incorporating improvised music into "classical" performance, performers can, in effect, remove the (perceived) judgmentalism of the audience. Improvisation serves to weaken the idea that music performance can be judged by predetermined outcomes (Allen, 2013). Finnish clarinetist Kari Kriikku has incorporated improvisation into his classical concertizing and as a result has perceived audiences as "listening to the music" rather than "listening to its execution" (Hill, 2017, p. 233).

Beyond asserting control over the conditions of their performance, musicians must focus on their preparation to effectively address situational stress. Of course, preparing for performance anxiety can be difficult as it typically occurs in public performance and *not* during practicing. In their preferred practice setting, musicians typically dress comfortably, they can take breaks as desired, and they do not have to deal with bright lighting and the openness of a stage. Considering this, musicians can better prepare themselves by incorporating performance aspects into their practicing.

Research suggests that musicians can do this in a variety of ways. A popular strategy for treating performance anxiety is the use of *mental rehearsal*, in which performers imagine what they will experience in an upcoming performance. As explained in Chapter 4, mental rehearsal is best suited for experienced and proficiently skilled musicians who can vividly imagine the sounds and their feelings of the music to be performed. Mental rehearsal can prepare the body and mind for the special conditions of performance so that these conditions do not feel so unexpected and disturbing when they occur during the actual performance. An effort to reduce one's reactivity to stimuli is what psychologists call *desensitization*.

Imaginal desensitization techniques have been shown to be effective with advanced musicians, including in the high-pressure context of auditions (Lazarus & Abramovitz, 2004; McGinnis & Milling, 2005; Spahn et al., 2016). In a study of Canadian university musicians by Gregg et al. (2008), mental imagery was more frequently used by performance majors (whose degree "hinged on the quality of their performances"). In discussing their results, this team of researchers explained how mental imagery can contribute to performance readiness:

> Though a piece may sound exactly as the musician wants it to in the prac-
> tice room, that can sometimes be little indication as to what will actually
> happen on stage. Musicians need to ready themselves for those experiences
> unique to performance alone in order to prepare for this disparity between
> quality of practice and performance. This preparation includes things like
> being impervious to distractions, recovering from a lack or slip of con-
> trol, maintaining mental toughness, demonstrating confidence, and over-
> coming fatigue. (p. 238)

One step better than imagined performance is simulated performance. It is, of course, common for music ensembles to hold dress rehearsals to become familiar with the performance hall. Such practice performances for solo musicians are probably not as routine, but they are a good idea. The success of a simulated performance depends on how well it includes the elements of a "real" performance that differentiate it from a typical practice session, such as the presence of an audience, more formal performance attire, and playing straight through the program without stopping to address errors. Such run-throughs give musicians opportunity to acclimate to the conditions of the coming performance while also monitoring their readiness (Chaffin et al., 2005; Williamon et al., 2017). Performance conditions can also be simulated through the use of media technology. Aufegger et al. (2017) asked conservatory musicians to perform before a virtual audience and virtual panel of judges (i.e., audio-video footage on a large screen in front of them) and found that the simulations *did* elicit symptoms of anxiety in performers. Based on musicians' feedback about their experiences in the study, the researchers concluded that virtual audience simulation can be a useful tool for enabling performers to adopt desensitizing strategies in a safe environment.

When working with performers whose anxiety is particularly crippling, some psychologists have employed the treatment approach known as *systematic desensitization* or exposure therapy. With this type of approach, which has been used to treat all sorts of phobias, a person attempts to maintain a relaxed state while being exposed to conditions that are increasingly stress inducing. This process may be carried out by having the person either imagine the situations or actually encounter them live. For example, after achieving a relaxed state, a musician might first think of an "easy" performance situation, such as playing a familiar piece for a friend in a practice room. If still feeling relaxed, the musician might then imagine an additional person in the room and then playing for the two people in a larger rehearsal room. The situations steadily intensify in terms of the elements that provoke anxiety. Of course, systematic desensitization can also be carried out with real performances, instead of imagined scenarios. Wilson and Roland (2002) suggested a self-directed strategy for systematic desensitization in which musicians build a personal *anxiety hierarchy*. In this exercise, musicians list many different performance situations so as to identify varying conditions that define performance (and anxiety), such as size of the performance venue, time of performance, proximity to audience, size of audience, etc. When they have a good-sized list, they then relist the performance situations in order of increasing stress production. Then comes the hard part: they set about vividly imagining performances in those situations (in increasing order of stress), or better yet, actually performing in them.

Understanding Source 3: The Task

A third source of stage fright is the performance task itself. Sometimes musicians go into performances questioning whether or not they truly possess the skills to play the music on the program. Some may believe that, to improve themselves, they must push their limits, to try to exceed what they think they are capable of. For some performers, however, best intentions of pushing limits can produce great dread and even nightmares in the weeks leading up to a big performance. Mastering the technical demands of a piece can consume all their practice time such that they feel unable to prepare an expressive interpretation of it. Ideally, musicians take the stage with confidence in the abilities they are about to put on display, but sometimes it seems that the music is just too difficult.

As pointed out at the very beginning of this chapter, "practice, practice, practice" is not a valid strategy for all forms of performance anxiety, but it is, in fact, a good solution when the source of musicians' anxiety is a lack of confidence in their performance musicianship (those needing to improve their practicing to alleviate performance anxiety are referred to Chapter 4 for a thorough discussion of quality practice). *Task mastery*, referring to musicians' command or proficiency of the skills needed to give a performance, is an important factor in managing performance anxiety. Obviously, increased practice generally leads to improved performance skills. More to the point here, though, is that musicians' greater mastery of musical tasks allows the tasks to be performed successfully under stressful circumstances.

Accepting the Challenge

Some musicians seem to perform better onstage for an audience than alone while practicing. Likely their general level of musicianship exceeds the challenge presented by the music itself, and only with the challenge of a public performance are they motivated to give their best performances. These musicians are not debilitated or even distracted by the arousal of a performance; they thrive on it. Performing is a rewarding experience for them.

Performing can be an "optimal experience" for musicians when it consists of the right musical tasks. As previously discussed in Chapters 3 and 7, the term *flow* describes the experience of being fully engaged in an intrinsically rewarding activity (Csikszentmihalyi, 1990; Miksza et al., 2012). According to flow theory, the first requisite for such an experience is a balance between task challenge and skill level. When a musician's skill level exceeds the challenge of a performing task (e.g., playing simple music alone in a practice room), apathy or boredom is likely. On the other hand, when the challenge is higher than a musician's skill level, the result is anxiety. Flow experiences while performing music—with or without an audience—are only possible when the challenge posed by a performance *matches* musicians' skill level.

According to research, musicians who struggle with stage fright would do well to focus on achieving flow rather than on avoiding anxiety (Cohen & Bodner, 2019). To assess their potential for experiencing flow (or anxiety) with a musical task, musicians should first examine their performance goal orientation. A goal orientation that is task involved, rather than ego involved, appears to be essential to achieving flow in performance (Fritz & Avsec, 2007; Stavrou et al., 2015). Genuine intrinsic interest in the music they are performing can also enable musicians to build the self-efficacy that supports skilled performance. Recall from Chapter 3 that self-efficacy refers to the confidence or trust musicians have in their skills. This point should remind musicians that the purpose of their practicing is not just to "learn the music" and be better prepared for their next performance but to improve their musicianship and to expand the confidence they have in it. Strong self-efficacy is based on a realistic appraisal of task mastery and belief in the ability to achieve performance goals.

Finding Balance

Realistic appraisal is critical in managing task-related performance anxiety. Musicians must work to attain the task mastery without overpracticing, the negative results of which can become even more troublesome sources of anxiety (Kenny, 2011; Kenny & Ackermann, 2016; Wilson, 2002). The task mastery that supports optimal performance likely includes some level of automaticity, such that simply producing the music does not demand too much concentration and effort of performers. As suggested by flow theory, an immersive experience in performance is characterized by keen awareness and responsiveness to feedback (i.e., what they hear of themselves and other performers). Some performers describe it as being "totally absorbed" or "lost" in the music. If task mastery has not been attained, musicians will expend much attention to physically producing the music and not have the mental resources available to fully engage in the musical moment. Wan and Huon (2005) provided evidence that the performances of novice musicians deteriorate under pressure due to exhausting their attentional resources to the production aspects of performance.

   Balancing the challenge of the task with skills they possess is a major consideration in the decision of what music to perform in a recital or concert. Unfortunately, musicians may not recognize this point of decision-making as a critical factor in performance anxiety. Choosing music to perform is different from choosing music to practice, especially for those who have struggled with performance anxiety. Here, the performer must be realistic in choosing music to perform and factor in the time and effort it will actually take to prepare for public performance. Some musicians have been known to intentionally program for performance music that is too difficult for their current skill level, thinking that the threat of looking foolish onstage will *compel them to practice more*. This is not an advisable approach for self-motivation, as it may lead to greater stress and self-handicapping rather than any increase in practice. If musicians are looking for a motivational hook, they should consider performing music that they personally like. All too often, student musicians relinquish the decision-making to a teacher, or they feel compelled to choose from a list of established repertoire. Music students (and their teachers), however, should strive for a balance between working on pieces they "should" perform and making music they actually enjoy. Student musicians who choose their own music gain an added incentive for learning to perform it well and are more likely to approach performance as an opportunity for musical sharing rather than a point of judgment.

This chapter has explained the symptoms of stage fright and emphasized the value of determining the primary source of a musician's performance anxiety as the person, the situation, or the task. Pinpointing the source can indicate the most efficacious treatment strategies. Of course, it must also be acknowledged that the categories of the person, the situation, and the task often interact. For example, the critical factor of self-efficacy refers not to some objective measure of musical skill, but to musicians' belief (source: the person) about their skill level (source: the task). Similarly, the research of Osborne and McPherson (2019) indicated that it is musicians' cognitive appraisal (the person) of the threat posed by consequential performances (the situation) that affects the levels of anxiety and confidence that musicians bring into performance.

Because sources of performance anxiety can overlap and interact, combining treatment approaches—so-called multimodal interventions—may be most effective (Brugués, 2011; Matei & Ginsborg, 2017). Based on their review of options for managing performance anxiety, McGinnis and Milling (2005) suggested that musicians incorporate both cognitive restructuring and exposure therapy. This is likely very sound advice; it recognizes that musicians' own beliefs and thought patterns are very influential and also acknowledges that the ultimate key to overcoming performance anxiety lies in performing more often.

Taking the Stage: Do More Informal Performing

The cruel irony of performance anxiety is that it motivates musicians to perform *less*, but ultimately overcoming the problem usually requires them to perform *more*. The more infrequent performance is, the more unfamiliar the conditions of performance are and the more unsettling the sensations of physiological arousal are to musicians. Further, performances will likely be infrequent if the only ones they do are those required of them (e.g., school concerts and recitals for student musicians, hired gigs for professionals). Musicians can make strides against stage fright by making their own performance opportunities, and ones in which they have more control over the performance circumstances. Musicians should consider volunteering to perform for local schools, nursing homes, and other community groups. Such organizations eagerly and gratefully accept performers donating their talents, so musicians can accomplish some career-advancing networking while simultaneously learning to better manage performance anxiety. They also can accomplish a similar effect by sharing their music making at informal gatherings with family and friends. Whether taking place in a library or their parents' living room, informal performances can offer musicians important opportunities to experience the act of performing as a simple sharing of their music and themselves. Without some of the most anxiety-inducing trappings of formal performance, musicians are more likely to have the cognitive wherewithal to fully engage in the moment and be aware and responsive to the feedback they receive while performing. The experience and insights gained in these informal settings can be taken with them into more formal performances in the future and likely allow them to better enjoy performing in those settings.

Leading Learning: Motivate Through Sharing, Not Showcase

Music is meant to be made and shared with others. Performance is a natural and necessary part of music learning. The youngest of music students often leap at opportunities to make music for their friends and family; they may even eagerly volunteer for solos in group performances. Teachers who enjoy this youthful enthusiasm likely find it disheartening to see their students grow up and gradually come to view performance as an experience to dread. As common as this change is, teachers can take heart knowing that they can help minimize the encroachment of performance anxiety into the musical lives of their students. One area of influence has to do with motivation. Teachers should carefully consider the means by which they motivate students to carry out individual practice and to take ensemble rehearsals seriously. To be sure, an imminent performance is a powerful motivator for musicians in the long run. It is probably a time-honored approach for teachers to give their students preperformance encouragement such as: "The concert next week is the one chance you have to show your parents and the public that all the time and effort put into the school music program is worth it. Take it seriously and finish strong with your practice and rehearsal. Don't let your peers down and don't let yourself down." Surely such encouragement is well intentioned. However, the benefit produced through increased practice and improved rehearsal can easily be negated by anxiety if young musicians' added preparation is carried out because of the *threat* represented by the looming performance. An alternative approach is to focus students' attention on learning outcomes that are more intrinsic to music. Students are better served in the long run if they understand their practice and rehearsal to be the means by which they acquire improved musical skills, and that by possessing better skills, they are more empowered to be expressive and use their music making to enrich the emotional lives of those for whom they perform. This way, young musicians can come to view the specialness of performance to be in the opportunity to share music with others, rather than as a high-stakes showcase event.

Chapter 8 Discussion Questions

1. Of the three broad sources of performance anxiety—the person, the situation, and the task—is there one that gets wrongly overlooked, in your experience? Is there one that gets too much attention?

2. Certain approaches that have been linked to performance anxiety— perfectionism, obsessive passion, and overpracticing—are actually encouraged by some musicians and music teachers. Have you experienced this in your musical life? What misconceptions may lead them to believe that these factors are somehow beneficial?

3. In your musical life, what situational factors most distinguish performance from practice? Are there simple ways that you could adapt your regular practicing to make it more performance-like?

PART III

MUSICAL ROLES

9

The Performer

This chapter opens the book's Part III on musical roles, extending beyond Part II, which focused on musical skills, including playing by ear, sight-reading, and memorizing musical works (Chapter 5); interpretation and expressive performance (Chapter 6); improvising (Chapter 7); and managing performance anxiety (Chapter 8). For most musicians, developing these music-making skills is their first priority. A certain level of skill mastery is required to be a performing musician.

These musical skills by themselves, however, are not enough to ensure success as a performer. Musicians who give live performances are also expected to skillfully use body gesture, facial expression, and other elements of stage presence to support their musical sound production. The visual aspects of live performance are influential to how audiences perceive the music, and therefore critical to performance. Further, outside of unaccompanied solo performing, musicians must know how to function effectively with coperformers, in terms of both musically coordinating performance (e.g., synchronizing multiple parts and performing in tune with each other) and communicating—both verbally and nonverbally—with each other.

Such factors have been called *extramusical skills* because, strictly speaking, they are not part of performers' musical sound production. Because they are so important to performance, however, a case can be made for considering them "*para-musical* (i.e., from the prefix *para*, meaning 'side by side' or 'closely related to')" (Woody, 2019, p. 83). Many formally trained musicians receive much instruction and devote much practice time focused on the music-making skills, such as technique, sight-reading, and interpretation; depending on the kind of performing they wish to do, others may also include playing by ear, improvising, or memorization among their target skills. Not nearly as many musicians give explicit attention to mastering the visual aspects of live performance and the interpersonal skills of musical collaboration. In fact, some highly trained musicians can find their early years as full-time performers to be a "crash course" in all the extramusical—or para-musical—skills required for a successful and rewarding performance career.

Psychology for Musicians. Robert H. Woody, Oxford University Press. © Oxford University Press 2022.
DOI: 10.1093/oso/9780197546598.003.0009

This chapter considers research that has examined aspects of being a performer that are sometimes overlooked. The results of these studies suggest the following:

1. What an audience *sees* in a live performance can heavily influence what it *hears*. A performer's physical appearance and stage behavior can affect listeners' judgments of the musical quality produced.
2. Musicians' bodily movements while performing have important communicative purposes. The most noticeable gestures often occur at key expressive moments in the music and can be more effective than sound for informing an audience about a performer's emotional intent.
3. Like any other group of people working together, musical ensembles are subject to powerful interpersonal dynamics and social processes. The success of a group can ultimately hinge on how the musicians handle among themselves leadership, individuality, and collaborative problem-solving.
4. Ensemble performance also requires specialized musical skills. The coordination of multiple parts into a unified musical whole is accomplished as musicians engage in some rather sophisticated perceptual and attentional processes.
5. For a music career to be most rewarding, performers must learn to deal with the unique challenges within it. Prioritizing their physical health and psychological well-being can help performers avoid potential hazards of the profession, including depression, substance abuse, and performance-related injuries.

Onstage: The Performer-Audience Relationship

There are many popular music entertainers who have been described as "not the strongest musician, but a great performer onstage." Also, outdoor musical events (e.g., at a street market, fair, or carnival) are often very well received because, regardless of whether the musicians are performing a style of music everybody likes, the live performance is so engaging that passersby and anyone in earshot feels compelled to take it in. All performing musicians should heed the object lesson provided by such scenarios and consider devoting some conscious attention to the visual aspects of the live performances they give.

First Impressions

In many social settings, people make judgments about other people based on how they look. This is true when audience members attend a live musical performance. They can start forming opinions and expectations quickly, even before any music is sounded. Performers' stage entrance can be very influential. Research conducted in a classical music performance context has indicated that audiences appreciate a strong stage entrance, characterized by a confident stride, repeated eye contact with the audience, a deep bow, and nods of appreciation for applause; on the other hand, a weak entrance—a narrow gate, limited eye contact, hands in pockets, and an abbreviated bow— tends to lower audience members' judgments of performance quality (Platz & Kopiez, 2013; Waddell & Williamon, 2017).

Listeners' opinions about the musical quality of a performance are also influenced by performers' physical appearance. In general, people tend to rate musical (sound) quality higher for performers who are judged to be physically attractive, as compared to those not judged as such (Iuşcǎ, 2020; Wapnick et al., 2009). It deserves mention, however, that physical attractiveness bias appears to be subject to other factors, including gender and musical genre. In Ryan and Costa-Giomi's (2004) study of young piano performers, the bias was found to favor pianists judged to be more attractive, but only among the female performers. Another study (Griffiths, 2010) provided evidence that audience members' judgments of female performers' musical quality are informed by opinions of what is appropriate performance attire; depending on whether the musician was performing classical, jazz, or folk music, opinions changed about whether jeans, a short nightclubbing dress, or a longer concert gown was appropriate for performance. More to the point, people's judgments of appropriate dress correlated with higher ratings of musicality and technical performance ability. The researcher applied her findings with the conclusion that perceptions of musical ability are influenced by physical appearance. She specifically stated that female classical performers "wishing to project a body-focused image should note that this may have a detrimental effect on perceptions of their musical ability" (Griffiths, 2010, p. 175).

Performers should also heed the psychological evidence that audience members can be predisposed to like (or dislike) a performance *even before* musicians take the stage. The *prestige effect* describes a phenomenon by which people are biased to think favorably of performers believed to be successful, famous, well respected, or otherwise of high status. The use of program notes may contribute to the prestige effect, as they typically list the greatest accomplishments of composers, which predisposes audience members to have favorable regard for works that may be unfamiliar to them (Waxman, 2012). In a recent study (Fischinger et al., 2020), listeners were found to enjoy a piece of music more and rate its characteristics more favorably when they believed it was written by Mozart rather than a lesser-known composer of the same era (who actually did compose it). Hargreaves and North (2010) categorized the prestige effect as a type of conformity, concluding that such social influences can have a powerful influence on people's aesthetic judgments of music. A more modern and real-world example of the prestige effect was found in research in which listeners considering musical recordings from the internet were found to be more likely to download a song if they knew it had been a popular download already (Salganik et al., 2006). In sum, performers may want to consider their "preparation" for a performance more broadly: it would appear that musicians' reputation, image, and professional credentials can have a significant effect on how their music is perceived by those for whom they perform.

Overall, the research indicates that performers can "win over" audience members, at least in part, based on their physical appearance and on their ability to signal confidence and connection with the audience. Audiences give higher appraisals of performance quality for musicians who are also judged favorably in attractiveness, dress, and stage behavior. The research does, however, acknowledge a diverse range of performance attire and stage mannerisms. In other words, the personal characteristic considered physically attractive and the stage behavior considered appropriate can vary across musical genres and cultural contexts. Performance etiquette is determined in large part by sociocultural norms. Within Western classical music, the expectation is formal attire, such as a dark coat and tie for men and an evening dress for women (black if they are playing in an orchestra). When walking onstage, featured performers are expected to greet the audience through facial expression and by bowing to applause. The strict compliance to such conventions suggests a psychological separation between performers and audience that is usually expected and valued. Even so, audiences seem to appreciate it when onstage musicians bridge the separation and speak comfortably and warmly to them during a concert, perhaps introducing pieces, providing interesting background information, or sharing anecdotes. Audiences sometimes take great delight when performers violate formal expectations, especially if done in a light-hearted way, as shown in Figure 9.1.

In recent years, some musicians within the Western classical tradition have shown greater openness to performance contexts other than its typical presentational style of concerts and recitals. Given the popularity of live performance in more vernacular music cultures, music scholars have considered

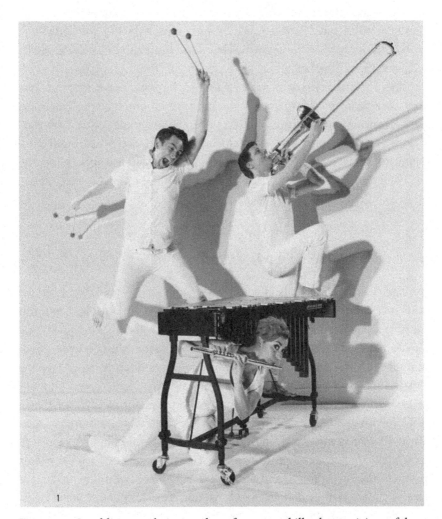

Figure 9.1 In addition to their superb performance skills, the musicians of the Fourth Wall ensemble enjoy violating formal expectations by incorporating elements of dance and theatrical stage practices to delight their audiences.
Photo used with permission of the Fourth Wall and Andy Batt, photographer.

borrowing from *participatory performance* traditions, defined as "a special type of artistic practice in which there are no artist-audience distinctions, only participants and potential participants" (Turino, 2008, p. 26). Classical musicians have taken chamber groups to coffee shops, bars, and clubs; those involved often report appreciating the greater interaction between audience members and performers and the overall "informal vibe" (Traasdahl, 2017, p. 1). Some performers make the most of informal settings to incorporate musical forms of audience participation. For example, a classical musician interviewed in one research study reported, "I've got a couple of compositions that take some cowbell beats and some shaker backbeat and [I] ask a couple audience members up to play them" (Robinson, 2013, p. 108). If considering human music making all around the world and throughout history, participatory performance is much more common than presentational performance models. Music educators have looked to participatory performance as a means of enhancing socioemotional outcomes (e.g., build community, nurture a sense of belonging) and building in learners an identity of "being musical" (Giebelhausen & Kruse, 2018; MacGregor, 2020; Reese, 2019; Shouldice, 2020; Woody et al., 2019).

Bodily Gesture and Movement

Research has also established that the bodily movements made by musicians while performing are an important part of the expressiveness and communicative aspects of performance as experienced by audiences. This finding should not come as a surprise, given the close relationship between music and movement. Consider how people use movement terms to describe the expressiveness of musical sound, such as calling staccato tones "bouncy" or saying that a repeated rhythm propels the music forward. People likely learn to connect music and motion from the earliest stages in life, as seen when a father bounces a young child on his knee while singing play songs or when a mother gently rocks an infant to the sounds of a lullaby. This basic connection of music and movement is further seen in the prominent role physical gestures play in expressive music performance (Davidson & Broughton, 2016). Romantic-era composer-pianist Franz Liszt was known for supplementing the musical communication of his piano performances with effusive bodily gestures (see Figure 9.2).

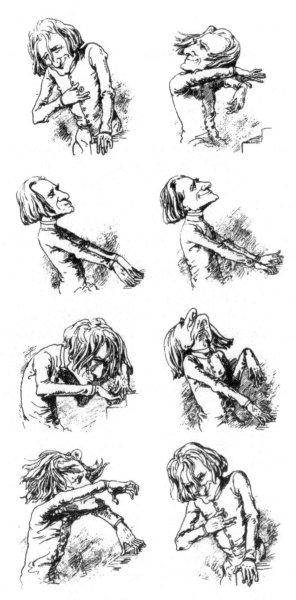

Figure 9.2 Caricatures of Liszt at the piano, attributed to A. Göschl, from magazine *Borsszem Jankó* (April 6, 1873).

Images courtesy of Electronic Periodical Archives & Database, National Széchényi Library, Hungary, http://epa.oszk.hu/01300/01338/00275/pdf/00275.pdf

There appear to be several functions and meanings of the body movements used by skilled performers. First is the production of musical sound itself. Obviously, the demands of the instrument (e.g., the slide mechanism of a trombone) and the music being performed (e.g., 16th-note scalar runs at a fast tempo) define the context within which a musician's body will move. In other words, performers' movements will reflect what they believe is the best way of achieving the desired sound in terms of rhythmic accuracy, timbre, and intonation. But beyond that, successful performers tend to use bodily movement to enhance their communication of expressive information. One general principle is: at the points during performance when musicians intend to be maximally expressive with their sound, they tend to also exhibit the most visually perceptible bodily movement (Dahl & Friberg, 2007; Davidson, 2005). In fact, the visual cues provided in a live performance can alter how the music would otherwise be perceived from the musical sound only (Bugaj et al., 2019; Krahé et al., 2015; Thompson et al., 2008; Vines et al., 2011; Vuoskoski et al., 2014).

Because a musician's expressive intentions are shaped by the musical structure of a piece (see Chapter 6), it follows that physical gestures during performance are often linked to structural features. Massie-Laberge et al. (2019) used motion capture video technology to analyze the expressive body movements of advanced pianists while performing Romantic-era excerpts under different conditions, including deadpan, normal, and exaggerated expression performance conditions; the researchers also interviewed the pianists about the consciousness with which they perform expressively. Their research found that skilled pianists employ a variety of strategies using body movement—especially movement of the head—to convey expressive intentions and structural parameters of a composition. Pianists tended to incorporate greater quantity of motion of the head when performing in the exaggerated expression condition. One plausible interpretation of this finding is that musicians strategically use visual aspects of their performance to "signal" to the audience when their sound is meant to be especially musically communicative.

Other types of performer movements are not as easily accounted for. The bodily rocking common among pianists has been of particular interest to some researchers (Davidson, 2007; Davidson & Correia, 2002). Although it surely can communicate expressive intentions to an audience, it has likely other functions as well. A pianist may carry out this movement for the comforting sensation it provides. This may put the musician at ease during the performance situation or engender what is believed to be the right mood for playing the music properly.

An alternative explanation of performer rocking is simply that it is a learned behavior. That is, musicians, sometime during their development, have observed it in more experienced performers and taken it on for themselves, believing it is simply what a performer should do. Much movement on the part of musicians surely falls under the category of learned behavior. This type of physical gesture is perhaps most common within popular styles of music known for their strong sociocultural links. The musicians of a rock band are expected to use bodily gesture to "assist in communicating the artistic message in and of the music (such as the lyrical narrative or rhythmical nuances)" (Pipe, 2019, p. 321). Analysis of popular musicians' performing has shown that many of the bodily movements of performance are learned behaviors that have expressive meaning or are triggered by emotions experienced (Davidson, 2001, 2005, 2009). The specific gestures used are largely culturally defined. For example, music with a sexual message is often performed with suggestive pelvic movements. Performers of rap and hip-hop music often use punching and jabbing arm motions reminiscent of boxing, thought to be related to the origins of the musical style (Ramsey, 2000). One entertainment writer, drawing on neuroscience research that theorized manual gesture as a deeply rooted companion to speech, suggested that "hip-hop hands" are much more communicative than decorative, offering as examples the back-up-off-me hand gesture, the one-finger chop, and not-having-it hand waves (Mudede, 2013).

Although the Western classical concert tradition usually prescribes a quiet and still audience, in other popular genres, musicians prefer to perform before a more active audience. Thus, some gestures from performers act as signals designed to elicit physical responses from those in attendance, perhaps clapping along to the music, dancing, and other kinds of movement. Finally, performers in all styles of music are known to use physical gestures to communicate with coperformers (see the section on ensemble performing later in the chapter).

Other Presentational Factors

When preparing for a concert or recital, many musicians do not spend much time practicing expressive body movements or considering how their physical appearance will affect the audience's perception of their music. After all, such extramusical factors may seem unimportant compared to practicing. This notion too can affect presentational aspects that affect an audience's experience; the degree to which performers are prepared and feel confident when the curtain rises is usually visibly perceptible by spectators. When musicians feel technical and expressive mastery over the music they are performing, they can approach the optimal state of flow and be fully engaged in a rewarding musical experience (see Chapter 8). There is no doubt audiences prefer musicians who are "into it" while performing.

Facial expressions are effective indicators of emotion, some being universally identifiable across cultures. Whether smiling to signal delight or furrowing one's brow to show consternation, a performer's use of facial expression (along with body movement) can enhance the communication of emotional intent (O'Neill & Sloboda, 2017; Thompson et al., 2008). Research has shown that singers' facial expressions can elicit similar expressions in observers (Chan et al., 2013) and can even affect how they hear the sound properties of music (Thompson et al., 2010).

One type of facial expression, closing the eyes while performing, is not available to musicians who are playing music from notation. Although it is extremely rare for vernacular musicians to use notation during performance, it is quite standard for classical chamber and symphonic musicians to perform from "sheet music" notation on music stands in front of them. Performing without notation necessitates special preparation through memorization. Research of memorized classical performance has suggested that performing without notation can afford a number of benefits to musicians (Kopiez et al., 2017; Williamon, 1999). First of all, preparing for a memorized performance typically requires greater practice and greater overall familiarity with the repertoire; additional preparation may improve the overall execution of the music performance. More likely, however, the positive impression made on audiences is due to "factors other than the objective performance quality" (Kopiez et al., 2017, p. 2). The main benefits may come from the absence of a music stand that can obstruct audience members' view of a performer. An unobstructed view may permit a more "direct psychological connection" between performer and audience (Williamon, 1999, p. 92). The impression, then, is that the music is coming from the performer, as opposed to coming from the printed page. Finally, it is possible that some audience members—especially those with greater musical training themselves—may simply be impressed by the fact that a performer expended the effort to memorize the music. Before even hearing a note, the listeners may be favorably predisposed toward the performance based on an admiration for the musician's diligence and authority shown through memorization.

The research is overwhelmingly clear that visual aspects of performance significantly impact audience members' listening experience. Behne and Wöllner (2011) concluded that "most listeners are prone to deceptions so that they believe that they hear what in fact they are seeing." In a research experiment that used as stimuli performances of finalists in prestigious international classical music competitions, people were asked to identify the eventual winners (Tsay, 2013). Although a vast majority (83%) stated that sound mattered most to them in evaluating music performance (left panel of Figure 9.3), they were significantly better able to identify competition winners from video-only recordings (53%) of the performances than with audio-only recordings (25%) of the performances (right panel of Figure 9.3).

Although there is consensus in the research about the impact of visual aspects of performance, there is far less agreement among musicians about whether they should embrace the effect. Some musical traditionalists may decry the idea that music is anything but a purely aural experience and worry it has "produced an aesthetic economy that threatens to privilege visual over aural aspects of music," which may lead to a "stifling" of serious musical forms and a proliferation of more popular "visual styles" of music (Thompson et al., 2005, p. 221). From a psychological standpoint, however,

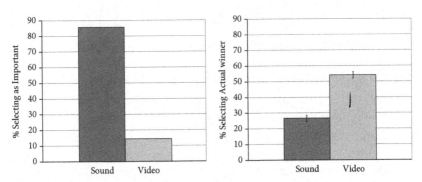

Figure 9.3 Comparison of reported importance of sound versus visuals (left) with actual ability to identify competition winners in sound-only or video-only conditions (right).

From Tsay, C. (2013). Sight over sound in the judgment of music performance. *Proceedings of the National Academy of Sciences of the United States of America, 110*(36), 14580–14585. https://doi.org/10.1073/pnas.1221454110

rather than faulting potential audience members for the way they naturally perceive music, it seems wise for performers of all styles to acknowledge the reality that vision is an important mode of musical communication and prepare for their performances accordingly.

Sharing the Stage: The Skills of Ensemble Performers

Whereas solo performing can offer a special satisfaction to some musicians, virtually all enjoy the rewards of group music making. In some cases, the group effort begins at the compositional level, as several musicians collaborate in creating music to be performed or recorded later. In other settings, a group of musicians who have never before worked with one another may be assembled together for the first time onstage to present a coordinated ensemble performance with no prior rehearsal. Group music making presents specialized challenges to musicians and involves a variety of social factors.

Social Processes of Collaborative Rehearsing and Creating

For many musicians, public performance of an ensemble is always preceded by rehearsal. In these rehearsals, musicians coordinate their multiple parts into a single musical product and create some interesting social dynamics. Music ensembles bear out some of the findings of general research into group processes (often conducted in workplaces, schools, and social organizations). For example, the productivity or quality of work produced by a group can be related to individual members' feelings of affiliation and cohesion. Also, leadership and status are important issues that affect a group's activities.

Some musical ensembles, such as professional orchestras and school bands, have a conductor or teacher as the designated leader. Although many other musical groups have no official authority structure, even chamber groups or rock bands may have leadership structures that are best described as informal, shared, or rotating (Ford & Davidson, 2003; Gilboa & Tal-Shmotkin, 2010). Regardless, successful collaboration depends not only on the musical but also on the social coordination between members. "Ensemble performance is about teamwork," one researcher wrote. "Half the battle of making music together (and ultimately staying together as an ensemble) is fought on social grounds" (Goodman, 2002, p. 163). In rehearsals, interpersonal dynamics between players take shape through social exchanges around the music. As a newly formed group rehearses and discusses their music making, leadership tends to emerge. In a study of musicians' roles in instrumental quartets, King (2006) reported that there was general agreement among group members about who served as leader and other team roles. The researcher identified eight common roles that were observable in quartet rehearsals: leader, deputy-leader, contributor, inquirer, fidget, distractor, joker, and "quiet one." The quartet musicians filled two, and occasionally three, roles in rehearsals, and though some musicians shifted roles from rehearsal to rehearsal, others fulfilled the same role consistently across sessions. Group leadership was found to remain fairly consistent across rehearsals, but leaders' moods changed and affected the musical progress made in rehearsals. Exactly who emerges as a leader can sometimes be linked to the personnel makeup of the group and performance demands of the music. These can be affected by the instrumentation of the group and certain associations or even stereotypes connected to the instruments. Related to this, Glowinski et al. (2012) identified three common leadership dynamics:

1. *Social statute*—for example, the first violin of a string quartet has a tradition of leadership in Western classical music. Also, a piano accompanist is often presumed to be subservient to soloist.
2. *Musical structure*—the musician who is playing the main part of a piece (i.e., the most prominently heard or thematically important) often emerges as a leader.
3. *Performance techniques*—musicians with special expertise important for the music being rehearsed (e.g., expertise keeping time with a piece that is particularly rhythmic or challenging tempo-wise) may assume a leadership role for rehearsal.

Yet other research has suggested that leadership in chamber music groups is subject to a variety of social factors, including interpersonal dynamics, communication styles, and gender stereotypes (Berg, 2000; Blank & Davidson, 2007; Davidson & Good, 2002; Keller, 2014, Lim, 2014).

Regarding improvement of individual musicianship, a group that shares leadership responsibilities and values each member may be most advantageous to musicians. Based on her research of peer-managed high school chamber music ensembles, Berg (2000) concluded that those members within a group who contribute to the decision-making (e.g., on matters of interpretation) are more likely to grow musically from the ensemble experience. This conclusion is corroborated by the empirically well-supported self-determination theory of motivation (see Chapter 3), which presents learner autonomy as a key psychological need that can determine whether people choose to continue or cease musical involvement (Evans, 2015; Evans et al., 2012).

An especially critical time in rehearsal, during which musicians' roles are perhaps clearest, is when performance problems are encountered. Depending on the music being rehearsed, the ensemble may have difficulty coordinating tempo, articulation, dynamic balance (loudness), and harmonic intonation, to name but a few aspects. Success in solving such performance problems depends largely on how well a group identifies and deals with individual performer idiosyncrasies (Davidson & Good, 2002; Ragert et al., 2013). Thus, with musicians' egos potentially on the line, the group cohesion felt by members is an important factor. Based on their research, Ford and Davidson (2003) advanced the idea that a group can better achieve its goals when all members feel free to address issues in rehearsals.

Other research suggests that ensembles progress musically while simultaneously addressing and working through social challenges (Parker, 2018). This may be more likely to occur in ensembles whose members have gained familiarity and trust by working together for some time (Gritten, 2017; Waddington, 2017). Seddon (2005) showed that a particularly well-functioning group, through openness to each other's musical ideas—what social psychologists call decentering—can become empathetically attuned, which facilitates creative risk taking and optimal flow experiences during music performance. Feeling a "sense of belonging" and an emotional connection with others can be important components of the "musician's identity" (Woody & McPherson, 2010, p. 404); groups in which members do not feel a strong sense of cohesion are less likely to be successful and risk having some members discontinue their involvement (Ford & Davidson, 2003; King, 2013).

Because the functioning of the group is so dependent on sociocultural factors, it follows that group music-making enterprises are affected by traditions related to musical genres. Allsup (2003) studied high school band students who formed two small groups (four or five members each) and met regularly to make original music together. One group decided to put aside their primary concert band instruments and instead work with a rock band instrumentation of electric guitar, bass, keyboard synthesizer, and drums.

The other group, rejecting rock music as too easy and formulaic, chose to create music for their "classical" concert band instruments. The creative sessions of the rock band were characterized by peer learning, collective generation of ideas, and productive peer critiquing. One participant described the process this way: "One person would come up with an idea, and we'd just kinda like work off the idea. . . . If someone didn't like it, they'd say so right away. It works pretty well" (Allsup, 2003, p. 30). The classical group, however, struggled with what they believed the compositional process should be and often separated from each other to work individually, usually notating their ideas on paper. The researcher concluded that once ideas were on paper, students were resistant to changing them to accommodate the contributions of others. The frustration of the students in this group ultimately led them to abandon the classical style in favor of jazz, at which point they began to experience greater collaboration.

More recent research has explored the processes of peer-led collegiate a cappella ensembles (Berglin, 2015; Paparo, 2013). Several qualities have emerged as important contributors to the positive experiences offered by such groups. First, without a designated teacher or ensemble director, group members demonstrate shared responsibility for decision-making. Berglin (2015) described this as musicians "stepping up" in the group's context of "equality of opportunity" (p. 60). Also, a cappella ensembles, in general, show a shared sense of values and group identity, which was knowingly transmitted from older members (and alumni) to newer members. Finally, the genre of popular music is an important element of a cappella ensembles. Paparo (2013), quoting a musician participant in his study, described popular music as what group members "are drawn to" and "the music that drives" them (p. 33).

Processes During Group Performance

As discussed, given that social factors are influential in group music making, interpersonal skills can be important in ensemble functioning. There is also a set of musical skills unique to group performance. After all, the many musicians of a large band or orchestra may sound great playing their independent parts while in individual practice, but they can still fail to "put it all together" to form a whole ensemble work. The skills required to do this center around musicians' abilities to coordinate the aspects of their own performing (e.g., pitch, rhythm, articulation, loudness) with those of other performers. Multiple psychological processes are involved as performing musicians monitor, evaluate, and anticipate their own parts while simultaneously doing the same with the music being produced by others.

Because music occurs across time, synchronization of performance is perhaps the most important effort undertaken by an ensemble. According to Keller (2008, 2014), coordinating the timing of performed music involves three anticipatory perceptual-motor skills, which allow ensemble members to plan and produce their own musical sounds in coordination with the sounds produced by their coperformers (see also Keller & Appel, 2010). First is *anticipatory auditory imagery*. This skill includes goal imaging (explained in Chapter 4), which involves mentally representing the performance of one's own part but also includes predictive imaging of others' music making. The second skill of ensemble performance is *prioritized integrative attention*, with which musicians pay attention to both their own performance and that produced by others. This split attention is "prioritized" in that musicians decide moment to moment whether the higher priority is focusing on their own part or tracking the aggregate sound of the ensemble, and it is "integrative" because what they hear from each source informs how they perceive the other. The third skill of ensemble performance is *adaptive timing*, which Keller (2008) explained as the requirement for musicians to "constantly adjust the timing of their movements in order to maintain synchrony in the face of expressively motivated deviations in local tempo (rubato), large-scale tempo changes, and other—often unpredictable—events" (p. 212). King & Gritten (2017) described ensemble performance as utilizing "dialogical skills of prediction and reaction," (p.315) drawing upon the concept of dialogue that refers to interactive communication between musicians accomplished via aural, visual, and kinesthetic cues.

Similar processes occur as musicians work to fit other qualities of their individual performing with those of a group, such as bringing their own single pitch in tune with the chord created by the ensemble or balancing the loudness of their note with the production of the rest of the ensemble. It becomes clear that skilled ensemble playing is a sophisticated cognitive activity. As pointed out by Keller (2007), ensemble performance requires complex multitasking of musicians who are limited in how much attention they can devote to simultaneous tasks. The two general tasks involved are the primary task of paying attention to one's own part and the secondary task of monitoring the aggregate ensemble sound (i.e., all parts). Attending to one's own performance alone involves accessing relevant musical knowledge from memory and carrying out the component cognitive skills of music performance (see Chapters 4 and 5). Additionally, tracking the aggregate sound production of the ensemble requires similar processes (Keller, 2008). Problems in coordinated ensemble performance frequently arise when musicians are forced to devote virtually all their attention to their own parts (perhaps due to the difficulty of the music) and are unable to attend to the aggregate ensemble sound. Thus, it is helpful for musicians to come to rehearsal with their individual parts already well practiced. If they can rely on some degree of automaticity in their own musical production, then they can allocate more attention to processing other musicians' parts and the overall ensemble sound. Attentional strain is further exacerbated when musicians are unmotivated or suffering from anxiety. Such conditions diminish the total "resource supply" that musicians have to allocate to the multiple performance processes.

The attentional resource demands of ensemble performance are more manageable for an expert musician who possesses an extensive generalized musical knowledge base. Drawing upon such knowledge and experience can allow more immediate mastery of one's own part and a more efficient understanding of the aggregate ensemble sound. This explains how certain advanced musicians are able to effectively perform together as an ensemble with little or no rehearsal. Such collaborative enterprises are called "zero history groups" by social psychologists (Myers & Anderson, 2008). Zero history music groups are a part of music traditions that include "jam sessions," such as jazz, folk, and bluegrass. Such groups are able to deliver a high-quality performance because of a shared knowledge base and performance expectations among members. In explaining what he called collective musicking, Duby (2020) offered:

> At expert level, the cognitive requirements of musicking are very demanding, entailing not only the coordination of fine motor responses and a high degree of responsiveness to environmental signals, but also resilience and adaptability. Obviously, such motor responses are not deployed anew on each occasion but draw from a storehouse of memory acquired over time through practice, such that the execution of musical tasks becomes "second nature." . . . [It] requires integrating individual skills with those of others and interpreting responsively a wealth of musical and extra-musical cues, such as gestures ("Continue in the same vein," "Fade out," "Next soloist," and so on). (p. 6)

The in-performance communication of jazz musicians has received considerable research attention, likely because of how common zero history performance is. Jazz musicians are often hired for a "gig" and expected to appear onstage without rehearsal with other performers whom they do not know. To do so successfully, they rely on a mutually known song repertoire, structural conventions, and performance practices of jazz. In other words, musicians know that the group will play songs they all know and that the performance of each song will rely on "stock" material and a quickly determined "roadmap" of the sectional form, such as (1) piano playing the song's melody, or "head," as introduction (the "in-head"); (2) improvised solos by multiple group members; and (3) guitar playing the head as an ending (the "out-head") (Doffman, 2012, p. 214). Also underlying shared information are established social practices, such as that the soloist at any given time has license to determine certain qualities of performance for the group (e.g., overall loudness level, style and texture, rhythmic complexity) and that the other musicians are expected to follow. Performers usually communicate such musical decisions in real time using physical gesture or via musical cues, such as signaling the "winding down" of an improvised solo by lowering the loudness and rhythmic activity of their playing (Davidson, 2012; Doffman, 2012; Eerola et al., 2018).

Eye contact is critical in the communication of coperformers. It may be used to supplement musical communication cues. One musician might look at another as if to say, "I'm expressing a certain musical idea. Try to match it." Eye contact is common at points in the music that are important as far as coordination, such as entrances and exits of individual parts (Williamon & Davidson, 2002). Goebl and Palmer (2009) found that when auditory feedback is not available, musicians use more visual cues to coordinate ensemble performance.

Furthermore, the importance of eye contact is related to musicians' prevalent use of physical gesture to communicate with each other. Sometimes the way a musician is carrying out the movements needed just to play an instrument can serve as a visual cue to coperformers. The height of a pianist's hand lifts or the size of a violinist's bowing motions can indicate how the music should sound. Otherwise, musicians may add to their performance body movements to convey information to others. Davidson (2005) has organized physical gestures of performers into categories: adaptor, regulator, illustrator, emblem, and display. *Adaptors* are movements musicians make for themselves, such as the aforementioned self-stimulating rocking of pianists or performers' gestures that reveal their inner emotional state. *Regulators* are movements made to coordinate performance with coperformers; for instance, to coordinate a synchronized group attack at the beginning of a piece, one performer might use a head nod to signal the downbeat (wind players commonly use the bells of their instruments). *Illustrators* are self-explanatory gestures that can serve communicative purposes; for example, a musician might use a full-face smile to communicate approval to a coperformer's musical choice made during performance. *Emblems*, on the other hand, are gestural symbols whose meaning must be learned. Consider, for instance, a jazz combo like the one mentioned earlier. A musician who thinks a coperformer may be "winding down" the current solo prematurely might make a circling gesture with a finger—an emblem—as if to say, "Keep soloing." *Display* refers to performer gestures done to draw attention to oneself or show off to impress audience members (dancing is an oft-used form of display).

Instructors within formal music education do not always explicitly teach the principles of ensemble performance to their students. It is even less common in formal training to address the social skills that facilitate collaborations between musicians. Music students often learn these through the enculturation provided by participation in school performance classes, community youth ensembles, and informal music-making ventures with friends.

Offstage: The Psychological Demands of the Performer Life

Musicians often wear many "hats" in their professional lives, reflecting their diverse roles and responsibilities. Few musicians as young adults are able to work exclusively as performers. It is common for musicians to find themselves filling multiple roles, both within and outside of music (Coulson, 2010; Smilde, 2009). Especially early in a musician's career, when he or she is trying to "make it" as a performer or composer or songwriter, time spent rehearsing and writing music may not directly result in any income. To make a living, some musicians may seek employment in music merchandising (e.g., as a salesperson at a local music store) or may establish a private teaching studio. Other times, aspiring performers hold down nonmusical jobs while simultaneously trying to further their music careers. As musicians diversify, they may not fully appreciate that different lines of work—even within the broader field of music—require the development of specialized skills to be successful. Even when a person is able to work exclusively as a performing musician, there are still important extramusical skills involved in having a successful career. Oftentimes, performers must be their own agents, publicizing and promoting their music and handling legal issues of copyright law, licensing, and contract negotiations.

Throughout their lives musicians deal with expectations and psychological demands that are quite different from those in the rest of the population. Some musicians, as young children, are put on a track toward full-time involvement in musical experiences and receive special attention. Research suggests that, compared with people in other walks of life, musicians more closely identify with their chosen profession and find it more difficult to detach themselves from their work (Spahn et al., 2004). For many musicians, life never arrives at any real place of stability. For example, it is common for a classical musician, after decades of focusing on work as a performer, to try to transition later in life to working primarily as a teacher.

The Performer Profile

Given the demanding nature of a musician's life, one might wonder whether only a "special type of personality" can be successful as a performer (López-Íñiguez & Bennett, 2020, p. 6). Is a certain type of person drawn to the life of a musician? Or might the pursuit of a musical career shape the defining qualities of those in the profession? Although it is likely impossible to know to what extent personality traits are set predispositions as opposed to consequences of life experiences, psychological research has revealed a number of personality tendencies among populations of musicians.

Musicians as a whole tend to score higher in measures of openness and neuroticism, that is, emotional instability (Corrigall et al. 2013; Greenberg et al., 2015; Miranda, 2020; Swaminathan & Schellenberg, 2018; Vaag et al., 2018). Consequently, one might think that a person with a "more sensitive personality" might be predisposed to be especially musical (Miranda, 2020, p, 58). That is possible, but it must also be recognized that as young people develop into skilled musicians, they likely take on the traits that accommodate the demands of musical involvement. For example, higher levels of introversion, independence, and conscientiousness have been found among musicians who learned their skills through formal instruction rather than through informal means (Gjermunds et al., 2020; Güsewell & Ruch, 2015; Rose et al., 2019). The traits of introversion, independence, and conscientiousness would seem facilitative of the self-sufficiency and dedication required to carry out the deliberate practice that is commonly expected in formal music education settings.

Related to the finding that personality traits of formally trained performers may not be shared by other musicians, research also suggests that personality traits likely differ according to music genre. Rock performers do not show as much introversion as their classical counterparts, and they tend to be more enthusiastic and comfortable in loud environments (Gillespie & Myors, 2000). Also, given the emphasis placed on improvisation and originality in jazz, it is not surprising that jazz musicians scored higher in measures of creativity and openness to new experiences, as compared to classical counterparts (Benedek et al., 2014).

The fact that research has revealed personality variations among musicians suggests that there is no single "performer personality." Moreover, aspiring musicians should not feel unequipped if their personalities do not line up with the trait tendencies described here. There are, of course, many successful musicians whose personalities are notable exceptions to the general trends. Additionally, there is evidence that, with respect to how they approach their activities and function in the field, successful musicians continually adapt or evolve across a career in response to experiences (López-Íñiguez & Bennett, 2020; Scarborough, 2017).

Openness to new experiences can be a critical trait when young musicians begin working as performers because they will likely receive a good amount of "on-the-job training." Being a professional musician can involve a variety of freelance activities that require "facility with numerous skills that are only tangentially related to music, if at all" (Pike, 2015). This includes the skills of entrepreneurship. Although entrepreneurship has long been of interest to researchers in economics, only more recently has it received much study from a psychological perspective (da Silva Veiga et al., 2017; Georgievski & Stephan, 2016). An entrepreneurial orientation for musicians involves developing a mindset of adaptability and flexibility (musically and otherwise) and acquiring interpersonal skills that allow for professional communication and effective promotion with potential audiences (Beeching, 2016; Dobson, 2011; MacNamara et al., 2006; Pike, 2015). In recent years, music conservatories and other institutions that train advanced musicians have begun providing entrepreneurship education to students targeting careers as performers (Bennett, 2016; de Reizabal & Gómez, 2020; Smith, 2014).

Prioritizing Health and Wellness

Expanded professional preparation has also begun to address musician health and wellness, perhaps in response to research that has shown that musicians can experience high levels of occupational stress and struggle to cope with the emotional and mental health issues they may face. Working musicians often deal with financial strain and, as a result, time pressures and difficulty balancing the demands of work and other personal commitments. In rehearsals and performances, musicians can experience interpersonal conflict with colleagues, which may arise from intense and criticism-filled working conditions. Additionally, as detailed in the previous chapter, performance anxiety afflicts many musicians, meaning that some may not experience music making as an enjoyable retreat from the stressors of life.

Although the general public may view music as an intrinsically rewarding profession, research has shown that this is not always the case. Amateur performers report enjoying many benefits of musical activity, including intellectual engagement, physical fitness, and social relationships (e.g., Hallam & MacDonald, 2016; Perkins & Williamon, 2014). Among professional-level musicians, however, "music activity has typically been considered a threat to holistic wellbeing" (Ascenso et al., 2017, p. 66). The physical demands and psychological pressures of a music performance career can be high (Parry, 2004; Vervainioti & Alexopoulos, 2015). Failure to adapt to these can have serious ramifications for musicians, including depression and other emotional disorders. Depression may be a special risk for individuals who are highly perfectionistic and self-critical, two qualities that, ironically, some musicians consider keys to success in the field (Diaz, 2018; Kapsetaki & Easmon, 2019; Kenny et al., 2004; Williamon et al., 2009; Wristen, 2013). Drug and alcohol abuse is a well-documented coping mechanism for anxiety and depression, and it is a problem among some musicians (Forsyth et al., 2016; Miller & Quigley, 2012).

Stress is also a significant contributor to the physical injuries that musicians can encounter. Performers who carry out repetitive motions with their hands and arms in playing their instruments are at risk for musculoskeletal problems (Kaur & Singh, 2016; Narducci, 2020; Rosenbaum et al., 2012). Another occupational hazard is hearing loss, especially among musicians working in electronically amplified performance environments (Di Stadio et al., 2018; Greasley et al., 2020). Hearing loss, like performance-related injuries, can be difficult to deal with because it constitutes a direct threat to the livelihood of performing musicians. Many musicians fail to recognize their health care needs and may not avail themselves of medical or psychological services, perhaps fearing that a doctor's prescription would include limiting or prohibiting certain music activities (e.g., practicing) that they feel compelled to do (Roy & Zhang, 2019).

Performers need to increase awareness and understanding of potential threats to their health and well-being (Chesky et al., 2002; Ginsborg et al., 2009; Heyman et al., 2019; Matei et al., 2018). Many are better able to cope as they become more accepting of the challenges of the music profession and form more realistic expectations for themselves and their careers. As such, mindfulness training has been shown to offer potential benefits to performers' managing of anxiety and to their overall well-being (Czajkowski et al., 2020; Diaz et al., 2020; Farnsworth-Grodd & Cameron, 2013; Juncos & Markman, 2016; Steyn et al., 2016). Ascenso et al. (2017) sought to understand musician well-being through a lens of positive psychology, suggesting that rather than focus on "alleviating symptoms of ill-health and coping with problems," research should study what can be done to help people "flourish and live to their fullest potential" (pp. 65–66). This team of researchers found that the music profession can offer opportunities related to all components of the Seligman (2008, 2011) PERMA model of well-being:

1. Positive emotions
2. Engagement (in intrinsically rewarding activity)
3. Relationships
4. Meaning (for one's life and experience)
5. Accomplishment (of important goals)

The research also indicated that musicians reporting high well-being, in addition to working hard musically, tend to be "wider achievers" who explore multiple identities and meaningfulness both within and outside the musical domain (Ascenso et al., 2017, p. 77).

Performance expertise in a strictly musical sense—that is, skill at producing musical sounds with one's instrument or voice—is not enough to ensure success as a performer. Musicians are more likely to succeed if they possess a variety of extramusical skills, such as those described throughout this chapter. The idea that these competencies are required for a career in music may challenge some who struggle just to find the time to practice their music making, let alone figure out how to develop additional skills. Others, however, embrace the great versatility that is demanded of a performing musician and thrive.

Taking the Stage: Bridge the Divide

In Western society, many music performance settings make a clear distinction between performers and audience members: the performers are the "doers" and those in the audience take a decidedly passive role. The performance space itself may further reinforce the distinction with a physical separation between the stage and audience seating. Perhaps because this distinction is so common, audiences seem to greatly value opportunities to have special "access" to performers that affords insights into performers' perspective of music. Some performing musicians have won great approval by regularly incorporating "audience participation" into their concerts. Whether by leading a sing-along activity or teaching a rhythm to be clapped at certain points, including audience members in the music making can boost the level of engagement and enjoyment for all involved. Performers who are uncomfortable leading audience participation can still bridge the divide simply by giving a special glimpse of the performer perspective. It is quite common in classical music to provide audiences with program notes. Typically, this text in a program gives background information about pieces of music being performed and perhaps biographical information about historically significant composers. What may be of more interest to audience members is background information about the very performers who are onstage, including an explanation of why they have chosen the music they are presenting. Such insight can help audience members feel closer to the musicians onstage, both metaphorically and emotionally. This connection will likely enhance the expressive and communicative experience.

Leading Learning: Facilitate Chamber Music Experiences

In many educational settings in which music is taught, students are provided group instruction in a large ensemble context and receive one-on-one tutelage related to solo performance. While these experiences are no doubt valuable, they are likely not enough for students to build a musicianship that is flexible and self-sustaining. Music teachers should consider providing chamber music experiences for their students; and here the term *chamber music* is used broadly to describe any small ensemble, including groups like a jazz combo, a singing quartet, and a rock band. In such small groups, students can naturally develop interpersonal skill, artistic decision-making, and collaborative creativity, all within a practical music-making context. While a chamber music ensemble does not have a conductor, the student members' music teacher still plays a critical role. As a more experienced musician with adult-level organizational skills, a teacher can offer much to help small ensembles be successful in their learning and performance ventures. Music teachers can oversee the formation of groups (i.e., the selection of membership) to ensure that good group dynamics will be likely. They can also guide students in choosing music to rehearse and perform and in finding performance events and venues in which they can eventually perform. Finally, music teachers should make themselves readily available to serve as mentors or coaches for students when they inevitably face challenges related to emergent leadership and shared goal setting and decision-making.

Chapter 9 Discussion Questions

1. Critically examine how you (and musicians like you) typically prepare for a public performance. To what extent do you think about, plan, and deliberately practice the visual elements (body movement and facial expression) of your performance? Can you identify specific ways that preparations could improve in this respect?
2. Consider small groups you have been a part of as a musician (e.g., chamber music ensembles, sections within large ensembles, informal music-making gatherings). In these settings, do leaders tend to emerge

according to who is the best musician, who has leadership-oriented personality traits, or something else altogether?

3. Recall the need for musicians to actively attend to their health and wellness to stave off potentially damaging effects of stress and fatigue. What do you do to appreciate and enjoy the positive rewards that can come to performing musicians?

10

The Teacher

Most accomplished musicians can readily identify music teachers whose encouragement and instruction were instrumental in their skill development. Truth be told, the so-called self-taught musician is likely a misnomer, as virtually nobody becomes musically skilled without the contribution of those who came before. Although many music teachers work with students within the formal setting of a school or music studio, other people serve more unofficially in the role of teacher for aspiring musicians. For example, parents supervise their children's home practicing, musical peers provide challenges and motivation, and professional musicians act as role models. Parents, peers, and performers all may possess one or two qualities that foster music learning in those with whom they come in contact, but music teachers by trade must have many of these qualities to be effective.

An old saying contends that "Those who can, do; those who can't, teach." This quippy adage finds no support from psychological research. Just as musicians must acquire a diverse set of skills to be successful performers (as shown in the previous chapter), effective music teachers develop their own range of specialized skills. While there is surely some overlap between the skillset of a performer and that of a music teacher (e.g., advanced knowledge about the subject matter of music), the two skillsets are largely distinct from each other. Prospective teachers usually receive professional training in education and psychology as a basis for advancing the effectiveness of their instructional skills.

Over the course of their careers, most musicians find themselves occupying the role of teacher—successful or not—at some time or another. Even those who are never employed on a full-time basis as instructors still encounter many situations in which they are asked to explain musical concepts and techniques or demonstrate their musicianship for the benefit of others. Many factors influence how fruitful musicians' instructional efforts will be. The principles offered in this chapter are derived from research on the functions, instructional strategies, and attributes of effective music teachers:

Psychology for Musicians. Robert H. Woody, Oxford University Press. © Oxford University Press 2022.
DOI: 10.1093/oso/9780197546598.003.0010

1. Effective teachers do more than just select performance repertoire for students and critique them as they work on it. For students to retain their learning for future musical ventures, teachers must build their instruction around specific learning objectives and deliberately teach generalizable music concepts.

2. Because the teacher-student relationship can greatly affect the learning process, building a relationship marked by mutual respect and exchange of ideas can aid students in realizing the highest levels of music preparation and performance.

3. Developing musicians rely on teachers for quality musical models, instruction for music making, and feedback on student performance. Over the course of their studies, students ideally become less dependent on teachers and learn to carry out these teacher functions for themselves.

4. Music teachers who support learners' autonomy can empower their students to have musically rich lives, including beyond the confines of their educational experience.

5. People are not simply born great teachers. The drive, behavior patterns, and personal qualities that support effective teaching are acquired by individuals through the process of developing a music teacher identity.

Teacher Effectiveness

Instructional Planning

Among the primary responsibilities of a teacher are the tasks of determining *what* students should learn and *how* to accomplish the learning. In education, a *curriculum* indicates what content is to be taught and in what order. Components of a formal music curriculum can include rationales for studying music, broad educational goals, more detailed learning objectives (related to specific musical concepts), instructional materials, teaching strategies, learner activities, means of assessing achievement outcomes, and a prescribed sequence for implementing these components. Some curricular direction is provided to those who embrace established music teaching methodologies (e.g., Orff, Kodály, Suzuki) or use a series of graded published music materials. Whether or not they use a written, formal curriculum, all teachers make decisions as to what their students will study and how to implement this content. Taken together, the individual decisions they make define the long-term music learning experiences of their students.

In the classical music tradition, much teaching occurs within the context of students' learning repertoire assigned by a teacher. Accordingly, many teachers believe that the selection of music is one of the most important decisions they make. For students whose music education focuses exclusively on the rehearsal of music for performance, the sequence of repertoire in fact forms a curriculum. Some have challenged the effectiveness of this approach, especially when it involves a student working with only a few pieces of music at a time. Extended practicing for a polished performance develops a limited set of musical skills and strategies that differs from that required for performing less familiar music. To what extent do students take what is taught and learned with one particular piece and apply it to the context of a new piece assigned later? Research suggests that little transfer of learning will occur from piece to piece unless teachers deliberately teach generalizable music concepts drawn from the repertoire and involve students in decision-making while preparing performance (Bazan, 2011; Price & Byo, 2002; Tan, 2017). Many exemplary teachers consider the rehearsal and performance of music literature not an end but a means for students to develop comprehensive musicianship. This goal is understood to include a variety of supplemental music learning activities, because simply rehearsing " 'high quality' literature does not guarantee a higher level of musical understanding" (Sindberg, 2012, p. 95). Research suggests that building a broader, more versatile body of musical knowledge can benefit performance, allowing musicians to more efficiently learn the music they practice.

Effective instructional planning involves teachers in identifying learning objectives for their students and preparing strategies with which to deliver their instruction (Schiavio et al., 2020). Some teachers' preparations result in written lesson plans; for others, however, it is a mental process of planning that contributes to the effectiveness of their teaching (Bazan, 2010; Shaw, 2017). Without adequate planning, instruction may default to an approach in which teachers merely listen to students perform assigned repertoire "line after line, waiting for students to make an error before they react" (Brittin, 2005, p. 36; see also Duke & Simmons, 2006; Karlsson & Juslin, 2008). Planning instruction around student learning objectives appears to be a hallmark of expert teaching. Bauer and Berg (2001) found that novice music educators, in deciding what to teach, tend to rely heavily on their own experiences (rather than student needs) and give much weight to the limitations of their situation with respect to the facilities and equipment available. The result can be that their teaching is driven more by performance events than by curricular needs.

Without adequate planning, teachers may not give instructional time to the knowledge and skills that they consider most important for their students to learn. For example, many teachers spend the bulk of instructional time addressing only technical aspects of performance, despite believing that expressivity is a paramount aspect of performance (Karlsson & Juslin, 2008; Laukka, 2004; Williamon, 2014). A technique-heavy teaching approach may be most common in a master-apprentice model of instruction, which appears to be especially prominent in one-to-one conservatoire teaching (Carey, 2010; Hyry-Beihammer, 2011; Young et al., 2003).

Rapport and Learning Environment

The master-apprentice model is just one archetype of the teacher-student relationship. It is perhaps the most traditional in music learning cultures. In a master-apprentice relationship, the role of teachers is to tell of their experiences and demonstrate their craft, and students are expected to listen, emulate, and seek teacher approval (Burwell & Shipton, 2013; Carey, 2010). This relationship is marked by one-way communication from teacher to student, often resulting in the direct copying of the teacher's musical models.

In contrast, the mentor-friend model reflects greater exchange between teacher and student. Through two-way dialogue, teachers facilitate students' musical exploration and discovery and encourage more individualized development (Bjøntegaard, 2015; Gaunt et al., 2012; Haddon, 2011). Rather than dispensing knowledge, teachers guide students in augmenting their own musical experiences. The mentor-friend model allows for greater contribution on the part of students and, as a result, can engender stronger feelings of autonomy.

The master-apprentice and mentor-friend models are conceptual archetypes of the teacher-student relationship. Real-life relationships may not closely resemble either or may incorporate aspects of both. What both models have in common is the element of *respect*. The student in a master-apprentice relationship typically respects the teacher for his or her performance expertise and professional accomplishments. A mentor-friend relationship includes the key component of mutual respect (Creech

& Hallam, 2011); the student may offer respect primarily because of the teacher's demonstrated investment in the student (and for reciprocating the respect for the student's investment in the learning process). Regardless of the exact form of the teacher-student model and whether the teacher is tutoring a single student or working with a larger class, the teacher-student relationship is usually a critical factor in determining the effectiveness of students' learning. In fact, that relationship can affect a young person's decision to continue in music or to quit. One participant in a study by Evans et al. (2012) explained unceremoniously: "The conductor was pretty much a bastard and I just started to hate it, so I stopped." (p. 87).

The two-way communication of the mentor-friend model may be a very important contributor to musical skill development. Rostvall and West (2003) have pointed out that when teachers dominate the verbalizations of music lessons with instruction and critical evaluation of student performance, the result can be a communication imbalance that inhibits learning:

> The strong asymmetric distribution of power was shown to have negative consequences for the students' opportunities to learn. When teachers ignored students' perspectives, they lost many opportunities to obtain information about the students' performance of tasks. This lack of information rendered teachers incapable of analysing many situations where students had problems. As a consequence, teachers did not provide their students with the help and support they needed during many observed situations. Instead, students were left alone with regards to many aspects of their musical development, especially motor learning and expressive aspects of musical performance. (p. 220)

Teaching Methods

Verbal instruction usage varies among music teachers, for example, in content. Many teachers lead students through a progression when working on a piece of music, starting with technically oriented aspects of performance and proceeding to more expressive considerations. They also reveal different musical priorities in their verbal instruction to students. Less proficient teachers, who are known to spend more time talking during lessons, are inclined to address technique predominantly, whereas expert teachers focus more efficiently on tone quality, intonation, and expression (Cavitt, 2003; Silvey, 2014;

Young et al., 2003). Expert teachers also tend to talk less overall, which allows for more instructional time for student music making (Duke & Simmons, 2006; Juchniewicz et al., 2014; Warnet, 2020). Figure 10.1 shows a number of the most important behavioral traits that distinguish expert teachers from less accomplished ones, as reported by Juchniewicz et al. (2014).

The verbal music instruction that teachers give can also be divided into two categories, depending on whether it is made up of (1) imagery and metaphors or (2) direction pertaining to concrete musical sound properties. When using an imagery- or metaphor-based strategy, a teacher might encourage a student to perform a musical phrase to reflect a soaring eagle, a weighty anxious mood, or the feeling of losing a loved one. Research attests to music teachers' widespread use of metaphors and figurative language, especially those that reflect motion and moods (Arrais & Rodrigues, 2007; McPhee, 2011; Meissner, 2017; Wolfe, 2019; Zorzal, 2020). Teachers may offer extramusical images and metaphors most often when working on expressive performance, intending to intimate a desired sound or to incite emotion in students. This approach is used to bring about certain sound qualities in students' performing, often in conjunction with other modes of

Important Conductor/Teacher Behavioral Traits Recurrently Mentioned by Successful American Middle and High School Band Directors

Effective planning
High expectations
Clearly defined goals
Organization and time management
Diagnosis/rehearsal of musical problems
Score study
Gives feedback
Teacher modeling
Energy/passion
Conducting

Note. Size of font above roughly represents the frequency of mention in study by Juchniewicz et al. (2014) Tables 1 & 2.

Figure 10.1 Important conductor/teacher behavioral traits recurrently mentioned by successful American middle and high school band directors.
Based on findings of Juchniewicz, J., Kelly, S. N., & Acklin, A. I. (2014). Rehearsal characteristics of "superior" band directors. *Update: Applications of Research in Music Education, 2*(2), 35–43. doi:10.1177/8755123314521221

instruction. For example, McPhee (2011) provided the example of a brass teacher discussing with a young trumpeter how to convey a gentle breeze, describing it as a "calypso sort of thing" and "on an island boat . . . with a breeze, sailing," and conducting for the student to show the desired amount of rubato and advising him to not be afraid to slow down (p. 338). Teachers who teach exclusively via figurative language may run the risk of frustrating students if they use metaphors and imagery that students do not understand (e.g., due to cultural differences) or cannot apply to their specific musical context (Woody, 2006a, 2006b).

Perhaps for this reason, other music educators advocate verbal instruction that focuses on concrete musical sound properties. Teachers using this approach may describe the qualities of a model sound or point out weaknesses in a student's performance, directly addressing elements such as note duration, tempo, intonation, dynamics, and articulation, among others. Most teachers would see the value of this kind of instruction when dealing with technical aspects of performance (i.e., playing the correct pitches and rhythms), but they can also find this approach effective when working on expressivity. Research has shown, with considerable consistency, that instruction addressing the sound properties of performance can effect change in music students' performing (Arrais & Rodrigues, 2007; Juslin et al., 2004; Woody, 2006b). As explained in Chapter 6 (see section "Approaches to Learning and Performing Musical Expression"), music students tend to perform more expressively when they form explicit mental representations regarding the sound properties of their desired performance. When provided with an extramusical metaphor or imagery example by a teacher, many students may need to consciously "translate" it into such explicit performance; this translation process is not needed if the teacher's instruction explicitly describes the sound properties of the musical goal.

In addition to teaching performance technique (i.e., *how* to perform on one's musical instrument), teachers serve two other broad functions in developing their students' musical skills. First, they often provide a source of musical models for students, including aural models of what well-performed music sounds like. Second, teachers offer specific feedback on student performances. These functions of the teacher allow young musicians to build the cognitive skills needed for musical performance (see Figure 4.3 in Chapter 4).

Aural modeling is a commonly used approach among music performance teachers (Lisboa et al., 2005; Meissner & Timmers, 2020; Sheldon

& Brittin, 2012). An instructor will perform a musical excerpt and ask listening students to then imitate it as exactly as possible in their own singing or playing. This process represents a skill set that expert performers have been shown to do with considerable accuracy and consistency, although they may philosophically reject imitation in favor of originality (Lisboa et al., 2005; Woody, 2006b). With modeling, student performance learning can be made more effective by having students immediately imitate the model and by alternating between teacher model and student imitation, rather than a longer "block" of teacher modeling followed by extended time of student performance (Simones et al., 2017). Through the modeling of teachers, students come to discern the desirable sound qualities of performance on their instruments and learn which kinds of variations in sound (e.g., timing, dynamics, and intonation) make for effectual music expression. Teachers may also refer students to sound recordings, which can serve as effective aural models.

Providing feedback to students is another critical task of teachers. General psychology has shown that knowledge of results is necessary for improving a skill. Advanced musicians are able to self-critique their performances, but developing music students rely on teachers to supply evaluative feedback. The most constructive feedback is that which expresses the discrepancies between a student's rendition of a piece of music and an optimal version. Expert teachers give more detailed feedback (about specific properties of performance) than general appraisals (e.g., "Good job!"), and music educators generally recognize that more specific teacher feedback facilitates student performance improvement (Biddlecombe, 2012; Duke & Simmons, 2006). Researchers also have explored whether the feedback of effective teachers is more often positively or negatively expressed, that is, constituting praise or criticism. One might intuitively think that positive comments are more motivating to students and, as a result, are more associated with effective teaching. The research, however, paints a slightly different picture. Although positive feedback is likely more helpful with younger learners and in one-on-one instruction, more advanced music students seem to accept and benefit from greater levels of criticism in lessons (Blackwell, 2020; Cavitt, 2003; Duke & Simmons, 2006; Henninger, 2018).

This may be especially true at the secondary school level, at which most music teachers primarily serve as directors of performance ensembles, such as concert bands, orchestras, and choirs (this is especially true in the United States). The role of conductor is viewed as requiring a set of specialized skills in addition to the competencies (described earlier) expected of all music teachers. Varying uses of posture, gesture, and facial expression are all associated with judgments of ensemble performance quality, in part because of their role in eliciting expressivity from performers. Research has shown that music students of all ages readily identify high-intensity conductors, whose behaviors on the podium contain marked contrasts to those of low-intensity conductors (Bender & Hancock, 2010; Morrison & Selvey, 2014; Poggi et al., 2020; Price et al., 2016). Nonverbal behaviors are the means by which conductors try to communicate with their musicians while they are performing. There is the need both to instruct them how they should play or sing and to provide them feedback on how they are actually performing. However, with regard to the ability to effect specific changes in student musicians' performances, nonverbal conducting behaviors by themselves are no alternative to verbal instruction.

A conductor's head movements, facial expressions, and gaze are also used to communicate with performers in an ensemble. Poggi and Ansani (2018) analyzed these nonverbal communications of conductors and concluded that these conveyances are not obscure and understandable only by specially trained musicians but more of a recognizable language. These researchers' analysis produced a lexicon that connects specific conductor gaze expression signals with their meaning to performing musicians (see Table 10.1). As part of instructing an ensemble *how* to perform, conductors may, for example, raise their eyebrows during the performance of phrase to ask musicians to perform softly or display a frowning facial expression to evoke a louder dynamic level. Conductors can also provide feedback this way. For instance, by closing their eyes, they seem to communicate that the performance is proceeding enjoyably, or by staring at a musician with wide open eyes, they express disapproval for a mistake and warn that it must not happen again.

Of course, also included among conductors' effective rehearsal techniques are more general music teaching proficiencies, such as efficient verbal instruction, quality modeling, and "closing the loop" on instruction given with teacher feedback (Warnet, 2020). Conductors' instruction must allow for ample opportunity for student performance. Even the best-expressed instruction of a conductor is useless unless the ensemble musicians can apply it to their performing. As compared with less experienced ensemble directors, experts stop the playing or singing of their groups more often in rehearsals, but the stops are shorter in duration because they deliver their instruction so efficiently. Stopping and starting during a rehearsal usually center on the

Table 10.1 Lexicon of the Conductor's Gaze (Selected Portions)

Gaze Item	Literal Meaning	Indirect Meaning	Type
Gazes at X	Request for attention	Prepare to attack	Technical (attack)
Gazes around at all musicians	Broadcast request for attention		Interactional
Raised eyebrows with oblique gaze	Warning gaze	I warn you about a difficult passage	Interactional
Raised eyebrows with wide open eyes	Emphasis	I ask for higher attention	Interactional
Wide open eyes fixing X	Threatening gaze (to prevent similar behavior)	I reproach you for your mistake	Interactional
Raised eyebrows (plus nodding)	Appreciation plus approval	I praise you	Interactional
Raises eyebrows all along the musical fragment	Imitation of light movement	Play/sing soft	Technical (intensity)
Raises eyebrows (plus head in the shoulders)	Caution gaze	Be accurate and precise	Attitude
Internal parts of eyebrows raised	Sad gaze	Play/sing in a sad way	Emotional
Frown	Angry gaze	Feel/express anger ∧ play aloud	Technical (intensity)
Squints eyes	Imitation of effortful movement	Play/sing "*sforzato*"	Technical (intensity)
Closed eyes	Concentration	I want (you) to enjoy the pleasure of music	Emotional (motivational strategy: nonmusical)
Squeezed eyes (plus trunk retracting backward)	Disgusted gaze	Outcome emotion ∧ negative feedback	Interactional

From Poggi, I., & Ansani, A. (2018, June). The lexicon of the Conductor's gaze. In *Proceedings of the 5th International Conference on Movement and Computing* (pp. 1–8). New York, NY: Association for Computing Machinery. https://dl.acm.org/doi/pdf/10.1145/3212721.3212811

detection and correction of performance errors. A conductor's precision in detecting errors is affected by a number of rehearsal variables, such as the texture and tempo of the music, as well as the attention devoted to conducting versus listening (Bergee, 2005; Price & Byo, 2002; Waggoner, 2011). More generally, however, error detection appears to be a skill that is developed through training, practice, and long-term rehearsal experience. Obviously, a musician's aural skills are of critical importance. Because conductors can use the music notation of a score to generate an auditory goal image of an ensemble's performance, score study is an accepted rehearsal preparation strategy (Henninger, 2018; Manfredo, 2008; Silvey, 2011). The error detection abilities of experienced ensemble teachers are likely enhanced by a knowledge of student musicians' performance tendencies (weaknesses), which explains how the teachers target errors for correction even prior to rehearsals (Cavitt, 2003; Henninger, 2018). These experts also show persistence in their correction of identified errors, utilizing a variety of approaches in prescribing solutions (e.g., verbal instruction, teacher and student modeling) and multiple repetitions of target passages in the music.

Linking Teaching to Learning

Over the course of their training, successful music students ultimately learn to function as their own teachers. Until this advanced level of musical expertise is attained, teachers are critical in supporting their developing student musicians to build the mental representations for music performance, especially in practice. The cognitive skills of music (as presented in Chapter 4) allow young musicians to ultimately self-regulate their skill development. The building of these critical cognitive skills depends heavily on teachers:

- *Goal imaging*, the ability to mentally represent what a piece of music *should* sound like, is developed as students work with the aural models provided by teachers and technical media.
- *Motor production* representations enable musicians to execute the movements and physical responses needed to play an instrument and to know how those movements feel. Instruction directed to technical and bodily aspects of performance are crucial here.
- *Self-monitoring*, the ability to accurately hear one's own performance (i.e., receive feedback), is also primarily acquired from a music teacher.

Young musicians especially rely on teachers for this because so much of their attention is devoted to the production of the music, not to monitoring the resulting sound.

Equipped with these skills, musicians can compare the sound image (of their own performance) with the goal image, identify discrepancies therein, and then correct them by adapting the representations for motor production. Research suggests that expert teachers, especially one-on-one teachers, guide students in this diagnostic process during their lessons (Woody, 2003), and that such instructor guidance can allow even young musicians to "begin pairing actions with outcomes to teach students how to make those associations independently" (Parsons & Simmons, 2020, "Conclusions and Limitations" section, para. 6).

Supporting Learner Autonomy

Unfortunately, not everyone in education considers student learning to be the ultimate indicator of effective teaching. For example, in a keynote address at a conference on assessment in music education, Lehman (2007) recalled reading a newspaper story about how students had performed on a standardized achievement test:

> The story reported that the local kids had done badly on one section of the exam, and a school official was explaining why this had happened. The problem wasn't that the teachers didn't teach that material, he said; they taught it. The problem was that the students didn't learn it. (p. 19)

Lehman added that teaching without learning is comparable to an automobile salesman claiming to have sold the car, even though the customer did not buy it. In fact, it may be somewhat common for some music teachers to try to separate teacher delivery of instruction from student learning (MacLeod & Napoles, 2015; Napoles & MacLeod, 2013).

An especially important trait of effective music teachers is being *autonomy supportive* with their students. Autonomy-supportive teachers involve students in instructional decisions (e.g., choosing music materials to use in their studies) and are open and responsive to students' opinions and questions (Bonneville-Roussy et al., 2020). A teaching approach that supports learners' autonomy sharply contrasts with one of psycho-logical control, in which teachers are "centered on their own agenda rather than being focused on their students' needs" (Bonneville-Roussy et al., 2013, p. 23). There is some indication from research that teacher-controlling approaches may be common in classical studio music teaching (Evans, 2015), but there are many reasons for music educators to move away from this type of teaching. Compared to students of psychologi-cally controlling teachers, learners with autonomy-supportive teachers are more likely to possess a harmonious passion for music, exhibit per-sistence in their studies, and enjoy better overall well-being (Bonneville-Roussy & Vallerand, 2020; Bonneville-Roussy et al., 2020; Freer & Evans, 2018).

Recall from Chapter 3 that autonomy is one of the three psychological needs identified in self-determination theory (SDT), which has been used effectively to explain the motivation behind human behavior and learning. The psychological need for autonomy, as defined by SDT, is seen in the added effort given—and rewards enjoyed—by music students when they choose repertoire, select an individualized creative medium, or otherwise "take ownership" of a music learning project of theirs. This point suggests that one of the greatest contributions that music teachers can make is to nourish their students' own motivations for music, even if those motivations differ from the teachers' own.

Lasting Student Musicianship

Autonomy-supportive teachers provide *student-centered instruction,* which contributes to advanced students ultimately becoming able to serve as their own teachers. This is a matter of musical independence. *Teacher-centered in-struction* may feed the ego of some teachers. Although good teachers right-fully enjoy a sense of reward with their students' accomplishments, the orientation is different for a teacher-centered instructor. They feel important and needed when their students show a dependence on them. But student dependence on a teacher—beyond the early stages of learning a skill—should decrease in teaching and learning, not be reinforced.

A lack of musical independence seems to be a chief reason so many young people cease their musical involvement, both during school age and immedi-ately after (O'Neill, 2011; Pitts, 2007; Woody et al., 2019). A student-centered instructional approach reflects the point of view that music education should equip students with a musicianship they can use for the rest of their lives, outside of the specific context of school music rehearsals and lessons (Weidner, 2020). The research findings of Woody and Parker (2012) raised concerns about whether certain traditional approaches can produce a debilitating dependence in some music students:

> But one might question whether such a teacher-centered curriculum, so common in American secondary music education, detracts from the attainment of an independent musicianship that would foster continued musical involvement after high school. The worst-case scenario is that music students graduate believing that they are simply unable to make music without a leader to select music, organize rehearsals, and instruct them how to perform. (p. 201)

The research of Weidner (2020) found support for his theory that musical independence can be attained by students in a large ensemble instructional context. Figure 10.2 shows an illustration of this theory. Its three interrelated outcomes are student agency (similar to autonomy), decision-making skill, and a musicianship for life. These outcomes are facilitated when teachers deliberately use student-led instruction, scaffolded coaching (e.g., posing questions, giving students choice), and cognitive modeling (i.e., sharing cognitive strategies for independent music making). Such approaches are characteristic of student-centered instruction.

Drawing on past research in music instruction, Carey and Grant (2014) made a case that even one-to-one conservatoire studio teaching can become more effective and meaningful to students by incorporating an open, collaborative, and exploratory approach. Teachers who use such a "transformative pedagogy" focus more on facilitating student learning than critiquing student performance and show flexibility as they choose teaching approaches that are individualized to student needs. The overriding objectives are for students to attain "expansive excellence" and "take ownership of their own learning" (" 'Rethinking' One-to-One" section, para. 3).

The logical conclusion is that excellent music teaching ultimately produces self-sufficient musicians capable of continuing to grow beyond the confines of their educational experience. A *lifelong* perspective on music learning is concerned with equipping music students with the knowledge, skills, and

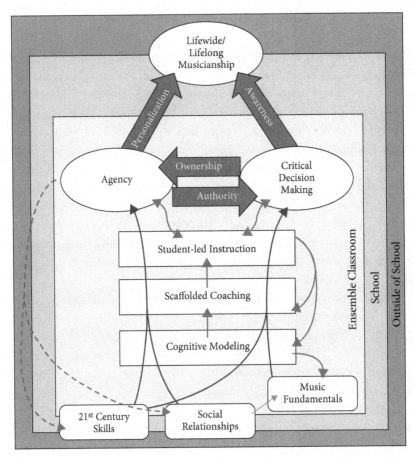

Figure 10.2 Weidner (2020) grounded theory of musical independence in the concert band.

From Weidner, B. N. (2020). A grounded theory of musical independence in the concert band. *Journal of Research in Music Education, 68*(1), 53–77. doi:10.1177/0022429419897616

confidence to be musical across their lifespan, including after their school years (Myers, 2008; Woody et al., 2019). Additionally, *lifewide* music learning allows people to be musical in a full range of life settings, including formal, informal, academic, personal, social, occupational, and recreational (Jones, 2009). Teachers who strive to provide their students with lifelong and lifewide musicianship value musical breadth and seek to individualize their instruction because each student "brings a very different blend of musical selves" to the learning experience (Jones, 2009, p. 205).

Building Music Teacher Identity

The ways a teacher implements effective instructional strategies depends partly on who he or she is as a person. In addition to musical expertise and teaching expertise, personal traits determine exactly how individuals fill the role of music teacher (McClellan, 2017). Much 20th-century research sought to identify personality characteristics that were associated with effective music teaching; an extensive list of attributes of successful teachers compiled by Pembrook and Craig (2002) included extroversion, conscientiousness, self-confidence, enthusiasm, flexibility, and proactive leadership. Also included in their list of successful teacher attributes were a number of traits categorized as "relating to others." An orientation toward others seems to be an important personal quality found in effective teachers and certainly relates to why so many teachers strive for student-centered, rather than teacher-centered, instruction.

More recent research has moved away from studying personality and focused more on the construct of *music teacher identity*, that is, how people come to be committed to teaching music as an important part of the essence of who they are. Young people typically first show interest in pursuing music teaching as a career upon entering adulthood and seeking music teacher education at a college or university (Austin et al. 2012; McClellan, 2014; Rickels et al., 2019). Music teacher identity, like other forms of occupational identity, develops through interaction with important people, especially former teachers who served as role models. In addition to highly valuing their subject matter of music, those who aspire to be teachers also tend to have had prior experience working with children; they experience reward in helping others learn and grow and may see teaching as a particularly honorable pursuit (Rickels et al., 2013).

Music education graduates continue to build and refine their teacher identities as they work in the profession. Chua and Welch (2020) offered important insight into how this can occur through transformative experiences in a music teacher role. Music educators often bring their whole being—including their personal self—into their teaching. For many, this includes an activist identity, in that they are committed to advocating for and empowering their students, and they believe in the power of music to contribute positively to their school and to the lives of their students. Indeed, the valuing of others appears to be an important component of music teacher identity; this includes being attentive to the responses of students to gauge one's effectiveness as an instructor, leader, and motivator, and belonging to a teacher community in which role models, mentors, and peers can share experiences.

Being an effective teacher clearly requires much more than expert-level musical knowledge and performance skill. This fact challenges the traditional idea (among some) that teaching makes a good "fallback job" for people who leave a performance career. In fact, exceptional performing musicians may be at a distinct disadvantage when it comes to reaching music students as a teacher. Although elite musicians surely learn a lot through the experience of their own advanced skill development, there is usually reason to doubt whether they can effectively guide the musical growth of other musicians who are different from them. With reference to the broad stages of skill acquisition explained in Chapter 4, among exceptional musicians, many of their performance skills have become highly automatized, such that they may not remember when those skills required more conscious attention or effortful learning strategies. They may not readily draw upon their own experiences in guiding others at the early stages of skill development. This is the same reason some psychologists working in the sports world have suggested that the best athletes are usually not good youth coaches (Bleilock, 2011; see also Flegal & Anderson, 2008).

Nobody is born a great musician, nor is anyone born a great music teacher. Musical people *become* proficient music teachers by choosing teaching as an enterprise and pursuing the knowledge and skills that teaching demands. College and university music teacher education programs provide young musicians with opportunities to develop important teacher dispositions and improve their instructional skills. Whether obtained through a teacher education program or gained through more informal means, it is likely only through extensive experience and deliberate effort that a musician can come to expertly carry out the role of the teacher.

Taking the Stage: Be a Performer and Performance Coach

Performers readily credit past music teachers for contributing meaningfully to their success. Many advanced performers speak of internalizing the tutelage they received, such that they become able to serve as their own performance coach from knowing how their past mentors would instruct them in the performance situations they encounter. When taking the stage, all musicians would do well to consider themselves both performers and performance coaches, as such a mindset can help them feel more empowered. Musicians who have never served as a performance coach should consider taking on this role for less experienced musicians. Whether or not they have any formal teacher credentials, musicians serving as performance coaches can do a lot of good—for others and themselves. Experts in many fields attest that they did truly understand their craft until they tried to teach it to someone else. For many, coaching another musician will likely come more naturally than coaching oneself. Performance coaches should draw from what is known about effective teaching and lead coaching sessions by communicating goals for the experience rather than simply listening for errors to be corrected. They should also seek to understand the cognition underlying performance by asking questions and listening to the musicians they coach. Such coaching experience can benefit musicians' own performing—especially if they struggle with stage fright—as they may become better able to see performances as experiences in which they can apply their learning, as opposed to circumstances that are happening to them.

Leading Learning: Use Questioning to Check Student Understanding

The research finding that expert teachers talk less than novices underscores this point: *teaching is not telling*. Effective teachers do not merely broadcast wisdom that students may or may not receive. Rather, the quality of teaching is defined by the learning that takes place. Accordingly, experienced music teachers make an effort to ensure that students are following their instruction and are applying it to their own musicianship. A good way to do this is to ask students questions. Consider, for example, teachers helping students whose performance of a solo lacks expressiveness. If the teachers believe they have already taught a number of strategies for expressive performance, instead of telling students what to do, they can instead ask the *students to identify* what can be done to increase expressivity. When students decide or discover for themselves how to improve their musicianship, this learning is more likely to become permanent. Questioning also is a great support strategy for teachers who do a lot of modeling. After providing a musical model for listening students to emulate in their own performing, teachers can ask them to describe the expressive qualities heard in the model. This way, teachers can have greater confidence that students will actually know *how* to change their performing to make it more like the teacher model. Finally, expert teachers are also expert questioners. They know their students very well and can also adapt their own verbalizations as needed. These qualities allow them to ask questions in such a way as to practically ensure that responding students will provide the correct answer. Students therefore essentially instruct themselves, with the result of making their learning more meaningful.

Chapter 10 Discussion Questions

1. As you think of past music teachers who were especially important to you, what qualities of theirs prompted you to value their guidance?
2. When a teacher, mentor, or music expert evaluates your performing, what kind of feedback do you value most? Have you found it easy to offer that kind of feedback yourself when you have evaluated others?
3. In addition to receiving formal teacher training (i.e., majoring in music education) at a college or university, what experiences in the "music world" can allow musicians to develop a teacher identity?

11

The Listener

Listening to music is such a common activity in everyday life today that it may seem strange to consider the listener as a musical role, let alone to regard music listening as a skill that people develop, even to specialized expert levels. Be that as it may, listening is an extremely important topic in the psychology of music, if only because it is a form of musical engagement done by virtually all human beings. Even those who would never consider themselves "musicians" readily fill the role of serious music listeners, and often quite enthusiastically.

In a very practical sense, listening is *the primary reason* music exists at all. Sound is the "stuff" of music. Thus, providing a meaningful sonic experience for others is largely the reason that composers work so hard on their creations and music performers enter the stage or recording studio. While live performance is an ancient universal listening activity, music recordings offer a listening experience to the modern technological world. In the words of famed inventor Thomas Edison, his phonograph was so popular because it stimulated "the speculative imaginations of all thinking people" with its potential for the "gathering up and retaining of sounds hitherto fugitive, and their reproduction at will" (Edison, 1878, p. 527). It is interesting to consider that before this invention, performed music was indeed "fugitive" because it could not be captured anywhere but in the minds of listeners. Still, music flourished and evolved well before any technology existed to record sound. When sound recording technology became available, many people focused on its use for documenting the spoken word. Edison himself did this, emphasizing the phonograph's use for letter writing, dictation of books, and teaching (of language). However, he also had the foresight to predict that "the phonograph will undoubtedly be liberally devoted to music" (p. 533).

Research suggests the following about music listening, which will be the focus of this chapter:

1. The physiological process by which acoustic sound properties become meaningful music is quite remarkable. Even beyond the intricate

Psychology for Musicians. Robert H. Woody, Oxford University Press. © Oxford University Press 2022.
DOI: 10.1093/oso/9780197546598.003.0011

mechanisms of human hearing, a number of perpetual processes are carried out for the mind to understand music.

2. The nature of a music-listening experience is largely determined by how listeners direct their attention. The resulting different ways of listening include having music in the background while doing other things, analytical and critical listening, and focused listening to have an emotional response.

3. In addition to the sound qualities of the music heard, people's listening experiences are greatly influenced by situational factors (e.g., when, where, and with whom they take place) and characteristics of the listeners themselves. These factors account for why seemingly similar listeners can have different responses to the same piece of music and have dissimilar musical tastes more generally.

4. Music's capability to evoke emotional responses in listeners is well documented. Although some responses may defy simple labeling with emotion word descriptors, the same listener reactions can be so intense as to elicit physiological responses, such as tears, shivers, and a racing heart.

Hearing: The Handling of Sound

The human auditory system is continuously receiving information and, unlike the eye, cannot be closed off to the environment. Although a multitude of sounds (even noxious ones) are present simultaneously and compete for attention, human beings can allocate attention selectively and psychologically filter what is heard. Thus, the difference between hearing and listening can be understood as the difference between perception and cognition, that is, the difference between having sensory contact with stimuli in one's environment and seeking to understand and find meaning in those stimuli. The following paragraphs describe the path of acoustical stimuli from their origin to where they are processed in the brain (see Figure 11.1).

Peripheral Auditory System

As introduced in Chapter 2, hearing starts very early in human development. As early as the first trimester of gestation, parts of the ear emerge. The

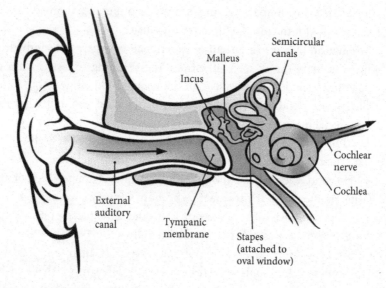

Figure 11.1 Human auditory system.

From Chittka, L., & Brockmann, A. (2005). Perception space—the final frontier. *PLoS Biology, 3*(4), e137. https://doi.org/10.1371/journal.pbio.0030137

cochlea, the primary site of hearing in the inner ear, reaches its final size by the 20th week. As early as the 24th week, fetuses have shown responses to auditory stimulation, including motor movements, heart rate changes, and auditory evoked potentials (electrical signals indicating brain activity; Lecanuet & Schaal, 2002). Although the uterine environment muffles perceivable sound and includes background noises of respiratory, gastrointestinal, and cardiovascular function, the fetus can hear intelligible speech and musical sounds produced by the mother and nearby external stimuli, especially in the third trimester of gestation. Fetuses have been shown to detect and respond to their mothers' voices and may also be sensitive to the rhythmicity of sounds heard (Provasi et al., 2014).

Once children are born and their ears are free of amniotic fluid, they hear sound as any other human being does. The intricacies of hearing, it should be noted, are complex and fascinating, beginning with the physics of sound, which is remarkable in its own right (and the topic of many other books). Suffice it here to say that produced sounds result in waves of vibrations traveling through the air to the ear, first reaching *the outer ear*. Figure 11.1 shows the anatomy of the human auditory system. From the outside, ears may not look like much, but even the visible pinna plays an important role in human hearing and listening. The pinnae help listeners identify from where a sound is originating; this process of sound localization is accomplished through the infinitesimal time difference between when sound waves reach the right versus left ear. As soundwaves make their way through the auditory canal, they are amplified before reaching the tympanic membrane (eardrum), which vibrates sympathetically with the soundwaves.

The vibrating eardrum moves the perception of sound into *the middle ear*. The vibration of the membrane sets three tiny bones—that is, ossicles—into motion (Vetter, 2008). These three bones, called the malleus (Latin for hammer), incus (anvil), and stapes (stirrup) based on their shapes, are connected and function like a lever system to mechanically boost the force of the movement as the stapes interfaces with the cochlea, in *the inner ear*. Inside the fluid-filled cochlea are tens of thousands of hair-like nerve endings. The piston-like action of the stapes sets into motion the fluid, and the motion of the nerve endings creates electrical impulses that travel to the brain via the auditory nerve (composed of the cochlear nerve and the vestibular nerve).

It should be pointed out that what is described in the previous two paragraphs—sound transforming from (1) sound waves in the air to (2) a vibrating membrane to (3) mechanically moving bones to (4) liquid motion to (5) electrical impulses—all happens *before* arriving in the brain for processing. In fact, the ear is called the *peripheral auditory system*, because the central auditory system is considered to begin in the cochlear nerve going to the brain (Staecker & Thompson, 2013). Only then can a listener understand or find meaning in the sound heard. The auditory cortex of the brain seems to handle most processing of music, especially with respect to pitch. Other parts of the brain can be activated by music as well; rhythm perception can involve motor cortical areas, and the cerebellum and/or basal ganglia, two parts of the brain associated with temporal processing (Nozaradan et al., 2017). When music elicits emotional response in listeners, it has been shown to activate other areas of the brain that have been linked to highly rewarding stimuli, including food and euphoria-inducing drugs (Peretz & Zatorre, 2005). Detailed study of the musical brain is beyond the scope of this book but has been covered very accessibly by Levitin (2006) and more comprehensively by Thaut and Hodges (2019).

Psychoacoustics and Processing Sound

Recall from Chapter 9 that listeners' appraisals of musical quality are influenced by what they see in a live performance. This illustrates that what listeners hear is not necessarily a veridical representation of the "objective" acoustical properties of musical sound. The anatomical features of a person's auditory system (Figure 11.1) can affect how an individual perceives sounds. For example, the size of the auditory canal affects which pitch frequencies are amplified as they reach the eardrum (a person with a smaller ear canal will receive more natural amplification of higher-frequency sounds). Also, exposure to loud sounds can cause irreparable damage to the inner ear that results in distorted hearing. In addition to such physiological characteristics, there are powerful psychological factors in play. Indeed, when listening to music, the mind essentially constructs a mental version of the music that is sounding. In addition to being informed by the acoustic stimuli of the music, the mental version is affected by characteristics of listeners themselves. It is this mental version of the music—rather than the sounded music physically in the air—that listeners understand and to which they respond.

In other words, what people psychologically hear is not the same as the musical sound that is physically present. This fact is well illustrated in musical illusions. Examples of these can be found in audio and video recordings readily available on the internet. Some of the more common musical illusions are the continuous scale and the tritone paradox. The continuous scale is a sequence of tones that evokes the sensation of continuous ascent or descent over many octaves while really remaining in a middle-frequency range. The tritone paradox presents simple intervals (diminished fifths) that some people hear as ascending and others perceive as descending (Deutsch, 2010, 2019). Yet all listeners have the clear impression that what they are hearing is unambiguous and true. Given that viewers can learn to see some optical illusions "the right way," obviously perceptual input requires interpretation. By analogy, the same applies to hearing and listening. The veridicality of auditory input is limited by and dependent on the physiology and psychology of hearing.

In many sound environments, there is a massive amount of incoming information for a listener to attend to and process. There are certain basic processes of perception that human beings use to organize sensory input. With respect to navigating the world of sound, people do this quite commonly, hence the classic phenomenon known as the cocktail party problem: how do people in a noisy or otherwise auditory complex environment manage to listen to the sound presented by only one source? This aspect of *auditory scene analysis* (Bregman, 1994) is accomplished through *auditory stream segmentation*, that is, the ability to associate certain sounds from the same source and segregate that stream of sounds from others (Lotto & Holt, 2011). Of course, this ability is not only useful at cocktail parties but also has many musical uses as well.

Auditory segmentation is an example of Gestalt principles of perception, which help make sense of and find meaning in sensory stimuli. Specifically, auditory segmentation reflects the principle of similarity, by which listeners can, for instance, group together musical tones that are similar in timbre and separate out those that are dissimilar (Deutsch, 2013). This explains how listeners can follow a solo flute melody against a background of orchestral instruments, and how a percussion aficionado, when listening to the recorded music of a rock band, might specifically listen to the bass drum use of the set drummer. This kind of listening—and Gestalt principles more generally—can also be described as categorical perception. This term is most often used in research in speech perception, which obviously has common ground with music perception. Just as listeners can identify the voices of different speakers in a group discussion, they can identify certain musical qualities, especially with experience.

In most cases when people listen to music, they focus their attention on certain auditory elements of the music, thereby leaving other elements ignored. This focus can account for why the same music—indeed, the same "hearing" of a piece of music—can have very different effects on different listeners. This result is especially true as listeners seek to make sense of and find meaning in music to which they listen. Although experienced musicians possess the capability to listen to music in a more analytical way (see the following section), the natural inclination of human beings is to listen to music more holistically, subjectively, and personally. In a review of past music listening research, Williams (2008) concluded, "It appears that the stimuli encountered are processed as a single, complex event that is perceived on the basis of *what the listener brings to the experience*" (p. 27, emphasis added).

Ways of Listening

As mentioned at the outset of this chapter, technological developments in electronic media have made it possible for people to listen to recorded music virtually any place and at any time of the day or night. Perhaps for this reason alone, many people who do not consider themselves particularly musical still say that music is an important part of their lives. People listen both alone and with others (Juslin et al., 2008; North et al., 2004), often while engaged in other activities, such as getting ready for the day, traveling, carrying out routine tasks at home or at work, exercising, and socializing with family or friends (Fuentes et al., 2019; Greb et al., 2018; Hu et al., 2021; Lamont et al., 2016; Landay & Harms, 2019). Listening is frequently carried out in private settings (e.g., one's home), but between car stereos and portable audio devices, individualized listening in public is increasingly common (Heye & Lamont, 2010; Juslin et al., 2008; North et al., 2004).

Of course, for many people, music listening serves purposes other than providing a "soundtrack" in the background while doing other things. Having *choice* in what one listens to is an important factor in the effect the experience has on a person (Greasley & Lamont, 2011; Krause et al., 2014; Lynar et al., 2017). In addition to choosing *what* music they will listen to (a privilege readily afforded by modern recording technology), people can choose *how* they will listen, that is, the manner in which they engage with the "subject matter" of the music (Clarke, 2005).

Learning to Listen, Listening to Learn

Although hearing is an innate biological function, *listening* is an ability that is developed. Thus, listening can be considered a skill, and as such, it can improve through experience and training. To appreciate listening as a function of learning, one need only try listening to the music of an unfamiliar ethnic culture, such as that of the San people of southern Africa, and experience the seeming lack of meaning for the uninitiated ear or try to follow multiple voices in a Baroque fugue. Whereas the first example addresses the learning effect of enculturation, the latter likely results only with formal study and practice.

When people have sought to improve their ability to listen to music and when music students have been taught how to listen, traditionally the emphasis has been on instructing listeners to pay attention to certain musical elements. For example, famed American composer Aaron Copland's (1939) book on listening, titled *What to Listen for in Music*, featured entire chapters on the elements of rhythm, melody, harmony, and tone color, among others. More recently, Gioia's (2016) *How to Listen to Jazz* recommended that listeners attend to rhythmic swing, phrasing in improvised melodies, and expressive tone created through altered timbres and pitches.

Attentional focus is a defining factor in music-listening experiences. At issue is *how much* attention listeners pay to the music (i.e., versus other activities they are doing, in the case of music in the background), as well as to *what musical element(s)* they focus their attention. As is true about music listening in general, attentional focus seems to depend on characteristics of the music, the listener him- or herself, and the situational context of a listening experience (Figure 11.2). Psychological research has indicated that with much Western music, melody seems to be the priority in listeners' attention (Ragert et al., 2014). Schmuckler (2016) suggested that this is because melody is the most ubiquitous form of musical structure and the first that infants encounter from being sung to by parents. In popular music, a song's "hook"—the feature most salient and easily remembered by listeners—is very often the melodic material that is repeated throughout the song (Deutsch, 2019; Honing, 2010; Margulis, 2014). Tunes can be so "catchy" that they can lead to an "earworm" or having a song "stuck in one's head" (see Deutsch, 2019, Chapter 8). Margulis (2014) described a particularly disruptive version of this somewhat common phenomenon:

> Few people are spared the at least occasional experience of being gripped by the obstinate unfolding of an imagined line of music. Although the sound might not exist at the present moment in the real world, or be audible to anyone else, it can seem compellingly, maddeningly real. An episode of this sort often seems more like the reliving of a tune than the simple remembering of it. (p. 75)

As this comment shows, repetition is a compositional aspect of music that can command the attention of listeners. Repetition reflects the fact that the presentation of a musical work to listeners occurs *across time*, and rhythm is the primary music structural element related to timing. Jones (2010) described listening to melodic content as attention "focused on the 'what'

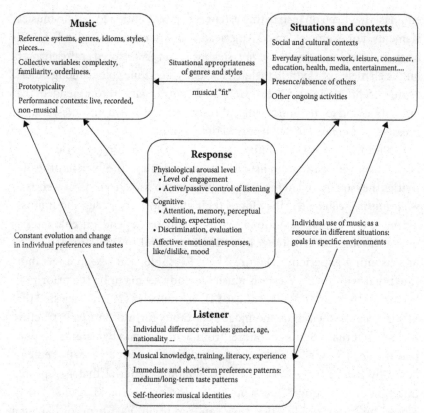

Figure 11.2 Reciprocal feedback model of musical response.

From Hargreaves, D. J., Hargreaves, J. J., & North, A. C. (2012). Imagination and creativity in music listening. In D. Hargreaves, D. Miell, & R. A. R. MacDonald (Eds.), *Musical imaginations: Multidisciplinary perspectives on creativity, performance, and perception* (pp. 156–172). Oxford, UK: Oxford University Press. Reproduced with permission of the Oxford University Press through PLSclear.

of forthcoming sounds" and suggested that listeners "tacitly 'use' event timing to attend" (p. 326). Thus, although listeners' conscious attention may often be directed to melodies in the music they hear, they are nevertheless entrained by timing and intensity (e.g., changes in loudness to create driving rhythms) to develop expectancies about what may happen next in the music. The resulting "anticipatory attending" can elicit more focused attention of listeners (Jones, 2010, p. 327).

Expectancy is an important contributor in music listening being such a rewarding experience for human beings (Huron & Margulis, 2010; Salimpoor et al., 2015). Largely through enculturation, people become familiar with music of certain styles, musicians, and performance contexts. This musical experience, once internalized, results in listeners having expectations when they hear music (Curtis & Bharucha, 2009). In effect, their exposure to past musical events facilitates their making predictions about future music events, that is, predicting what will happen in the music they are listening to (Koelsch et al., 2019). Music elicits feelings in listeners as their expectation are met, are denied, or result in musical surprises (Margulis, 2005). In the moments of a listening experience, musical events—for example, an appoggiatura, a variation on a melody—are emotionally impactful to listeners because of the expectations around them. The ITPRA theory of Huron (2006) explains musical expectancy as follows: approaching a musical event, a listener's expectations exist as *imagination* (anticipating future musical sounds or emotional states) and *tension* (a musical buildup to or dramatic delaying of the anticipated event); the moment of the musical event is experienced on the basis of the listener's *prediction* of what would musically occur and his or her immediate *reaction* to what did occur; and finally a more lasting and contextual *appraisal* response is felt as an assessment of the entire experience of the musical event. Figure 11.3 illustrates how expectancy occurs across time according to the ITPRA theory.

Musical events cannot interact with a listener's expectancies if that individual is not inclined to attend to the music or if situational circumstances prevent it (Krause et al., 2016). As alluded to earlier, oftentimes when people listen to music, the music serves as a kind of soundtrack in the background of what they are doing. When music listening *is* the main activity, the primary

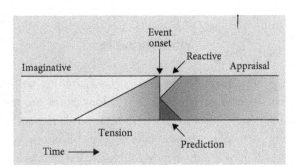

Figure 11.3 Illustration of Huron's ITPRA theory of musical expectation.

From Huron, D., & Margulis, E. H. (2010). Musical expectancy and thrills. In P. N. Juslin & J. A. Sloboda (Eds.), *Handbook of music and emotion: Theory, research, applications* (pp. 575–604). Oxford, UK: Oxford University Press. Reproduced with permission of the Oxford University Press through PLSclear.

purpose is often to affect listeners' emotions or moods, cope with problems, or gain self-awareness (Greb et al., 2018; Schäfer et al., 2013). In such situations, listeners' attention may be applied broadly to the music, as opposed to any specific musical element such as lyrics, melody, or rhythm. Although relatively rare, sometimes listeners engage in "pure music listening," that is, while doing no other activity and with no ulterior motive for the listening. In such cases, listeners focus the bulk of their attention to the musical sound itself and by doing so can gain intellectual stimulation and improve their musical knowledge (Greb et al., 2018).

Listening for the defined purpose of music learning is, of course, common among musicians. As was mentioned in Chapter 5, listening (to recordings) is a key strategy for musicians of all kinds as they prepare music for performance.

As explained in detail in Chapter 4, mentally representing music— including auditory "imaging" of musical sound—is a cognitive skill that underlies virtually all music making. As such, aural skills instruction (so-called ear training) is a standard component of formal music education, and multiple types of music listening are prominent in the informal learning of vernacular musicians (e.g., those in popular music and jazz). The many learning experiences—formal and informal—that people gain en route to becoming musicians seem to result in their listening to music differently than nonmusicians. Musicians have demonstrated superior ability in differentiating concurrent musical streams (Johnson et al., 2020; Ragert et al., 2014; Zendel & Alain, 2009). Overall, they more often engage in attentive music listening (Dellacherie et al., 2011).

Critical Listening

Judging a musical performance is a specialized listening task that is fairly common. There exist many music competitions, from the multiple popular singing television shows to contests and festivals in which all levels of music students participate. Additionally, a very common responsibility of music educators is to assess the development and performance competency of their music learners, including for the purpose of assigning grades. In these common music performance settings, much of the listening is done with a "critical ear," that is, with the specific purpose of critically assessing the quality of the music performed.

In music, as it is in life, whenever judges are involved, the chief concern is to carry out their role in a proper and impartial manner. Their opinions and appraisals should be well founded and unbiased. With this in mind, it may be surprising or disappointing to know that research has shown musical judging can be quite unreliable (across multiple judges). This result is common especially when judges do not use well-established assessment techniques that can help ensure consistency.

A lack of reliability in performance judging can be explained by two basic mechanisms. First, as mentioned in Chapter 9, observer judgments of a musical performance are susceptible to sources of bias, including physical appearance, performer attractiveness, and the prestige effect (Griffiths, 2010; Hargreaves & North, 2010; Iuşcă, 2020; Tsay, 2013; Wapnick et al., 2009). It should be noted that these biases have been found among experienced music listeners and highly educated musicians serving as performance judges. Second, as mentioned earlier in this chapter, a listening experience is in large part determined by what people themselves bring to the experience and how they allocate their attention while listening.

In light of this, certain techniques are often used to strengthen the reliability of music adjudication and performance assessment in education. One is to identify in advance specific musical criteria on which performances will be evaluated (Hash, 2012; Latimer et al., 2010; Wesolowski, 2016). In effect, using predetermined criteria constrains and directs the attention of judges while listening. This not only helps with agreement between multiple judges but also can ensure consistent assessment of music offered by multiple performers who are similarly skilled (Norris & Borst, 2007). If specific criteria are identified for judging, judges must have the requisite musical expertise to direct their attention (i.e., audio stream segregation) to the musical elements designated for focus (Kinney, 2009).

Determining the musical criteria for judging may result in structuring the performance conditions for the musician contestants. For example, a decision to focus on musical sound qualities at the exclusion of visual presentation factors may lead adjudicators to require that musicians give live performances behind the screen (Mitchell & Benedict, 2017). This structure was used to address sex-biased hiring among American orchestras that excluded female musicians from orchestral membership through much of the 20th century; the use of a screen for "blind" auditions increased by 50% the probability that a woman would advance beyond preliminary rounds and increased "by several fold the likelihood that a woman will be selected in the final round" (Goldin & Rouse, 2000, p. 738).

Making Meaning: Musical Emotion

The superior listening skills developed by musicians and devoted music connoisseurs equip them with superior perception of the sound qualities of music. Such musical experts are able to track individual parts or instrument groupings within polyphonic music and to identify specific musical devices used by composers and performers. The most important perceptual advantage of musical expertise, however, is increased sensitivity to the emotionally expressive properties of music (Dellacherie et al., 2011; Mikutta et al., 2014). After all, being moved to an emotional response is the primary motivation for listening to music among all people.

Emotional Response to Musical Expressiveness

Sound is universally expressive, especially with respect to certain basic emotions. Therefore, although listeners' perception and cognition of music rely heavily on enculturation, sometimes listeners can emotionally understand music of unfamiliar cultures to the extent that the music's acoustic properties include universal sound qualities that are reflective of human emotional behavior and language use (Patel & Demorest, 2013). For example, across cultures, sorrowful people tend to behave at a low activity level; thus, listeners may be more likely to hear sorrow in music that has low rhythmic activity. Similarly, because cross-culturally people tend to yell when they are angry, listeners may be more likely to hear anger in loud music. In addition, research has shown that infant cries and human screams occur in a pitch frequency range to which human hearing is especially sensitive, and that professional singers may exploit this auditory sensitivity to elicit frisson (i.e., a sudden thrilling or chilling feeling of excitement) in listeners (Beeman, 2005; Huron & Margulis, 2010).

    To study how music engenders emotions in listeners, researchers have had to grapple with the words people use to describe emotional states. At the most basic level, human emotions can be defined by two dimensions: valence (positive or negative) and activity level (low or high;

Posner et al., 2005). These two dimensions can be combined to produce four broad emotions that were shown in Figure 6.2 in Chapter 6: tenderness (positive valence, low activity), happiness (positive valence, high activity), anger (negative valence, high activity), and sadness (negative valence, low activity). More specific emotion words have also been useful to researchers. As early as the 1930s, American psychologist Kate Hevner (1935, 1936) investigated the range of emotions expressed in music by asking listeners to choose from a list of adjectives. Schubert (2003) updated Hevner's work, producing a list of 46 words in nine clusters. Figure 11.4 presents these clusters and shows how they can be mapped onto the two dimensions of valence and activity level (see also Myint & Pwint, 2010).

Based on an exhaustive review of empirical research findings, Gabrielsson and Lindström (2010) provided a thorough account of how specific human emotions are linked to certain sound properties in Western tonal music. Gabrielsson (2016) offered an abridged version of this review updated with the insights of more recent research. The most distinct results (of musical properties' effect on emotional expressiveness) can be linked to variables most basic to human hearing, namely loudness, timbre, and pitch, as well as the musical variable of tempo. Also, the common associations of major mode as happy and minor as sad are not absolute; these can be overruled by certain uses of variables, including tempo and pitch. More findings include the following:

- Mode/key. Major mode may be associated with positive valence emotions such as happiness, gracefulness, or serenity, or possibly with solemnity. Minor mode may be associated with sadness, anger, or disgust, or may be heard as dreamy, dignified, or tense. According to Temperley and Tan (2013), the church modes have been judged expressive of happiness in this order (from most to least expressive of happiness): Ionian, Mixolydian, Lydian, Dorian, Aeolian, and Phrygian (Locrian was judged to be too problematic for composing melodies and excluded from the research). (p. 219)
- Tempo. Fast tempo may be associated with expressions of activity/excitement, happiness, potency, surprise, whimsicality, anger, uneasiness, or fear. Slow tempo may be associated with expressions of calmness, peace, sadness, dignity/solemnity, tenderness, longing, boredom, or disgust. (p. 218)

Emotion Cluster	Adjectives describing the dimension
A	Bright, cheerful, happy, joyous
B	Humorous, light, lyrical, merry, playful
C	Calm, delicate, graceful, quiet, relaxed, serene, soothing, tender, tranquil
D	Dreamy, sentimental
E	Tragic, yearning
F	Dark, depressing, gloomy, melancholy, mournful, sad, solemn
G	Heavy, majestic, sacred, serious, spiritual, vigorous
H	Dramatic, exciting, exhilarated, passionate, sensational, soaring, triumphant
I	Agitated, angry, restless, tense

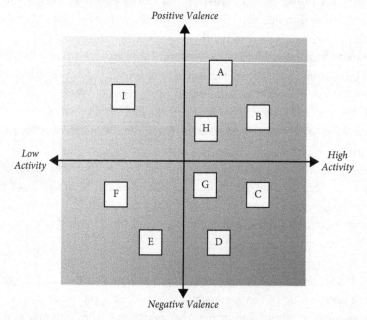

Figure 11.4 Emotion clusters mapped onto dimensions of valence and activity.
Based on research of Schubert, E. (2003). Update of the Hevner adjective checklist. *Perceptual and Motor Skills, 96*, 1117–1122. https://doi.org/10.2466/pms.2003.96.3c.1117; and Myint, E. E. P., & Pwint, M. (2010, July). An approach for multi-label music mood classification. In *Proceedings of the 2010 2nd International Conference on Signal Processing Systems* (Vol. 1, pp. 290–294). Piscataway, NJ: Institute of Electrical and Electronics Engineers.

- Pitch. Music with high pitch content may be heard as happy, graceful, serene, dreamy, or exciting, or suggestive of surprise, potency, anger, fear, or activity. Low pitch may suggest sadness, dignity/solemnity, strength, boredom, or pleasantness. Large pitch variation may be associated with happiness, pleasantness, activity, or surprise, and small pitch variation with disgust, anger, fear, or boredom. (pp. 219–220)

- Loudness. Loud music may be associated with excitement, joy, intensity, power, tension, or anger, and quiet music with peace, tenderness, sadness, or fear. Crescendos and diminuendos may be associated with increasing and decreasing activation/potency, respectively. Large variations of loudness may suggest fear. (p. 219)
- Articulation. Staccato articulation may be associated with gaiety, energy, fear, or anger. Legato articulation may be associated with sadness, longing, solemnity, or tenderness. (p. 221)
- Timbre. Tones with many and higher harmonic frequencies may be associated with higher activity emotions such as power, anger, disgust, fear, or surprise. Tones with few and low harmonics may be associated with lower activity emotions such as pleasantness, boredom, happiness, or sadness. (p. 219)

Whereas these findings report emotion associations for separate musical sound properties, with real music, listeners cannot emotionally attend to one property (e.g., tempo) separately from others (e.g., mode, pitch, harmony). Thus, it is important to understand the individual properties listed as co-contributors to the expression of emotion in music.

As shown here, some important insights have come from research in which listeners describe or label the emotions induced by music. This approach, however, is not entirely adequate, in part because of what philosophers have referred to as the *ineffability of art*. That is, experiences with the arts can induce moods, emotions, or aesthetic responses that defy labeling or description with words. In fact, music listeners have reported especially strong responses to music, experiences that they characterize as being powerful and unforgettable, yet "inaccessible to verbal description" (Gabrielsson et al., 2016, p. 750). Therefore, in some situations, assigning certain words to describe emotional responses to music may not accurately capture the experience. In this spirit, instead of studying listeners' experiences of certain emotions, some researchers have investigated more general responses. One such response, affect *arousal*, has received a good deal of attention from researchers in the behavioral sciences (Niven & Miles, 2013). Music researchers have found listeners able to indicate their arousal induced by music on a sliding scale of less to more, and they seem to indicate it similarly whether the response of interest is labeled *arousal, aesthetic response,* or *felt emotional response* (Geringer et al., 2004). Research results indicate that listeners' arousal responses are particularly sensitive to variations in loudness within the music (Dean et al., 2011; Schubert, 2004, 2010).

Emotions elicited by music can be so intense that listeners experience physical and physiological responses (Hodges, 2016). Some of the more common ones are tears, shivers, and a racing heart. According to Sloboda (2005b), some musically sophisticated listeners have been able to identify specific musical features by which they think their physiological responses were provoked: melodic appoggiaturas and certain harmonic sequences were thought to prompt crying and "lump in the throat" responses, new and unprepared harmonies were often credited for producing shivers or "goose pimples," and rhythmic syncopation and the arrival of earlier-than-expected musical events were associated with a racing heart and "pit-of-the-stomach sensations" (p. 210). Khalfa et al. (2008) found that listeners' physiological responses are significantly different between "happy music" (i.e., major mode, fast tempo of 110 to 154 bpm) and "sad music" (minor mode, slow tempo of 40 to 69 bpm), specifically in terms of cardiovascular and respiratory function. Further, through experimental manipulation of the musical stimuli, the research team was able to demonstrate that tempo alone could not account for the finding that "happy music" produced higher levels of blood pressure, skin conductance, and heart and respiration rate.

Physiological response may also be key in understanding why people find it rewarding to listen to music that is expressive of negative emotions, such as sadness or anger. So-called sad music can engender the physical response of crying, which can lead to the body's secretion of prolactin, a "feel-good" hormone that can have the psychological effect of consoling the person (Huron, 2011; Lamont et al., 2016, p. 717). Listening to sad music appears very common with people in the aftermath of suffering loss or significant emotional pain. In fact, among many people, music listening may be *the most important* personal strategy for finding consolation (Hanser et al., 2016).

Mood management is one of the most common uses of music among people (Hays & Minichiello, 2005; Lamont et al., 2016; Saarikallio et al., 2013; Schäfer et al., 2013). Music that induces positive emotion is often used to reinforce a good mood caused by favorable life circumstances and events or to relax in order to fall asleep or regain energy. Mood management plays out differently with music that is expressive of negative emotions. Listeners report a mix of emotions—including positive ones—when listening to "sad music"; Peltola and Eerola (2016) found that the emotional responses comprise a range of emotions, broadly categorized as *grief, melancholia,* and *sweet sorrow.* Such music-listening experiences can trigger memories of painful past events and cause listeners to re-experience negative feelings from the past. A result may be the experience of *cathartic grief,* described by one participant in the Peltola and Eerola (2016) study, who spoke about how sad music brings up memories:

> I remember just how sorrowful and desolate I was back then . . . and those feelings attack me again; instantly I feel just as sad, anxious and sorrowful as I did then. . . . On the other hand, if I let myself go through those feelings, I usually feel relieved afterwards. (p. 91)

Because the grieving process is thought to include the emotions of anger, fear, despair, and guilt (Bonnano et al., 2008), it may be that listening to "angry music" can also have a positive cathartic effect (Baker & Brown, 2016). A young adult participant in a study by Sinclair and Dolan (2015) explained that angry music "sort of vents it and that would actually calm me down I would find" (p. 431).

Tastes and Preferences

In addition to what music people choose, their musical preferences are borne out in their motives for listening to music in the first place. Research has shown that listeners' emotional responses to music are affected by much more than the music itself; also very influential are situational factors around a listening experience (e.g., where, when, and with whom it takes place) and personal and emotional traits of listeners themselves (Gabrielsson, 2010; Hargreaves et al., 2012; Juslin et al., 2008). The three factors—the music, the listener, and the listening context—can interact to produce widely varied responses among people. Hargreaves et al. (2012) called this the reciprocal model of musical response and illustrated it with the diagram shown in Figure 11.2. Research of Sloboda (2005b) has indicated that many listeners use music as a "trigger or an outlet" to release emotions that would otherwise be "bottled up," leading him to conclude that sometimes "music does not create or change emotion; rather it allows a person access to the experience of emotions that are somehow already 'on the agenda' for that person, but not fully apprehended or dealt with" (p. 204).

Personal factors can interact with (past) situational factors in a principle of musical emotion amusingly called the "Darling, they're playing our tune" theory, explained here by Lamont and Hargreaves (2019):

> Specific pieces of music have connections to the wider sociocultural context through association with popular culture, and we all have individual memories associated with different pieces of music, which both affect memorability and thus preference. For instance "Eye of the Tiger" was used on the soundtrack of *Rocky III*, and has become synonymous with the trope of training against the odds and physical endurance. Thus it has become an extremely popular song for athletes and sportspeople (Hallett and Lamont, 2015), whatever their age when the track was first released. Following the "Darling they're playing our tune" theory first coined by Davies (1978), specific pieces will also have highly personal connections, such as one's first dance at a wedding, or one's first important breakup. (p. 111)

Thus, listeners' musical memories and emotional agendas largely drive what they like and choose to listen to. Having choice in their listening is extremely important to people. As mentioned earlier, music-listening experiences are influenced by what listeners bring to the experience as much as or more than the sound properties of the music itself. Being made to listen to music not of their choosing can produce "negative emotions such as irritation, disapproval, and dislike" (Sloboda, 2010, p. 498). In fact, it could be said that one's tastes must be accommodated for music to serve the function that a listener desires it to serve (Greb et al., 2018; Schäfer, 2016).

Especially in the modern technological music world, people's listening behavior clearly reflects their choices of music, and hence their tastes in music. Consequently, some psychologists consider music preference as a meaningful indicator of personality. In something of a landmark study, Rentfrow and Gosling (2003) presented a four-dimension model of music preferences, based on personality and attitudinal traits. The four dimensions were (1) Reflective and Complex, (2) Intense and Rebellious, (3) Upbeat and Conventional, and (4) Energetic and Rhythmic. More recently, Dunn et al. (2012) conducted similar research but relied on an industry-standard *All Music Guide* for categorizing, which yielded a different four-factor model.

The following four categories show the closest Rentfrow and Gosling (2003) dimension and personality trait correlations:

- Acoustic foundation (Reflective and Complex). Classical, blues, and folk. Preference for classical music correlated with the Neuroticism facet of "self-consciousness."
- Hard rock (Intense and Rebellious). Alternative, rock, heavy metal. Preference for rock music correlated with the Extraversion facet of "excitement seeking."
- Soft rock (Upbeat and Conventional). Pop, soundtracks.
- Bass foundation (Energetic and Rhythmic). Rap/hip-hop, soul/rhythm and blues/funk, electronica/dance.
- Additional genres not corresponding well with Rentfrow and Gosling dimensions. Whereas Rentfrow and Gosling placed jazz in their Reflective and Complex dimension, Dunn et al. found jazz to be in their Bass foundation factor, and a preference for jazz correlated with the Openness to Experience personality trait facets of "aesthetics" and "ideas." Also, Rentfrow and Gosling placed religious music and country music in their Upbeat and Conventional dimension, but Dunn et al. found these two genres to be in their Acoustic foundation factor.

As communicated by the word *correlated* earlier, the research stops short of identifying whether music preference is a cause or an effect in its relationship with personality. Generally, psychological research has yet to produce conclusive evidence to explain precisely how an individual's personality is formed. Therefore, with respect to music, it is impossible to say with any certainty whether people's musical preferences are determined by their personalities or, alternatively, their personalities are formed as a result of their experiences, including their musical exposure, engagement, and chosen listening experiences.

Clearly people's music preferences are affected by their exposure to music, perhaps especially at a young age through enculturation. Past research led Levitin (2006) to propose that the age of 14 is a "sort of magic age for the development of musical tastes" (Levitin, as quoted in Hajdu, 2011). Although not all research has corroborated the specific age of 14 as a peak year establishing musical taste (Gerlich et al., 2010), it is difficult to refute the idea that listeners' tastes are shaped by songs from their teenage years "because those years were times of self-discovery, and as a consequence, they were emotionally charged" (Levitin, 2006, p. 231).

While it is generally true that increased exposure to a type of music will ultimately result in increased liking of it, this principle is not absolute. As shown with the example of teenage music tastes, exposure during certain stages of life and in certain contexts can be highly influential in the long term. Also, just as people are disinclined to like unfamiliar music, they tend to respond similarly to overexposed music. Thus, a moderate level of familiarity with music seems to produce the optimal level of emotional engagement or arousal in listeners (Chmiel & Schubert, 2017, 2019). Not all types of exposure are equal, however, and musicians and music teachers should take heed. It seems possible that young children who are put to sleep to soothing classical music may come to experience the genre as nonarousing or even boring (Green, 2014; Mindell & Williamson, 2018). Also, certain types of music exposure in formal educational settings—perhaps especially those involving public performance—may foster negative attitudes about the genres used in school music (Sloboda, 2005d).

Alternative Ways of Listening

To this point, the chapter's explanations of music listening have pertained to individuals with typical hearing capability. There are, of course, many people who perceive music in atypical ways. This includes deaf people and neuro-atypical individuals whose brains process music differently.

Although many assume typical intact hearing to be the "bare minimum" for music listening, this assumption is refuted by the fact that "deaf people have long engaged with music through tactile, visual, and kinesthetic stimuli as an alternative to normal hearing" (Holmes, 2017, p. 173). People's experiences of deafness vary considerably. It is typically categorized as ranging from mild to profound. Regardless of level of deafness, people seek to enjoy music listening in whatever ways they can (Nanayakkara et al., 2009). Among people who are Deaf—the capital D indicating they identify with deaf culture—most were either born deaf or lost hearing early in childhood, before acquiring spoken language; as a result, emotional responses of Deaf listeners tend to differ from those of typically hearing listeners, likely because they have not learned or assimilated emotional cues of music and spoken language (Darrow, 2006). The human brain shows compensatory plasticity;

that is, when the sense of hearing is unavailable, it adapts to accommodate the experiencing of music through visual and vibrotactile modalities (Good et al., 2014). This alternative type of listening can support a high level of musical expertise, as seen in the case of renowned percussionist Evelyn Glennie, who is classified as profoundly deaf. She has described the human body as a "resonating chamber" and has explained that she hears music through sounds vibrating in her hands, arms, cheekbones, scalp, stomach, chest, legs, etc. (Glennie, 2003). Further, adaptational technology offers aid by, for example, amplifying vibrations or generating an abstract animated visual display. Such adaptations have been found to enhance music listening for deaf individuals in meaningful ways (Borowiec et al., 2019; Nanayakkara et al., 2013).

The nature of individuals' listening experiences is also affected by neurological and developmental characteristics. Like deafness, however, disorders of this kind do not preclude the enjoyment of music. For example, autism spectrum disorder (ASD) is said to be characterized by varying but often marked difficulties in communication. Yet, people with ASD have shown the ability to recognize emotional expression communicated through music in ways comparable to those of typical development (Whipple et al., 2015). Individuals with the neurodevelopmental disorder Williams syndrome often show exceptional interest in and receptivity to music; as listeners, they often display heightened emotional responsiveness to music (Thakur et al., 2018).

Synesthesia is a particularly fascinating neurological condition, in which stimuli perceived by one sensory system (e.g., sound) triggers sensation in another (e.g., vision). Although having isolated synesthetic experiences is not uncommon—perhaps associating certain musical sounds with a color or other visual image—true involuntary perceptual synesthesia is rare, with incidence estimates ranging from 0.05% to 4.4% of the population (Johnson et al., 2013; Simmonds-Moore et al., 2019; Simner et al., 2006). Some historically famous composers are said to have been synesthetes (Rimsky-Korsakov and Scriabin among them), but there remains some debate as to whether their sound-to-color associations were neurological, metaphorical, or even "deliberately constructed" (Gawboy & Townsend, 2012; see also Galeyev, 2007). It is believed that synesthesia may occur with greater incidence among musicians and artists, suggesting that it can be used to some creative advantage in some cases (Brang & Ramachandran, 2011; Merter, 2017).

No matter how people experience music, listening is a favorite activity of a great many people. Music-listening experiences can be intensely personal because, in large part, they depend on what listeners bring to the experience, in the form of their current emotional state, experienced-based associations, and music-related memories. The emotional responses induced by music appear to be a reward that is remarkably powerful for human beings as a species.

Taking the Stage: Listen to Yourself as You Listen to Others

One of the most empowering qualities of a performer is adaptability. Those who can perform only one style of music or can be successful only in very specific performance settings have a limited musicianship indeed. Flexibility in listening is also valuable for musicians.

It is always a good idea for performers to at least occasionally record their practicing or performing to assess how they sound to others. Of course, that option is readily possible now with the great accessibility of recording and playback technology on smartphones, tablets, and laptop computers. Little is accomplished, however, if one simply makes a recording and "gives it a listen." Rather, *how* musicians listen to themselves is critically important, and again, flexibility is key. That is, musicians will gain the most insight when they listen in multiple and different ways.

Musicians seeking maximum improvement may be inclined to listen critically to themselves and simply try to identify moments in the music that don't sound "good" or how they had hoped it would. Recall, however, that listening for predetermined criteria enables music adjudicators to provide better (more reliable) appraisals. In this vein, before listening to *themselves*, performers should consider first listening to recordings of other performers and make note of to what musical qualities they direct their listening attention. These qualities can then make up the criteria they use as they judge their own recorded performances.

Leading Learning: Teach Music Appreciation Toward Emotional Response

Many music teachers identify as an educational objective exposing their students to styles of music to which they may not otherwise be exposed.

This goal implies that young people should expand their musical tastes to appreciate less popular genres that teachers deem worthy of recognition and patronage. In formal education, music appreciation instruction has traditionally taken the form of (1) assigning students to listen to pieces of music and (2) providing information about the music and the historical and cultural circumstances around its creation.

Unfortunately, there is little evidence that such listening lessons lead students to increase their appreciation for previously unfamiliar styles of music. An alternative approach is to give students listening experiences in which they can respond to new music in ways that are more natural to them. Bearing in mind that it is common for people to have music playing in the background when they do other tasks, teachers should consider playing recordings—without drawing attention to the music—when students carry out routine tasks, such as entering the classroom to take their seat. If teachers later use the same recording in a music-learning activity, the earlier background experience may provide just enough familiarity to the music to give a helpful boost to the arousal and liking of the music.

Additionally, music teachers may want to consider different criteria for choosing the specific pieces of music they use in listening lessons. Instead of choosing pieces that scholars have deemed most historically significant or analysis-worthy, they can instead opt for musical selections that they think are most likely to evoke emotional responses from their students. A good starting place is selecting pieces that evoke strong emotional responses from themselves. If, while sharing the recording of a piece, the emotional effect on the teacher is visibly apparent, it will likely give weight to the emotionally expressive capacity of the music. If students experience an emotional response to a relatively unfamiliar style of music, there is reason to expect that they may come to appreciate or even *like* it in the future.

Chapter 11 Discussion Questions

1. When you first hear music that is unfamiliar to you, to what aspects of the music are you directing your listening attention?
2. Think of a situation in which two (or more) listeners had opposite appraisals of the same piece of music. Was this simply a matter

of different tastes, or is there another possible way to explain the inconsistency?

3. Think of a specific recording of music that you listen to regularly. Is your connection to it more attributable to the properties of the music itself or to personal and situational factors related to you?

12

The User

It can be a valuable exercise to examine the familiar with fresh eyes. For many of the readers of this book, the most familiar music performance practices are those of Western classical music and formal music education. Without trying to determine whether good or bad, of value or not, musicians can gain important insights by considering their most familiar music culture from the perspective of an outside observer, the way an anthropologist or ethnographer would. Researchers of this type have noted that music is an important aspect of human cultures around the world and that it functions as much more than a mere diversion or entertainment. In fact, people *use music* in their lives in very meaningful ways. Most people are music users in addition to the roles they may more readily identify for themselves—for example, as performers, teachers, or listeners.

The classical music culture faithfully carries out time-honored traditions that signal certain assumptions about how music should take place— traditions and assumptions that are quite different from those of other music genres, both past and present. Comparing classical concert settings to other musical settings brings into clear focus some of the assumptions that may limit performers' potential to function musically in different artistic and cultural situations. In a classical concert, performers and audiences enter by different doors; they are generally separated from each other by physical and psychological barriers. Performers produce all the music; audience members quietly observe and appreciate. Performers and listeners are also separated economically. By and large, listeners pay to hear the music, and performers get paid. Attendance at a classical recital or concert can require massive self-restraint on the part of an audience member. Conversation is forbidden during performance, and even coughing can attract hostile attention. Movement is discouraged (leaving one's seat is considered appropriate only in an emergency). Even facial expressions tend to be muted. Looking at the faces of the participants at a classical concert would suggest to an uninitiated observer that the audience was either in a trance or deeply sedated. Audience members are expected to maintain this silence and immobility

Psychology for Musicians. Robert H. Woody, Oxford University Press. © Oxford University Press 2022.
DOI: 10.1093/oso/9780197546598.003.0012

without complaint for long periods of time, and their response of approval to the performance can only be shown after it is over (Small, 2011).

Classical music venues all over the world have an essential "sameness" that reflects a historically grown and socially constructed consensus about the ideal settings for the reception of classical music. The concert auditorium is usually separated, both spatially and acoustically, from any disturbances, so there is no possibility of interference with the key activity, which is the music performance taking place onstage. Seating and room construction maximize comfort and are designed to allow everyone to have the most acceptable visual and acoustic experience possible. Everything possible is done to focus attention onto what is happening onstage. Lighting is dimmed in the auditorium, and decor is often sparse and soothing, with all lines converging on the performance stage. It is no coincidence that concert halls tend to resemble a cathedral because there is a strong sense of creating a "sacred space" where listeners can have their eyes and ears opened and minds and hearts stretched through "music that they may not otherwise experience in their ordinary lives outside concert halls, opera houses, and churches" (Jorgensen, 2020, p. 139). Influenced by the classical notion of aesthetics, performers and audience members alike expect the grand music to give them an experience that is beautiful, sublime, awe-inspiring, or even spiritual (Doğantan-Dack, 2014; Zentner et al., 2008).

Although some scholars have suggested that Western classical music has long exhibited a superiority complex and perpetuated elitism by exalting classical music above "all of the rest," a more reasoned perspective is to recognize it as one musical culture among many others (Asia, 2018, p. 424; Kertz-Welzel, 2020). In fact, a great number of diverse musical cultures around the world have existed and thrived. Many, such as Argentinian Tango, Indian raga, Celtic music, and Venda call songs (of the South African Bantu people), boast long-enduring and sophisticated music traditions, in which music is learned, performed, and consumed very differently from Western classical music (Mamlok, 2017; Sturman, 2019). More specifically, in many music cultures, boundaries between performers and audience members are virtually nonexistent—nobody fills the role of a quiet spectator; rather, everyone present contributes to the music making. In fact, around the world, most music performance takes place outside formal settings like a concert hall.

An important premise for this chapter is that classical music does, in fact, represent a culture, and it is one of many in the musical world. Furthermore, it is only one of many music cultures within Western civilization. This point must be made at the outset of this chapter because classical music, as compared to other musical genres and cultures, has received a disproportionate amount of attention within musical academic study. Because this is an academic book, it is reasonable to assume that many readers have been enculturated into classical music, perhaps even at the expense of exposure to other musical traditions. In this spirit, this chapter explains the following principles about how human beings use music in their lives:

1. Although focusing on the musical works of composers and performers—the "work-focused approach"—is very important among those who study music, the "person-focused approach," which emphasizes the effect music has on people, is much more common all over the world and throughout human history.
2. Musical styles and skills emerge in cultures as a function of what the group members value, consume, and nurture in their people. Worldwide, groups of people (of various sizes) use music to express their identity and to accomplish many other social purposes.
3. People commonly use music to try to influence behavior—both their own and others'. Because music can so powerfully affect arousal and emotion, many human activities can be enhanced by using music.
4. With portable music technology so prevalent now, many people have music playing for themselves as a soundtrack of life. Even though the music plays in the "background" while they do other things, rather than considering music incidental, they tend to count it as a very important part of their emotional lives.

Work-Focused and Person-Focused Approaches to Music

Although many music scholars will assert that a piece of music can be analyzed and evaluated in and of itself, from a more human perspective (i.e., that of the behavioral sciences), the significance of a piece of music is inextricably linked to its cultural context and who its participants are—with that extending beyond musicians to all people who have any interaction with the music. Take, for example, a Beethoven piano sonata. A classical music lover, who is a Beethoven enthusiast in particular, is likely to pay a substantial sum of money and travel a considerable distance to sit in an upscale city concert hall and hear an internationally renowned concert pianist perform the piece.

Contrast this to the situation of two parents sitting in a suburban school auditorium listening to their daughter perform the sonata in her first solo recital. Even different still is a third scenario in which a rideshare driver plays a recording of the Beethoven piece because he hopes that hearing classical music will calm the riders whom he picks up after a night of carousing. While all of these scenarios feature the same Beethoven piano sonata, the function and meaning of the music differ significantly between them.

One way to think about music, which is prominent in musical academic study and within the classical tradition, is the *work-focused approach*. With this perspective, the musical work—the composition or, in the case of the audiophile, a particular musical recording—is the most important factor in understanding musical meaning and significance. The work itself can be considered as a pure object, detached from any specific performance of it or any specific context in which it might be heard. Traditional musicology has applied this way of thinking by analyzing musical works, in terms of their structure and content, without making explicit reference to any actual performances of compositions or any effects of the music on actual listeners. Analysis typically focuses on musicians' uses of composition sectional form, harmonic progression, and instrumentation and orchestration techniques. The value system of the work-focused approach tends to have particularly high regard for compositional sophistication and innovative uses of musical properties.

An alternative way of thinking about music is the *person-focused approach*, in which music is primarily defined by the "purpose assigned to the activity by the person using it" (Browning, 2017, p. 33). The perspective of this approach is that every musical object or event is situated in a sociocultural context involving human actors, with their backgrounds and motivations. Musical objects and events thus have rich social meanings and functions for all of the people involved—composers, performers, listeners, and others. No music happens unless it is fulfilling a purpose for people (i.e., people *use* it for their reasons). With the person-focused approach, music is regarded for its different meanings and purposes among people and as a symbol of the people it represents. Within the ethos of the person-focused approach, music is valued for its power to affect the emotional, social, and personal lives of the people who interact with it.

Both the work-focused and person-focused approaches to music are valid and can yield important insights into music and its significance. However, the work-focused approach has been very dominant in the music education world during most of the 20th century and has influenced the way people think about music in quite profound ways. It has framed conventional aesthetics, philosophy, and musicology. Scholars in these areas have used the academic discipline of music analysis to study "the music itself" and to ostensibly examine the purity of a work or its musical autonomy. Bonds (2014) has sought to elucidate the often-overlooked values-based nature of this approach:

> The claims of purity and autonomy, qualities closely associated with absolute music, frequently mask their own ideological premises. We always listen to or think about music within a specific historical moment and cultural context, and the idea of "pure" music is itself an abstraction, for the "purely musical experience" is never purely musical. Ethnomusicologists have developed an entire discipline based on this premise. (p. 4)

This chapter explores the person-focused approach to music in more detail. This, of course, is not to suggest that there is no merit in the work-focused approach. On the contrary, deepening one's understanding of specific works is at the heart of effective musicianship. However, it is not adequate for fully understanding music, especially from a psychological perspective.

The work-focused emphasis of much music scholarship often reveals itself in discussions of musical *quality* by those who wish to dismiss musical styles outside of those traditionally studied in music education (i.e., Western classical and jazz). The objection is often raised that a popular musician having influenced the lives of many listeners "says little about the quality of her music" and that cultural relevance cannot make "bad music" worthy of being learned by music students (Rogers, 2007, p. 7). As explained previously, quality from the work-focused perspective is primarily determined through analysis of a musical work's compositional sophistication and innovation, as established by masterworks of classical music. Those adhering to this approach often fail to recognize that they are applying a particular value system and one that is not shared by the vast majority of music listeners. To this point, Woody and Adams (2019) reviewed research in popular music and vernacular music making and concluded that the work-focused versus person-focused approaches explain much of the divergence between classical and popular music traditions:

Should popular music be judged by classical music's expectation of compositional complexity, then popular music may easily be labeled "bad music" (i.e., poor quality); similarly, should classical music be judged by popular music's expectation of being influential in the everyday lives of a large portion of people worldwide, then classical music may be considered "bad music." (p. 895)

The purpose of the person-focused approach is *not* to devalue the styles of music that have been favored by the work-focused approach. No reasonable orientation to music can conclude that classical music is irrelevant or undeserving of people's attention and appreciation. Rather, classical music can be and is valued—even beloved—from a person-focused perspective. Further, a breaking down of rigid barriers between classical and nonclassical music is one of the most encouraging signs of contemporary musical life.

Social and Cultural Functions of Music

Major musical forms emerge because lots of people use them; that is, they serve cultural roles. The skills that are encouraged and developed in musical young people are totally a function of society's values and requirements for its musicians. As explained in Chapter 1, because skill development is culturally bound, a child born in 18th-century Europe was more likely to become a violinist, as compared to a 20th-century New Yorker, who may be more likely to develop as a freestyle rapper, hip-hop singer, or jazz musician. Different skills rise and fall as the need for them rises or falls. People with the potential to become skilled glass harmonica players were not more common in the 19th century than they are now (also mentioned in Chapter 1). Society institutionalizes skill according to changing need and fashion, and musicians change their skill profiles to suit. In this context it becomes clear again that the specific skills of music performance cannot be innate. Human biology and genetics cannot possibly select skills that come and go over periods of time measured in decades.

Among a group of people who are immersed in a particular music tradition, questions about its purpose are not often consciously considered. Especially in certain circles of music academia, people who consider themselves "musicians" rarely possess all the skills expected across all style genres. For example, it is extremely rare to find a conservatory-trained symphony musician who also actively produces rap music, or a jazz musician who is equally adept at operating a turntable, audio mixing console, and other hardware as a club DJ. Those whose musicianship is limited to what has been traditionally valued in formal education settings may gain valuable perspective by realizing that the genres long preferred by music academia account for a very small percentage of the music economy, as shown in Table 12.1.

Again, this is *not* to say that classical music is irrelevant because it is not popular. Such perspective should, however, prompt musicians of all types to embrace a broadened understanding of the uses and functions of music and acknowledge how these can vary markedly between different groups of people. Also, since musical meaning is largely assigned by the human mind, uses and functions of music can also differ between individuals who might otherwise be considered similar.

Table 12.1 Share of Total Music Consumption by Format and Genre for 2019

Genre	Total Volume	Physical Album Sales	Digital Album Sales	On-Demand Streams
R&B/hip-hop	27.7%	10.5%	15.9%	30.7%
Rock	19.8%	42.2%	32.4%	14.7%
Pop	14.0%	11.0%	11.0%	14.7%
Country	7.4%	10.4%	8.1%	5.9%
Latin	5.3%	1.0%	1.0%	8.2%
Dance/ electronic	3.6%	1.0%	2.2%	3.9%
Christian/ gospel	2.3%	4.8%	3.2%	1.8%
World music	1.5%	2.3%	1.7%	1.6%
Holiday/ seasonal	1.4%	3.3%	1.8%	1.0%
Children	1.2%	2.1%	1.9%	1.1%
Jazz	1.1%	2.7%	2.0%	0.7%
Classical	1.0%	2.0%	2.5%	0.7%

Selected top genres, from data reported by Nielsen Music (2020). *Year-End Music Report: U.S. 2019.* https://static.billboard.com/files/pdfs/NIELSEN_2019_YEARENDreportUS.pdf

Group Identity

Many of the world's musical situations involve people doing things together. In fact, a number of English idioms used to express togetherness or cooperation share musical terms, such as *harmony* and *in concert*. Worldwide, a fundamental function of music is the expression of group identity and solidarity (Clayton, 2016). People commonly use music as a symbol or *badge of identity*, to declare to themselves and others who they are and what they value and believe. Communal sharing of music reinforces cooperative and cohesive behavior—musical and social—and therefore establishes and rewards certain culturally acceptable practices (Cross, 2016). Because examples of this are so many and so diverse, several select cases in point, from the research literature, will have to suffice here:

- Choral singing can promote a sense of belonging and camaraderie and create important positive relationships. Research has linked choir participation—and the group singing in particular—to much-needed social support for people dealing with difficult times and life circumstances, including personal trauma and poverty (Bailey & Davidson, 2005; Barrett & Vermeulen, 2019; Kreutz, 2014; Parker, 2010). A sense of fellowship or *communitas*, developed among choristers, serves to advance "the centrality of the group," even over the individual's needs (Parker, 2016, p. 230). In a recent study of choir members' perceived losses when group gathering was prohibited during the 2020 COVID-19 pandemic, the social aspect of choral singing emerged as the element that participants missed the most (Theorell et al., 2020).
- Indigenous peoples use music for social support and a sense of community while they maintain and conserve their cultures (Laurila & Willingham, 2017; Salmon et al., 2019; Shanahan et al., 2016). Based on their research of the drumming circles of Aboriginal women in the Anishnaabe Ojibwe territory of northern Ontario, Canada, Goudreau et al. (2008) offered a framework for understanding the benefits of culturally supportive group music making, shown in Figure 12.1. The outermost ring shows the four broadest health-promotive benefits, the next ring in presents social-supportive benefits, and the innermost ring describes aspects related to four elements of being (mental, physical, emotional, spiritual), all of which exist around the center circle of culture.

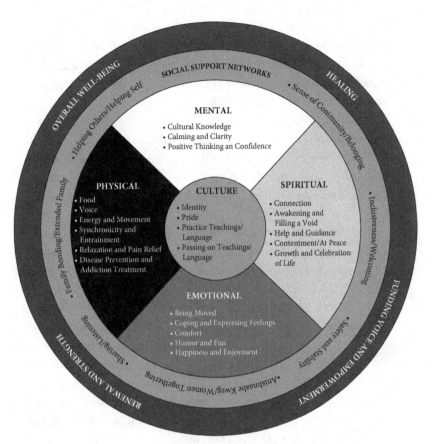

Figure 12.1 Model of the benefits of culturally supportive group music making.

Adapted from Goudreau, G., Weber-Pillwax, C., Cote-Meek, S., Madill, H., & Wilson, S. (2008). Hand drumming: Health-promoting experiences of Aboriginal women from a northern Ontario urban community. *International Journal of Indigenous Health, 4*(1), 72–83. Note: In their original figure, rather than "overall well-being," Goudreau et al. originally used the term *Mino-Bimaadiziwin,* which in the language of the indigenous Ojibwe people translates to "the good life."

- Fans of sports teams and clubs use songs and chants to proclaim their group identity, both to cheer on their athletes and to demoralize opponents (Clark, 2006; Collinson, 2009; Tamir, 2019). The collective and coordinated voices of fans are a key contributor to the affective atmosphere that makes sporting events so dramatic and popular worldwide (Ashmore, 2017).
- Social groups use music as symbols and rallying cries to support their causes of protest, resistance, and political upheaval. In geographic regions all around the world, the political environment has shaped music,

and people have used music to effect political change (Damodaran, 2016; Onyebadi, 2017; Pawłusz, 2018). The music itself varies and evolves interactively with the politics and people who use it. For example, an ethnographic account of American protest music in the 20th century was summarized as follows:

> The tradition of using song to express political ideas flourished in the first four decades of the century, declined due to political repression in the fifth decade, flourished again during the 1960–1980s, and moved to spoken poetry and rap toward the end of the century. (Seeger, 2018, p. 1029)

- Since antiquity, music has been believed to have healing power, a sentiment encapsulated by German Romantic philosopher Novalis's assertion that "every illness is a musical problem, its healing a musical solution" (Horden, 2017, p. 3). Modern research attests to the facilitative role music can have in psychological mourning and healing, including at a sociocultural level (Newberger, 2020). For example, after the 9/11 terrorist attack in the United States in 2001, popular music was identified as being used "in the service of mourning, healing, patriotism, and nation building" (Garofalo, 2012, p. 4; see also Forman, 2002, and Bodner & Gilboa, 2009). The same has been said of musical responses to tragedies in other parts of the world (e.g., see Knudsen, 2017, regarding healing after the Utøya massacre in Norway).

Although these examples feature music as a contributor to positive or prosocial outcomes, it must be pointed out that music is not always used as a "force for good." Indeed, music is used by groups to strengthen cohesion among their members. However, one well-established means by which *ingroup* bonding is accomplished is by members distinguishing or segregating themselves from others considered *outgroup*. For example, Pearce et al. (2016) reported that feelings of closeness among members in university fraternity singing groups increased when they *competed against* groups from other fraternities. Accordingly, just as music can be used to give people a sense of belonging so as to feel "part of something greater" (Gabrielsson, 2010, p. 566), it can also be used to hurt, exclude, and divide people (Kent, 2007).

For an example of music as a two-edged sword, one need look no further than how music has been used to show national identity. When the National Anthem Project was launched in the United States in 2005 by the National

Association for Music Education (then called MENC), it featured prominent governmental, educational, and corporate sponsorship and seemed to many people to promote a particular value system and way of life. What some defined as patriotic, others saw as propagandistic (Garofalo, 2010; see also Hebert & Kertz-Welzel, 2016).

One final phenomenon of contemporary society is so pervasive that it merits special mention. This is the way in which adolescents' overtly expressed musical choices and tastes function as statements about youth identity. Lamont and Hargreaves's (2019) literature review confirmed that the sociocultural roles that music plays in adolescence are central in understanding young people's identity formation, as well as their musical tastes, interests, and skill development, which in many cases remain stable (from adolescence) for a lifetime. Considering teenagers' well-known desire to have positive social status among peers, it is not surprising that the genres that make up so-called popular music are the most preferred by adolescents. Musical choices serve as indicators of values, which are also often very evident in adolescents' image (e.g., hair and clothing styles) matching those modeled by favorite musical artists. A teen group's preferences within popular music are often quite defining of it as a subculture or "clique." Many adolescent social groups rely heavily on accepted music preferences to reinforce their group's identity and to judge others outside of it. Accordingly, adolescents will sometimes hide from their peers individual music preferences that do not match the group's collectively valued music (Greasley et al., 2013).

Cultural Capital

Membership in any musical culture entails making discriminations and judgments that generally correspond with the consensus view. The same social dynamics that are responsible for the emergence of a distinct identifiable culture may also lead a group to become uncompromising in what is considered acceptable and even become hostile toward outsiders. For example, Burnard (2012) credited the cult of Beethoven for the high status and dominance of the music conservatoire and its "privileging of Western classical music above all other musics," preserved as "the canons of good taste" (pp. 1–2). Alternatively, some modern music subcultures assert themselves by virtue of their chosen art's lack of popularity or influence of mass culture. Hibbett (2005) explained a cultural characteristic of indie rock this way:

Obscurity becomes a positive feature, while exclusion is embraced as the necessary consequence of the majority's lack of "taste." Indie rock enthusiasts (those possessing knowledge of indie rock, or "insiders") comprise a social formation similar to the intellectuals or the avant-garde of high culture. (p. 57)

Among those who are insiders—be they indie rock enthusiasts or Beethoven connoisseurs—a less-than-laudatory comment by one of the uninitiated is likely to be met with disapproval or dismissal.

Group members with the greatest social status are those with the ability to engage knowledgeably and take part in informed interchanges about the relative worth of cultural objects and issues. The term *cultural capital*, usually attributed to 20th-century French sociologist and philosopher Pierre Bourdieu (1979), refers to possessing the knowledge, relationships, and skills that allow a person to be accepted as an expert within a domain. Cultural capital can facilitate comparisons and power struggles between individuals within a subculture and between musical genres more broadly. Many people who have no significant music-making skills have nonetheless become connoisseurs of particular styles of music. Sometimes connoisseurship, or "fandom," takes very specific forms, for instance, knowing details about every work written by a certain composer or owning every recording ever made by a particular singer. Some may even achieve the level of curatorship, in which uber fans serve as keepers of the culture and music around which the group is built and bear the responsibility of discriminating good from bad and valuable from vulgar (Barna, 2017). Acquiring this kind of detailed and highly articulated knowledge is a skill in its own right, including for musicians. Unless they become connoisseurs within their chosen styles and musical subcultures, they will not be able to exercise independent aesthetic judgment, but will simply recycle other people's cultural perspective. It is possible for some performers to be less musically informed than members of their audiences!

One issue on which cultural capital is expended is discussing and debating what is authentic or "real" within a musical culture. Many proponents of classical music accept a performance as authentic only if it sounds as it did at the time of the work's composition or premiere (Keen, 2020). In contrast, in rock and popular music, authenticity has more to do with how honest or genuine performers appear than with adherence to performance tradition. The precise definition of authenticity varies between genres, but there is general agreement on the importance of being authentic, whether it is classical music, jazz, or rock and roll (e.g., Dyndahl & Nielsen, 2014; Hibbett, 2005).

Obviously, individual group members' cultural capital affects how others within the group interact with them. Status changes, however, may result when group values shift or a group member's accomplishments increase his or her capital. Just as an individual's capital affects his or her ingroup status, the perceived status of a subculture—within a larger cultural context—can affect how members are treated by outsiders. If group membership is seen as desirable by those who are not in it, the result can be similar to how lower-status members of the group orient to higher-status members. The result is a type of prestige effect, in which people treat generally admired members with unconsidered favoritism and positive regard. One interesting illustration of this was reported by Bongard et al. (2019), who found that young adults' ratings of dating website profiles differed according to whether prospective dates described themselves as people who made music. Specifically, participants who were not music makers themselves gave higher attractiveness ratings to musicians who said they play instruments or sing in private settings. Moreover, in a study of musical improvisation skills, greater musicality generally boosted women's appraisals of men's desirability for dating, sex, and long-term relationships (Madison et al., 2018).

Influencing Group Behavior

Because music is known to be so well liked and emotionally affecting for people, some have utilized music to effect outcomes they desire among people. One area in which this is especially prominent—and there has been research conducted—is consumer behavior. The playing of music (usually from recordings) is a common means of creating an appealing multisensory atmosphere in retail businesses, with the intention of turning positive consumer thoughts and emotions into increased purchase behavior (Helmefalk & Hultén, 2017; Spence et al., 2014). As explained by one research team, ambient music that is well received "sounds like a healthy retail strategy" (Biswas et al., 2019, p. 37). Based on their thorough review of the extant research at the time, North and Hargreaves (2010) concluded that the effects that music can have on consumer behavior are "striking" and that "different types of music very clearly have different effects" (p. 924). More recent research has shown that musical fit—that is, consumers' perceptions of the music's relevance or appropriateness—affects consumer purchase intentions and choices within retail situations (Herget et al., 2020; Kontukoski et al., 2016).

Of course, music in the workplace is heard by employees as well as consumers, and the effects of music in occupational settings also has received a good amount of research attention. The origins of workplace music began with work songs sung by agricultural field workers and other physical laborers before the advent of sound recording technology (Gioia, 2006). Later, in industrial workplaces in the 20th century, the use of music (e.g., the radio played through loudspeakers) generally was thought to have a positive impact on employees (Korczynski, 2003; Prichard et al. 2007). As music technology became more personal and portable, music listening became more common in office work settings. Using various music-playing devices and headphones, employees tend to listen when carrying out solitary routine desk work (Haake, 2011; Lamont et al., 2016). In such contexts, music users are provided a private space within a public workplace with the potential to prevent distraction and interruption (Dibben & Haake, 2013). Landay and Harms (2019) succinctly explained the potential of music to improve productivity and employee morale, saying that, according to the research, "music works through the mediator of mood and emotion" (p. 371). As illustrated in their model, presented in Figure 12.2, the music interacts with other factors to ultimately affect the outcomes of task performance, organizational citizenship behaviors (OCBs), and job-related training. In this model, being able to choose one's own music (listening autonomy) is an important factor to modern workers, and their desired mood or mindset (to be induced by music) depends on the complexity of the work tasks for which they are responsible.

On the topic of influencing behavior, one question seems to persist in piquing popular interest: does listening to certain types of music incite socially delinquent or undesirable behavior? Concern often arises when popularity (among young people) is achieved by music that ostensibly has content that is illicitly sexual, violent, or suicide related. Upon reviewing the extant research on the matter, North and Hargreaves (2012) concluded that young fans of such music are more likely to come from home environments that "experience higher than normal levels of family dysfunction" and that this factor is a more probable cause of undesirable behavioral outcomes than the music they hear (p. 506).

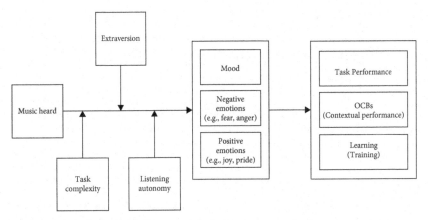

Figure 12.2 Effect of music on work behavior.

From Landay, K., & Harms, P. D. (2019). Whistle while you work? A review of the effects of music in the workplace. *Human Resource Management Review*, *29*(3), 371–385. https://doi.org/10.1016/j.hrmr.2018.06.003

Individualistic Functions of Music

Social uses of music, such as those described previously, create associations in the minds of individuals that can have their own personal functional power. Music associated with key people, groups, or events can invoke personal reminiscences of emotional relationships. It often has a memorial or nostalgic component; Davies (1978) aptly called this the "darling, they're playing our tune" effect. Among the many personal roles of music listening, serving as a reminder of valued past events has been shown to be one of the most common (Sloboda, 2005c). Although people are quite often alone when they use music in this way, the function is also social, as it points to a relationship or a group situation that was very memorable to the individual.

As alluded to in Chapter 1, there are a number of functions that music plays cross-culturally in human societies around the world, such as in institutional ceremonies and religious rituals. Such functions are found in many of the cultures of the world and across history. In more recent and industrialized societies, however, sounded music can be separated from the act of live performance through recording and playback technology. Accordingly, new and enhanced functions have emerged. Music can be used far from its originally intended setting, and an individual alone can engage with a very wide range of music. Portable music players allow people to hear music wherever they choose and during whatever activity they are engaged. For many people, it is possible in every moment of the day to hear music at the press of a button. Once the basic technology is in place, individuals need not relate to or interact with anyone else in their music consumption.

Soundtrack of Life

Research has shed light on how individuals use music as a private resource to manage and enhance everyday life (e.g., Batt-Rawden & DeNora, 2005; Krause et al., 2014, 2016; Saarikallio et al., 2013, 2020; Sloboda, 2010). Two very important general conclusions can be drawn from this research. First, people generally use music in everyday life as background to accompany something else that they are doing. The primary activities are varied and include domestic chores, commuting, studying, and other tasks of one's daily routine. This means that the concentrated and motionless focused listening is almost entirely absent from this everyday contemporary use of music. Rather than any close tracking of the melodies or structure, people generally use the music for a soundscape and the induced mood of the music (also see Chapter 11).

The second important conclusion to draw from the research is that listening to music in this way remains extremely valuable to people. Users of music widely credit it for improving their moods and helping them to handle or enjoy situations they are in. Therefore, rather than everyday listening as "background music," it is better understood as the "soundtrack" that people choose for their lives (Forman, 2002; Heye & Lamont, 2010; Lamont et al., 2016). Mood improvement is greatest in those cases in which people can exercise high degrees of choice over what music they hear and when they hear it. As shown in Chapter 3, the importance of personal autonomy in creating one's own musical life extends well beyond choosing music for listening.

Although music can be heard in almost any life context, the research suggests that travel is an especially common activity to be accompanied by music listening (Greb et al., 2018; Heye & Lamont, 2010; Saarikallio et al., 2020; Skånland, 2013). In industrialized societies, people spend huge amounts of time in cars, buses, trains, and airplanes. In all of these contexts, recorded music is not simply used to pass the time but very often chosen deliberately to assist a transition in mood or energy that is required during the journey. For instance, someone commuting to work in the morning may listen to upbeat, energetic music to obtain energy and focus for the day. The same person traveling home after a hard day's work may choose his or her favorite mellow, soothing music to detach from the stresses of work and prepare for a relaxing evening at home.

For many people, the setting in which they listen to music most consistently is driving a car (Dibben & Williamson, 2007; George et al., 2018). Drivers credit music for relaxing them and sometimes helping them to concentrate while driving and, accordingly, tend to believe that listening to music improves the quality of their driving. Compared to other potential contributors to distracted driving, music seems to be regarded as less dangerous than many others. In fact, research exploring smartphone apps to prevent distracted driving have left music playing intact, along with GPS navigation, as these functions are thought to support driving and require minimal visual-manual attention from drivers (Oviedo-Trespalacios et al., 2019). The research, however, shows that using music while driving can present possible risk factors (Millet et al., 2019). Likely the most dangerous moments are those when listener-drivers choose their music, such as searching for a radio station to their liking or scrolling through the available music on a smartphone (Lee et al., 2012; Millet et al., 2019). In addition, the listening itself can be distracting inasmuch as the music can attentionally absorb drivers into following and thinking about the musical sounds heard or emotionally engage them in reminiscing about past life experience. If the emotional effects of this are particularly intense, it is easy to see how listening could detract from the necessary attention to safely operate the vehicle. Another potential source of impairment to driving is when people engage in the music themselves, by singing along, drumming on the steering wheel, playing "air guitar," or dancing in their seat, which some drivers surely do (Brodsky, 2015; Dibben & Williamson, 2007). Still, listening while driving is an activity that few car-owning music lovers are likely to give up. Perhaps especially among young people, listening to music while driving constitutes much-valued time when they can assert their music preferences and express their identities. After Brodsky and Kizner (2012) specially designed music to be minimally distracting to drivers, subsequent research found that although younger and less experienced drivers preferred their self-chosen music, their driving was less aggressive and error-prone when listening to the researcher-designed less distracting music (Brodsky & Slor, 2013).

Physical exercise is another aspect of modern life in which music users hope to improve task performance. As with other areas of individual music use, having personal choice in what is heard has been found to be very consequential in the perceived effectiveness of the music (Hallet & Lamont, 2017). Enhanced athletic performance produced by music also largely results from its effect on exercisers' affective state, including their mood, motivation, and feelings about the physical exertion required of them (Clark et al., 2016; Karageorghis, 2020). Athletes of a variety of levels have reported that they most often listen to music during training and pre-event preparations and warmup. Their main reasons for using music involve increasing arousal, motivation, self-confidence, positive mood, endurance, and feelings of being "in the zone" (Karageorghis & Priest, 2012; Laukka & Quick, 2013).

Defining the User

It warrants reinforcing that although people use music to accompany other activities, they do *not* consider the music to be incidental. In television and film, the musical soundtrack is an important component of the emotional communication and message of the artwork. So too is the music for people who use it as soundtrack to their lives. In this way, they generally believe that having music during many moments of their days does not merely help pass the time, but makes their lives better.

The word *user* throughout this chapter demands acknowledgment that the word has two common referents: a person who operates a computer (or other machine) and one who takes illicit drugs. It is interesting to consider to which of these the music user is most similar. In fact, music has been compared to drugs for its potential analgesic effect, that is, the ability to relieve, reduce, or manage pain (Cepeda et al., 2006; Herbrand & Silverman, 2020; Lu et al., 2020; Richard-Lalonde et al., 2020). Reviews of the research on music-supported pain management have affirmed that music can have a significant effect on pain reduction, that personal choice of preferred music is an important variable, and that data are lacking to conclusively identify what musical characteristics contribute to perceived pain reduction (Martin-Saavedra, Vergara-Mendez, & Talero-Gutiérrez, 2018; Martin-Saavedra, Vergara-Mendez, Pradilla, et al., 2018; Mitchell & MacDonald, 2012).

Denora (2003) offered a different comparison of music use to drug use when she likened music lovers to drug addicts in how they often carefully set up the optimal conditions for using their product of choice and their desire for the experience to be one in which "the self is 'abandoned' or given over to sensation and/or emotion" (p. 171). Similarly, the pleasure-seeking functions of music suggest it compares to the human activity of sex. Taylor (2012) is one of the few researchers who has considered the matter, having noted that among scholars, "there has been little discussion of music's ability to evoke and choreograph erotic action." This point is surprising, "given that there are hundreds of websites that claim to rank 'the best music to have sex to' and thousands of online forum discussions concerning what music works best in sexual situations" (p. 607). In her small-scale survey study, people overwhelmingly acknowledged their belief that music is a useful—even essential—device in structuring sexual activity of varied types. Beyond simply "setting the mood," music was cited for its ability to cue the emotional intensity and determine the kind of sex to be had (e.g., "raw and frantic sex" or "I warn you I am emotional and this encounter comes with heartstrings," p. 608).

Coping Through Music

Research also has shown that people quite commonly use music to manage emotions during difficult circumstances of life. The field of music therapy, as a whole, has as its primary purpose presenting music as a resource that people can use to adapt and cope when they are "living with profound health problems, disabilities and difficulties, facing daily issues of struggle, loss and pain" (Bunt, 2012, p. 165). Among people who use music listening to cope, it seems likely that personality type interacts with the effectiveness of music as a coping strategy; listening to music may work best for those with high trait neuroticism but who are willing to face or engage with their problems and emotions (Miranda et al., 2010). Similarly, private music listening may be especially helpful to those who seek relief from stresses perceived to originate in the environment around them and who find comfort in feelings of solitude (Skånland, 2011).

For others, social interaction and inclusion are key to their needs for coping, healing, or recovery. Toward this end, psychological research has provided evidence that active music making may be especially efficacious in helping people cope with difficult life circumstances and pursue health and well-being (Hanser, 2010; Hargreaves & Lamont, 2017). For example, research has shown that group music making can provide social and emotional support for a variety of people in need, including individuals who are vulnerable to drug and alcohol addiction (Harrison, 2019), people with chronic mental health conditions (Williams et al., 2020), and spouse caregivers of people with Parkinson's disease (Forbes, 2020b). It is well known that adolescence can be a difficult time even in the best circumstances, so coping ability is even more critical when young people have to deal with special challenges, such as lack of family support, ethnic-based discrimination, or a physical, sensory, or cognitive disability. Research with youth facing such challenges has shown that participating in musical activities can be beneficial, including socially by making friendships with others (Cheong-Clinch, 2009; Lindblom, 2017).

Finally, in a large-scale questionnaire study conducted during the 2020 COVID-19 pandemic, music emerged as the best activity to cope with psychological distress (Mas-Herrero et al., 2020). The data, provided primarily from individuals in Italy, Spain, and the United States, showed that time spent engaged in music activities correlated with decreased symptoms of depression. The researchers concluded:

> Our results demonstrate that music is an important means of improving well-being, and suggest that the underlying mechanism is related to reward, consistent with neuroscience findings. Our data have practical significance in pointing to effective strategies to cope with mental health issues. (p. 1)

An understanding of the neurology and physiology of music's coping power has begun to emerge in the research. A study of group singing by Keeler et al. (2015) reported hormonal changes (specifically oxytocin and adrenocorticotropic hormone) indicative of reduced stress and increased social flow. Chanda and Levitin (2013) corroborated the positive effects of group singing and added that group drumming circles have been shown to increase lymphocyte cell activity and 5-DHA-to-cortisol ratio, both of which suggest enhanced immune system functioning. In an overview of the psychoneuroimmunology of music, Fancourt (2016) concluded that the research data suggest promising links between music and the immune system, but that much remains to be discovered.

Music as a Booster

Clearly, music is a beloved human phenomenon. Users quickly and freely avail themselves of music with designs to improve important aspects of their lives. Perhaps it is not surprising, then, that this context has given rise to speculation about the capacity of music to enhance nonmusical abilities in people. One prominent example of this was the Music Makes You Smarter movement that arose around the turn of the 21st century (e.g., Demorest & Morrison, 2000). When making such overreaching claims about the power of music, people often cite the "Mozart effect" as evidence. A closer look at the actual research, however, shows that the Mozart effect that was reported by the original researchers provides little support to claims that music boosts intelligence, IQ scores, or academic achievement. The original study of Rauscher et al. (1993) found that college students did better on a spatial rea-soning task—measured by a pattern analysis test, multiple-choice matrices test, and multiple-choice paper-folding and -cutting test—after listening to a 10-minute Mozart piano piece, as compared to sitting in silence or hearing a relaxation tape. The researchers also reported, though, that the effect was temporary and did not extend beyond 10 to 15 minutes. They also acknowl-edged that their research did not address other more common measures of general intelligence, such as verbal, math, or memory skills, or whether the effect could be generalized to music of other composers or styles; in fact, they explicitly theorized that different music "may interfere with, rather than en-hance, abstract reasoning" (p. 611).

Despite the limitations stated by the researchers, their very specific result somehow led many music stakeholders to proudly assert that exposure to music boosts general intelligence. A more carefully considered appraisal of the situation has explained that the music-for-intelligence movement was born out of a societal and political climate in which music had relatively low status as a discipline, making it vulnerable to elimination when budgets had to be cut. Therefore, in multiple ways, claiming "music makes you smarter" was an example of "the timeless and universal appeal of quick fixes to com-plex problems" (Schellenberg, 2016, p. 149). Further, since the time of the original 1993 study, other researchers have been largely unsuccessful in pro-ducing similar results. Pietschnig and colleagues (2010) conducted a compre-hensive meta-analysis of Mozart effect research, examining nearly 40 studies involving over 3,000 participants combined; their research concluded there was little evidence supporting the existence of a direct music-to-intelligence effect from music exposure through listening.

This is not to say, however, that music cannot indirectly contribute to enhancement in other activities and performance on nonmusical cogni-tive tasks. As explained in this chapter, as well as the previous one, music is unquestionably capable of affecting listeners' moods and levels of arousal, and changing people's feelings can, in turn, influence how they carry out physical and cognitive tasks (Schellenberg, 2012). Further, the research suggests much stronger links between music and nonmusical abilities when the type of music activity under consideration goes beyond mere exposure through listening.

More specifically, incorporating music into instruction can facilitate learning in other subject areas (e.g., Gaboury et al., 2020) and extended musical training can produce superior perceptual and psychomotor abilities that may transfer to other types of activities. Herholz and Zatorre (2012) have explained this from a neurological perspective:

> Musical training not only changes the structural and functional properties of the brain, but it also seems to affect the potential for new short-term learning and plasticity. Such interaction effects of long- and short-term training have been demonstrated in the auditory (Herholz et al., 2011), in the motor (Rosenkranz et al., 2007) and in the tactile domain (Ragert et al., 2004). (p. 493)

Again, however, one must temper applications of such transfer effects with a realistic understanding of music and psychology. For example, learning to play the piano from the notation of a traditional method book is very different from learning to play ear-based and improvisatory jazz saxophone through informal participation in jam sessions under the mentoring of more experienced players. Visuospatial and tactile benefits are more likely from notation-based experiences on the patterned layout of a piano keyboard, whereas auditory and socioemotional benefits seem more likely from the informal jazz saxophone experience. As shown throughout this chapter, the ways that people effectively use music to impact their lives are many, but "if a child is struggling with math, will thoughtful parents' response be to find more music opportunities for her? More likely, they'll look to get her some better math instruction" (Woody, 2019, p. 28).

Implications for Musicians

In summary, the psychological research on the music user indicates that music is a much-valued and consistently impactful element of many people's lives. Although in the case of music listening the music occurs in the "background" while people carry out other tasks, nevertheless, the music can powerfully affect people's emotion and level of physiological arousal, which can enhance how they experience the tasks they do and even improve the effectiveness with which they do them. On both individual and cultural levels, music commonly serves as a symbol or badge of identity for people to declare to themselves and others who they are and what they stand for. Indeed, throughout history and into current modern times, music has served many important functions for groups of people of all sizes and locations around the world.

Musicians can feel great comfort and pride knowing that according to the research, music is extraordinarily valued by virtually all people. By sharing their music with others, musicians actively contribute to an important domain that is distinctively human and, by all accounts, practically essential to health and well-being. Anyone who asserts that music is simply a distraction or "mere entertainment" does so from a place of ignorance (Woody, 2019, p. 27). In reality, music is a universally human phenomenon and one that is beloved and powerful, at that.

Finally, the person-focused approach to music, explained in an early section of this chapter, connects very meaningfully to the perspective of psychology as presented in Chapter 1 of this book. The person-focused approach to music emphasizes the impact music has and the purposes it serves for all people, the producers and the consumers alike. In the same vein, psychology as a whole seeks to understand all people: their thought processes, their emotions, and their behavior. As pointed out in Chapter 1, music is made *by* human beings *for* human beings, and *people* are the most important elements of music. Psychology is, therefore, an integral lens through which music must be considered. Similarly, the person-focused approach to music is not a perspective that musicians can afford to ignore in favor of focusing purely on music as an object for analysis. The field of psychology has provided much supporting evidence for the position that music is a fascinating yet indispensable facet of human life. People who identify as musicians should know that they can enhance their musical lives if they glean insight from the findings of psychology, and all other members of the human race should know that they can benefit meaningfully as they seek opportunities to become more musical themselves.

Taking the Stage: Connect with Community

Few people are members of only a single culture. Musicians wanting to connect with potential audience members and patrons should take stock of their own subcultures and communities of which they are a part. Most will find that they identify with quite a few groups based on, for example, their ethnic background, affiliations with schools or other institutions, or even places of business that they frequent. They may even be members of online communities, perhaps built around their preferred genres of music or instruments played. These groups, in which they already have some social standing, may be prime targets for performers' musical outreach rather than thinking of potential audience members as nameless, faceless strangers. Of course, performers also should not forget about the communities of which they are a part because of where they live. The other inhabitants of their cities, towns, and residential areas likely see their musician neighbors as interesting—if it is known they are musicians—and people whose activities they may want to support. Performers also can connect in their geographic communities by sharing their music as a service to vulnerable people and those in need of an emotional boost, such as residents of nursing homes and other care facilities. Such settings are ones in which it can be critical to apply the advice of the Chapter 9 "Taking the Stage" Sidebar Box: Bridge the Divide, in which performers are encouraged to incorporate "audience participation" into their performances, if only by having conversations with those in attendance before and after the performance. Also, while onstage, musicians can informally talk to the audience about the music and the music making and invite questions from audience members.

Leading Learning: Teach to the Music User

Teachers should always remember that the young people they teach are not only students but also human beings. Music is not simply a subject matter of study for them as outlined in a stated curriculum. Music is also a valued and meaningful part of their personal lives. In an article titled "Educating the Music User," Adams (2016) has offered suggestions and teaching strategies to prepare students for "lifelong participation in and enjoyment of music" (p. 64). To accomplish this, teachers need to understand what music truly means to their students. They can gain this insight through discussions, which can be initiated by inviting students to think deeply about the music they like and respond to questions about *why* they like it and what qualities of performers and pieces they consider characteristic of "good music." Instead of seeking to move students away from the music they currently like, teachers can help them grow within their tastes and preferences. For example, starting from a single song they love, students can be given the homework of listening to the rest of the album from which the song appears as a track or listening to other music by the same artist. If desired, they could be assigned to write a review as a music critic would in a newspaper or magazine. Alternatively, students could also be asked to find online and watch (e.g., on YouTube) a live performance of their favorite song and note the performance techniques they see and what elements contribute to the energy and spectacle of live music performance. Because most music teachers have extensive backgrounds as music makers themselves, asking their students to simply discuss and evaluate music may not feel like enough. Indeed, all students need music making experiences in their education. From the perspective of the music user, however, they also can benefit from opportunities to express and explore their own musical tastes and values. The ability to do so effectively will allow them to participate in and enjoy musical subcultures in which they come in contact in their lives.

Chapter 12 Discussion Questions

1. How much exposure and experience have you had with the work-focused and person-focused approaches to music? From your own background and having known other musicians who identify with one or the other, what do you think is the primary appeal of each?
2. How much of a connoisseur or curator are you with respect to the types of music you perform most?
3. What activities do you like to do with music playing in the background? Do you choose a particular style of music for this purpose? When you use music in this way, do you think it makes you more effective or productive in the main activity you are doing?

References

Abell, A. M. (2016/1955). *Talks with great composers*. Auckland, NZ: Pickle Partners Publishing.

Abril, C. R. (2013). Perspectives on the school band from hardcore American band kids. In P. S. Campbell & T. Wiggins (Eds.), *The Oxford handbook of children's musical cultures* (pp. 435–448). New York, NY: Oxford University Press.

Adams, M. C. (2016). Educating the music user. *Music Educators Journal, 103*(1), 64–69. doi:10.1177/0027432116651117

Adams, M. C. (in press). Songwriting and the importance of classroom community. In S. Burton (Ed.), *Engaging musical practices: A sourcebook for middle school general music* (2nd ed.). Lanham, MD: Rowman and Littlefield.

Akkermans, J., Schapiro, R., Müllensiefen, D., Jakubowski, K., Shanahan, D., Baker, D., Busch, V., Lothwesen, K., Elvers, P., Fischinger, T., Schlemmer, K., & Fieler, K. (2019). Decoding emotions in expressive music performances: A multi-lab replication and extension study. *Cognition and Emotion, 33*, 1099–1118.

Allen, R. (2013). Free improvisation and performance anxiety among piano students. *Psychology of Music, 41*(1), 75–88. doi:10.1177/0305735611415750

Allsup, R. E. (2003). Mutual learning and democratic action in instrumental music education. *Journal of Research in Music Education, 51*, 24–37. https://doi.org/10.2307/3345646

Arnett, J. J. (Ed.). (2016). *The Oxford handbook of emerging adulthood*. New York, NY: Oxford University Press.

Arrais, N., & Rodrigues, H. (2007). Cognitive feedback and metaphors in emotional communication instruction of musical performance. In A. Williamon & D. Coimbra (Eds.), *Proceedings of the International Symposium on Performance Science 2007* (pp. 265–270). Utrecht, The Netherlands: Association Européenne des Conservatoires, Académies de Musique et Musikhochschulen (AEC).

Ascenso, S., Williamon, A., & Perkins, R. (2017). Understanding the wellbeing of professional musicians through the lens of Positive Psychology. *Psychology of Music, 45*(1), 65–81. doi:10.1177/0305735616646864

Ashley, R. (2004). *All his yesterdays: Expressive vocal techniques in Paul McCartney's recordings*. Unpublished manuscript.

Ashley, R. (2016). Musical improvisation. In S. Hallam, I. Cross, & M. Thaut (Eds.), *The Oxford handbook of music psychology* (2nd ed., pp. 667–679). Oxford, UK: Oxford University Press.

Ashmore, P. (2017). Of other atmospheres: Football spectatorship beyond the terrace chant. *Soccer & Society, 18*(1), 30–46. doi:10.1080/14660970.2014.980743

Asia, D. (2018). Front and center: The place for Western Classical music in the curriculum. *Academic Questions, 31*(4), 424–431. doi:10.1007/s12129-018-9744-y

Aufegger, L., Perkins, R., Wasley, D., & Williamon, A. (2017). Musicians' perceptions and experiences of using simulation training to develop performance skills. *Psychology of Music*, 45(3), 417–431. doi:10.1177/0305735616666940

Austin, J. R., & Berg, M. H. (2006). Exploring music practice among sixth-grade band and orchestra students. *Psychology of Music*, 34, 535–558. doi:01.0077/1315735616167071

Austin, J. R., Isbell, D. S., & Russell, J. A. (2012). A multi-institution exploration of secondary socialization and occupational identity among undergraduate music majors. *Psychology of Music*, 40(1), 66–83. doi:10.1177/0305735610381886

Baer, J. (2018). The trouble with "creativity." In R. J. Sternberg & J. C. Kaufman (Eds.), *The nature of human creativity* (pp. 16–31). Cambridge, UK: Cambridge University Press.

Baer, J., & Kaufman, J. C. (2005). Bridging generality and specificity: The amusement park theoretical (APT) model of creativity. *Roeper Review*, 27(3), 158–163. doi:10.1080/02783190509554310

Bagert, M., Peschel, T., Schlaug, G., Rotte, M., Drescher, D., Hinirichs, H., Heinze, H., & Altenmüller, E. (2006). Shared networks for auditory and motor processing in professional pianists: Evidence from fMRI conjunction. *NeuroImage*, 30(3), 917–926. doi:10.1016/j.neuroimage.2005.10.044

Bailey, B. A., & Davidson, J. W. (2005). Effects of group singing and performance for marginalized and middle-class singers. *Psychology of Music*, 33(3), 269–303.

Baily, J. (1985). Music structure and human movement. In P. Howell, I. Cross, & R. West (Eds.), *Musical structure and cognition* (pp. 237–258). London, UK: Academic Press.

Bakan, M. B. (1999). *Music of death and new creation: Experiences in the world of Balinese gamelan beleganjur.* Chicago, IL: University of Chicago Press.

Baker, C., & Brown, B. (2016). Suicide, self-harm and survival strategies in contemporary heavy metal music: A cultural and literary analysis. *Journal of Medical Humanities*, 37(1), 1–17. doi:10.1007/s10912-014-9274-8

Bandura, A. (1977). Self-efficacy: Toward a unifying theory of behavioral change. *Psychological Review*, 84, 191–215.

Barna, E. (2017). "The perfect guide in a crowded musical landscape": Online music platforms and curatorship. *First Monday*, 22(4). https://doi.org/10.5210/fm.v22i4.6914

Barrett, M., & Vermeulen, D. (2019). Drop everything and sing the music: Choristers' perceptions of the value of participating in a multicultural south African university choir. *Muziki*, 16(1), 31–60. doi:10.1080/18125980.2019.1611384

Batt-Rawden, K., & DeNora, T. (2005). Music and informal learning in everyday life. *Music Education Research*, 7(3), 289–304. doi:10.1080/14613800500324507

Bauer, W. I., & Berg, M. H. (2001). Influences on instrumental music teaching. *Bulletin of the Council for Research in Music Education*, 53–66. https://www.jstor.org/stable/40319099

Bazan, D. (2011). The use of student-directed instruction by middle school band teachers. *Bulletin of the Council for Research in Music Education*, 189, 23–56. https://doi.org/10.5406/bulcouresmusedu.189.0023

Bazan, D. E. (2010). Planning and assessment practices of high school band directors. In L. K. Thompson & M. R. Campbell (Eds.), *Issues of identity in music education: Narratives and practices* (pp. 109–125). Charlotte, NC: Information Age.

Bean, K. L. (1938). An experimental approach to the reading of music. *Psychological Monographs*, 50, 1–80.

Beaty, R. E. (2015). The neuroscience of musical improvisation. *Neuroscience & Biobehavioral Reviews*, 51, 108–117. https://doi.org/10.1016/j.neubiorev.2015.01.004

Beeching, A. M. (2016). Who is audience? *Arts and Humanities in Higher Education, 15*(3–4), 395–400. doi:10.1177/1474022216647390

Beeman, W. O. (2005). Making grown men weep. In A. Hobart & B. Kapferer (Eds.), *Aesthetics and performance: The art of rite* (pp. 23–42). New York, NY: Berghahn Books.

Behne, K. E., & Wöllner, C. (2011). Seeing or hearing the pianists? A synopsis of an early audiovisual perception experiment and a replication. *Musicae Scientiae, 15*(3), 324–342. doi:10.1177/1029864911410955

Bender, T. S., & Hancock, C. B. (2010). The effect of conductor intensity and ensemble performance quality on musicians' evaluations of conductor effectiveness. *Journal of Band Research, 46*, 13–22.

Benedek, M., Borovnjak, B., Neubauer, A. C., & Kruse-Weber, S. (2014). Creativity and personality in classical, jazz and folk musicians. *Personality and Individual Differences, 63*, 117–121. http://dx.doi.org/10.1016/j.paid.2014.01.064

Bennett, D. (2016). Developing employability in higher education music. *Arts and Humanities in Higher Education, 15*(3–4), 386–395. doi:10.1177/1474022216647388

Berg, M. H. (2000). Thinking for yourself: The social construction of chamber music experience. In R. R. Rideout & S. J. Paul (Eds.), *On the sociology of music education: II. Papers from the Music Education Symposium at the University of Oklahoma* (pp. 91–112). Amherst, MA: University of Massachusetts.

Bergee, M. J. (2005). An exploratory comparison of novice, intermediate, and expert orchestral conductors. *International Journal of Music Education, 23*(1), 23–36. doi:10.1177/0255761405050928

Berglin, J. (2015). "It's much more collaborative": Democratic action in contemporary collegiate a cappella. *Bulletin of the Council for Research in Music Education, 205*, 51–69. https://www.jstor.org/stable/10.5406/bulcouresmusedu.205.0051

Bergreen, L. (2012). *Louis Armstrong: An extravagant life.* New York, NY: Random House.

Berkowitz, A. L. (2010). *The improvising mind: Cognition and creativity in the musical moment.* New York, NY: Oxford University Press.

Berkowitz, A. L. (2016). The cognitive neuroscience of improvisation. In G. E. Lewis & B. Piekut (Eds.), *The Oxford handbook of critical improvisation studies* (Vol. 1, pp. 56–73). New York, NY: Oxford University Press.

Berkowitz, A. L., & Ansari, D. (2008). Generation of novel motor sequences: The neural correlates of musical improvisation. *NeuroImage, 41*(2), 535–543. doi:10.1016/j.neuroimage.2008.02.028

Berliner, P. (2009/1994). *Thinking in jazz: The infinite art of improvisation.* Chicago, IL: University of Chicago Press.

Bernhard, C. (2010). A survey of burnout among college music majors: A replication. *Music Performance Research, 3*(1), 31–41.

Bernhard, H. C., II. (2004). The effects of tonal training on the melodic ear playing and sight reading achievement of beginning wind instrumentalists. *Contributions to Music Education, 31*(1), 91–107. http://www.jstor.com/stable/24133280

Biasutti, M. (2015). Pedagogical applications of cognitive research on musical improvisation. *Frontiers in Psychology, 6*, article 614. https://doi.org/10.3389/fpsyg.2015.00614

Biasutti, M. (2017). Teaching improvisation through processes. Applications in music education and implications for general education. *Frontiers in Psychology, 8*, article 911. https://doi.org/10.3389/fpsyg.2017.00911

Biasutti, M., & Frezza, L. (2009). Dimensions of music improvisation. *Creativity Research Journal, 21*(2–3), 232–242. doi:10.1080/10400410902861240

Biddlecombe, T. (2012). Assessing and enhancing feedback of choral conductors through analysis and training. *International Journal of Research in Choral Singing, 4*(1), 2–18.

Bisesi, E., & Windsor, W. L. (2016). Expression and communication of structure in music performance. In S. Hallam, I. Cross, & M. Thaut (Eds.), *The Oxford handbook of music psychology* (2nd ed., pp. 615–631). Oxford, UK: Oxford University Press.

Bishop, L. (2018). Collaborative musical creativity: How ensembles coordinate spontaneity. *Frontiers in Psychology, 9*, article 1285. https://doi.org/10.3389/fpsyg.2018.01285

Biswas, D., Lund, K., & Szocs, C. (2019). Sounds like a healthy retail atmospheric strategy: Effects of ambient music and background noise on food sales. *Journal of the Academy of Marketing Science, 47*(1), 37–55. https://doi.org/10.1007/s11747-018-0583-8

Bjøntegaard, B. J. (2015). A combination of one-to-one teaching and small group teaching in higher music education in Norway—a good model for teaching? *British Journal of Music Education, 32*(1), 23–36. doi:10.1017/S026505171400014X

Blackwell, J. (2020). Expertise in applied studio teaching: Teachers working with multiple levels of learners. *International Journal of Music Education, 38*(2), 283–298. doi:10.1177/0255761419898312

Blank, M., & Davidson, J. W. (2007). An exploration of the effects of musical and social factors in piano duo collaborations. *Psychology of Music, 35*(2), 213–230. doi:10.1177/0305735607070306

Bleilock, S. (2011). *Choke: What the secrets of the brain reveal about getting it right when you have to.* New York, NY: Free Press.

Blum, D. (1998). *Quintet: Five journeys toward musical fulfillment.* Ithaca, NY: Cornell University Press.

Bodner, E., & Gilboa, A. (2009). On the power of music to affect intergroup relations. *Musicae Scientiae, 13*(1), 85–115. https://doi.org/10.1177/1029864909013001004

Bogunović, B. (2019). Creative cognition in composing music. *New Sound International Journal of Music, 53*(1), 89–117.

Bonds, M. E. (2014). *Absolute music: The history of an idea.* New York, NY: Oxford University Press.

Bongard, S., Schulz, I., Studenroth, K. U., & Frankenberg, E. (2019). Attractiveness ratings for musicians and non-musicians: An evolutionary-psychology perspective. *Frontiers in Psychology, 10*, article 2627. https://doi.org/10.3389/fpsyg.2019.02627

Bonnano, G. A., Goorin, L., & Coffman, K. C. (2008). Sadness and grief. In M. Lewis, J. M. Haviland-Jones, & L. F. Barrett (Eds.), *Handbook of emotions* (3rd ed., pp. 797–810). New York, NY: Guilford Press.

Bonneville-Roussy, A., & Bouffard, T. (2015). When quantity is not enough: Disentangling the roles of practice time, self-regulation and deliberate practice in musical achievement. *Psychology of Music, 43*(5), 686–704. doi:10.1177/0305735614534910

Bonneville-Roussy, A., Hruska, E., & Trower, H. (2020). Teaching music to support students: How autonomy supportive music teachers increase students' well-being. *Journal of Research in Music Education, 68*(1), 97–119. doi:10.1177/0022429419897611

Bonneville-Roussy, A., Lavigne, G. L., & Vallerand, R. J. (2011). When passion leads to excellence: The case of musicians. *Psychology of Music, 39*(1), 123–138. doi:10.1177/0305735609352441

Bonneville-Roussy, A., & Vallerand, R. J. (2020). Passion at the heart of musicians' well-being. *Psychology of Music, 48*(2), 266–282. doi:10.1177/0305735618797180

Bonneville-Roussy, A., Vallerand, R. J., & Bouffard, T. (2013). The roles of autonomy support and harmonious and obsessive passions in educational persistence. *Learning and Individual Differences, 24*, 22–31. http://dx.doi.org/10.1016/j.lindif.2012.12.015

Borowiec, J., Hökelmann, A., & Osiński, W. (2019). The level of self-esteem of deaf children: Can participating in dance lessons with vibrational headphones improve it? *Arts in Psychotherapy, 64*, 34–38. https://doi.org/10.1016/j.aip.2019.03.004

Bourdieu, P. (1979). *Distinction: A social critique of the judgement of taste*. London, UK: Routledge.

Boyle, J. D., & Radocy, R. E. (1987). *Measurement and evaluation of music experiences*. New York, NY: Schirmer Books.

Brang, D., & Ramachandran, V. S. (2011). Survival of the synesthesia gene: Why do people hear colors and taste words? *PLoS Biology, 9*(11), e1001205. doi:10.1371/journal.pbio.1001205

Bregman, A. S. (1994). *Auditory scene analysis: The perceptual organization of sound*. Cambridge, MA: MIT Press.

Brittin, R. V. (2005). Preservice and experienced teachers' lesson plans for beginning instrumentalists. *Journal of Research in Music Education, 53*(1), 26–39.

Brodsky, W. (2015). *Driving with music: Cognitive behavioral implications*. Surrey, UK: Ashgate.

Brodsky, W., & Kizner, M. (2012). Exploring an alternative in-car music background designed for driver safety. *Transportation Research Part F: Traffic Psychology and Behaviour, 15*(2), 162–173. https://doi.org/10.1016/j.trf.2011.12.001

Brodsky, W., & Slor, Z. (2013). Background music as a risk factor for distraction among young-novice drivers. *Accident Analysis & Prevention, 59*, 382–393. https://doi.org/10.1016/j.aap.2013.06.022

Brothers, T. D. (2007). *Louis Armstrong's New Orleans*. New York, NY: W. W. Norton & Company.

Brown, R. M., & Palmer, C. (2012). Auditory-motor learning influences auditory memory for music. *Memory & Cognition, 40*, 567–578. doi:10.3758/s13421-011-0177-x

Browning, B. (2017). *An orientation to musical pedagogy: Becoming a musician-educator*. New York, NY: Oxford University Press.

Brugués, A. O. (2011). Music performance anxiety—part 2. A review of treatment options. *Medical Problems of Performing Artists, 26*, 164–171.

Bugaj, K. A., Mick, J., & Darrow, A. (2019). The relationship between high-level violin performers' movement and evaluators' perception of musicality. *String Research Journal, 9*, 23–33. doi:10.1177/1948499219851374

Bugos, J., & Lee, W. (2015). Perceptions of challenge: The role of catastrophe theory in piano learning. *Music Education Research, 17*(3), 312–326. doi:10.1080/14613808.2014.899334

Bunt, L. (2012). Music therapy: A resource for creativity, health and well-being across the lifespan. In O. Odena (Ed.), *Musical creativity: Insights from music education research* (pp. 165–181). Surrey, UK: Ashgate.

Burnard, P. (2006). Understanding children's meaning-making as composers. In I. Deliège & G. Wiggins (Eds.), *Musical creativity: Multidisciplinary research in theory and practice* (pp. 111–133). Hove, UK: Psychology Press.

Burnard, P. (2012). *Musical creativities in practice*. Oxford, UK: Oxford University Press.

Burnard, P., & Younker, B. A. (2002). Mapping pathways: Fostering creativity in composition. *Music Education Research, 4*(2), 245–261. doi:10.1080/1461380022000011948

Burniston, A. (2011). From Stanley Spencer's *Resurrection* to John Coltrane's *Ascension*. *Psychological Perspectives, 54*(2), 197–207. doi:10.1080/00332925.2011.573398

Burwell, K., & Shipton, M. (2011). Performance studies in practice: An investigation of students' approaches to practice in a university music department. *Music Education Research, 13*(3), 255–271. doi:10.1080/14613808.2011.603041

Burwell, K., & Shipton, M. (2013). Strategic approaches to practice: An action research project. *British Journal of Music Education, 30*(3), 329–345. doi:10.1017/S0265051713000132.

Butler, B. E., & Trainor, L. J. (2015). The musician redefined: A behavioral assessment of rhythm perception in professional club DJs. *Timing & Time Perception, 3*, 116–132. doi:10.1163/22134468-03002041

Campbell, P. S. (2016). Global practices. In G. E. McPherson (Ed.), *The child as musician: A handbook of musical development* (2nd ed., pp. 556–576). Oxford, UK: Oxford University Press.

Cantero, I. M., & Jauset-Berrocal, J. (2017). Why do they choose their instruments? *British Journal of Music Education, 34*(2), 203–215. doi:10.1017/S0265051716000280

Carafoli, E. (2017). The complex structure of the creativity process. *Rendiconti Lincei. Scienze Fisiche e Naturali, 28*(3), 449–462. doi:10.1007/s12210-017-0629-8

Carey, G. (2010, July). Performance or learning? Reflections on pedagogical practices within the conservatoire. In M. Hannen (Ed.), *The musician in creative and educational spaces of the 21st century: Proceedings from the International Society for Music Education (ISME) 18th international seminar of the commission for the education of the professional musician* (pp. 34–38). Nedlands, Australia: International Society for Music Education.

Carey, G., & Grant, C. (2014). Teachers of instruments, or teachers as instruments? From transfer to transformative approaches to one-to-one pedagogy. In G. Carruthers (Ed.), *Proceedings of the 20th International Seminar of the ISME Commission on the Education of the Professional Musician* (pp. 42–53). Nedlands, Australia: International Society for Music Education.

Cavitt, M. E. (2003). A descriptive analysis of error correction in instrumental music rehearsals. *Journal of Research in Music Education, 51*, 218–230. https://doi.org/10.2307/3345375

Cepeda, M. S., Carr, D. B., Lau, J., & Alvarez, H. (2006). Music for pain relief (review). *Cochrane Database System Review, 2*, article CD004843. https://doi.org/10.1002/14651858.CD004843.pub2

Chaffin, R., Imreh, G., & Crawford, M. (2005). *Practicing perfection: Memory and piano performance.* New York, NY: Psychology Press.

Chaffin, R., Imreh, G., Lemieux, A. F., & Chen, C. (2003). "Seeing the big picture": Piano practice as expert problem solving. *Music Perception, 20*(4), 465–490. https://doi.org/10.1525/mp.2003.20.4.465

Chaffin, R., Lemieux, A., & Chen, C. (2007). "It is different each time I play": Variability in highly prepared musical performance. *Music Perception, 24*(5), 455–472. https://doi.org/10.1525/mp.2007.24.5.455

Chaffin, R., Lisboa, T., Logan, T., & Begosh, K. T. (2009). Preparing for memorized cello performance: The role of performance cues. *Psychology of Music, 38*(1), 3–30. doi:10.1177/0305735608100377

Chan, L. P., Livingstone, S. R., & Russo, F. A. (2013). Facial mimicry in response to song. *Music Perception, 30*(4), 361–367. doi:10.1525/MP.2013.30.4.361

Chanda, M. L., & Levitin, D. J. (2013). The neurochemistry of music. *Trends in Cognitive Sciences, 17*(4), 179–193. http://dx.doi.org/10.1016/j.tics.2013.02.007

Chen, J. C. W. (2012). A pilot study mapping students' composing strategies: Implications for teaching computer-assisted composition. *Research Studies in Music Education, 34*(2), 157–171. doi:10.1177/1321103X12465515

Cheng, E., & Chew, E. (2008). Quantitative analysis of phrasing strategies in expressive performance: Computational methods and analysis of performances of unaccompanied Bach for solo violin. *Journal of New Music Research, 37*(4), 325–338. doi:10.1080/09298210802711660

Cheong-Clinch, C. (2009). Music for engaging young people in education. *Youth Studies Australia, 28*(2), 50–57.

Chesky, K., Kondraske, G., Henoch, M., Hipple, J., & Rubin, B. (2002). Musicians' health. In R. Colwell & C. Richardson (Eds.), *The new handbook of research on music teaching and learning* (pp. 1023–1039). New York, NY: Oxford University Press.

Chittka, L., & Brockmann, A. (2005). Perception space—the final frontier. *PLoS Biology, 3*(4), e137. https://doi.org/10.1371/journal.pbio.0030137

Chmiel, A., & Schubert, E. (2017). Back to the inverted-U for music preference: A review of the literature. *Psychology of Music, 45*(6), 886–909. doi:10.1177/0305735617697507

Chmiel, A., & Schubert, E. (2019). Unusualness as a predictor of music preference. *Musicae Scientiae, 23*(4), 426–441. doi:10.1177/1029864917752545

Chua, S. L., & Welch, G. F. (2020). A lifelong perspective for growing music teacher identity. *Research Studies in Music Education.* Advance online publication. doi:1321103X19875080.

Clark, E., Dibben, N., & Pitts, S. (2010). *Music and mind in everyday life.* Oxford, UK: Oxford University Press.

Clark, I. N., Baker, F. A., & Taylor, N. F. (2016). The modulating effects of music listening on health-related exercise and physical activity in adults: A systematic review and narrative synthesis. *Nordic Journal of Music Therapy, 25*(1), 76–104. doi:10.1080/08098131.2015.1008558

Clark, T. (2006). "I'm Scunthorpe 'til I die": Constructing and (re)negotiating identity through the terrace chant. *Soccer & Society, 7*(4), 494–507. doi:10.1080/14660970600905786

Clark, T., & Williamon, A. (2011). Evaluation of a mental skills training program for musicians. *Journal of Applied Sport Psychology, 23*, 342–359. doi:10.1080/10413200.2011.574676

Clarke, E. F. (2005). *Ways of listening: An ecological approach to the perception of musical meaning.* New York, NY: Oxford University Press.

Clauhs, M. (2018). Beginning band without a stand: Fostering creative musicianship in early instrumental programs. *Music Educators Journal, 104*(4), 39–47. doi:10.1177/0027432118768383

Clayton, M. (2016). The social and personal functions of music in cross-cultural perspective. In S. Hallam, I. Cross, & M. Thaut (Eds.), *Oxford handbook of music psychology* (2nd ed., pp. 47–59). Oxford, UK: Oxford University Press.

Cohen, S., & Bodner, E. (2019). The relationship between flow and music performance anxiety amongst professional classical orchestral musicians. *Psychology of Music, 47*(3), 420–435. doi:10.1177/0305735618754689

Collins, D. (2005). A synthesis process model of creative thinking in music composition. *Psychology of Music, 33*(2), 193–216. https://doi.org/10.1177/0305735605050651

Collins, D., & Dunn, M. (2011). Problem-solving strategies and processes in musical composition: Observations in real time. *Journal of Music, Technology and Education*, 4(1), 47–76. doi:10.1386/JMTE.4.1.47_1

Collinson, I. (2009). "Singing songs, making places, creating selves": Football songs & fan identity at Sydney FC. *Transforming Cultures eJournal*, 4(1). https://epress.lib.uts.edu.au/journals/index.php/TfC/article/view/1057/1060

Colvin, G. (2008). *Talent is overrated: What really separates world-class performers from everybody else.* New York, NY: Portfolio.

Connolly, C., & Williamon, A. (2004). Mental skills training. In A. Williamon (Ed.), *Musical excellence: Strategies and techniques to enhance performance* (pp. 221–245). Oxford, UK: Oxford University Press.

Copland, A. (1939). *What to listen for in music.* New York, NY: McGraw-Hill.

Corrigall, K. A., Schellenberg, E. G., & Misura, N. M. (2013). Music training, cognition, and personality. *Frontiers in Psychology*, 4, article 222. https://doi.org/10.3389/fpsyg.2013.00222

Coulson, S. (2010). Getting "Capital" in the music world: Musicians' learning experiences and working lives. *British Journal of Music Education*, 27(3), 255–270. doi:10.1017/S0265051710000227

Coyle, D. (2009). *The talent code: Greatness isn't born. It's grown. Here's how.* New York, NY: Bantam Books.

Coyne, S. M., Padilla-Walker, L. M., & Howard, E. (2015). Media uses in emerging adulthood. In J. J. Arnett (Ed.), *The Oxford handbook of emerging adulthood* (pp. 349–363). New York, NY: Oxford University Press.

Creech, A. (2016). Understanding professionalism: Transitions and the contemporary professional musician. In I. Papageorgi & G. Welch (Eds.), *Advanced musical performance: Investigations in higher education learning* (pp. 381–396). Abingdon, UK: Routledge.

Creech, A., & Hallam, S. (2011). Learning a musical instrument: The influence of interpersonal interaction on outcomes for school-aged pupils. *Psychology of Music*, 39(1), 102–122. doi:10.1177/0305735610370222

Crispin, D., & Östersjö, S. (2017). Musical expression from conception to reception. In J. Rink, H. Gaunt, & A. Williamon (Eds.), *Musicians in the making: Pathways to creative performance* (pp. 288–305). Oxford, UK: Oxford University Press.

Cropley, D., & Cropley, A. (2010). Functional creativity: "Products" and the generation of effective novelty. In J. C. Kaufman & R. J. Sternberg (Eds.), *The Cambridge handbook of creativity* (pp. 301–317). New York, NY: Cambridge University Press.

Cross, I. (2016). The nature of music and its evolution. In S. Hallam, I. Cross, & M. Thaut (Eds.), *Oxford handbook of music psychology* (2nd ed., pp. 3–17). Oxford, UK: Oxford University Press.

Csikszentmihalyi, M. (1990). *Flow: The psychology of optimal experience.* New York, NY: Harper and Row.

Csikszentmihalyi, M. (1996). *Creativity: Flow and the psychology of discovery and invention.* New York, NY: HarperCollins.

Csikszentmihalyi, M., & Sawyer, K. (2014). Creative insight: The social dimension of a solitary moment. In D. K. Simonton (Ed.), *The systems model of creativity* (pp. 73–98). Dordrecht, The Netherlands: Springer. https://doi.org/10.1007/978-94-017-9085-7_7

Curtis, M. E., & Bharucha, J. J. (2009). Memory and musical expectation for tones in cultural context. *Music Perception*, 26(4), 365–375. doi:10.1525/MP.2009.26.4.365

Czajkowski, A. M. L., Greasley, A. E., & Allis, M. (2020). Mindfulness for musicians: A mixed methods study investigating the effects of 8-week mindfulness courses on music students at a leading conservatoire. *Musicae Scientiae*. Advance online publication. doi:10.1177/1029864920941570

da Silva Veiga, H. M., Demo, G., & Neiva, E. R. (2017). The psychology of entrepreneurship. In E. R. Neiva, C. V. Torres, & H. Mendonça (Eds.), *Organizational psychology and evidence-based management* (pp. 135–155). Cham, Switzerland: Springer. https://doi.org/10.1007/978-3-319-64304-5_8

Dagaz, M. C. (2012). Learning from the band: Trust, acceptance, and self-confidence. *Journal of Contemporary Ethnography, 41*, 431–461. doi:10.1177/0891241612447813

Dahl, M. (2014, September 30). *The alarming new research on perfectionism.* The Cut. https://www.thecut.com/2014/09/alarming-new-research-on-perfectionism.html

Dahl, S., & Friberg, A. (2007). Visual perception of expressiveness in musicians' body movements. *Music Perception, 24*(5), 433–454. doi:10.1525/mp.2007.24.5.433

Damodaran, S. (2016). Protest and music. In W. R. Thompson (Ed.), *Oxford research encyclopedia of politics.* https://doi.org/10.1093/acrefore/9780190228637.013.81

Darrow, A. (2006). The role of music in deaf culture: Deaf students' perception of emotion in music. *Journal of Music Therapy, 43*(1), 2–15. https://doi.org/10.1093/jmt/43.1.2

Davidson, J., & Burland, K. (2006). Musician identity formation. In G. McPherson (Ed.), *The child as musician: A handbook of musical development* (pp. 475–490). New York, NY: Oxford University Press.

Davidson, J. W. (2001). The role of the body in the production and perception of solo vocal performance: A use study of Annie Lennox. *Musicae Scientiae, 5*(2), 235–256. https://doi.org/10.1177/102986490100500206

Davidson, J. W. (2005). Bodily communication in musical performance. In D. Miell, R. MacDonald, & D. J. Hargreaves (Eds.), *Musical communication* (pp. 215–237). Oxford, UK: Oxford University Press.

Davidson, J. W. (2007). Qualitative insights into the use of expressive body movement in solo piano performance: A case study approach. *Psychology of Music, 35*(3), 381–401. doi:10.1177/0305735607072765

Davidson, J. W. (2009). Movement and collaboration in musical performance. In S. Hallam, I. Cross, & M. Thaut (Eds.), *Oxford handbook of music psychology* (pp. 364–376). Oxford, UK: Oxford University Press.

Davidson, J. W. (2012). Bodily movement and facial actions in expressive musical performance by solo and duo instrumentalists: Two distinctive case studies. *Psychology of Music, 40*(5), 595–633. doi:10.1177/0305735612449896

Davidson, J. W., & Broughton, M. C. (2016). Bodily mediated coordination, collaboration, and communication in music performance. In S. Hallam, I. Cross, & M. Thaut (Eds.), *Oxford handbook of music psychology* (2nd ed., pp. 573–595). Oxford, UK: Oxford University Press.

Davidson, J. W., & Correia, J. S. (2002). Body movement. In R. Parncutt & G. E. McPherson (Eds.), *The science and psychology of music performance: Creative strategies for teaching and learning* (pp. 237–250). New York, NY: Oxford University Press.

Davidson, J. W., & Good, J. M. (2002). Social and musical co-ordination between members of a string quartet: An exploratory study. *Psychology of Music, 30*(2), 186–201. doi:10.1177/0305735602302005

Davies, J. B. (1978). *The psychology of music.* London, UK: Hutchinson.

Davis, S. G. (2005). "That Thing You Do!": Compositional processes of a rock band. *International Journal of Education & the Arts, 6*(16). http://ijea.asu.edu/v6n16/

de Reizabal, M. L., & Gómez, M. B. (2020). When theory and practice meet: Avenues for entrepreneurship education in music conservatories. *International Journal of Music Education. 38*(3), 352–369. doi:10.1177/0255761420919560

Deahl, L., & Wristen, B. (2017). *Adaptive strategies for small-handed pianists.* New York, NY: Oxford University Press.

Dean, R. T., Bailes, F., & Schubert, E. (2011). Acoustic intensity causes perceived changes in arousal levels in music: An experimental investigation. *PloS ONE, 6*(4), e18591. doi:10.1371/journal.pone.0018591

Dellacherie, D., Roy, M., Hugueville, L., Peretz, I., & Samson, S. (2011). The effect of musical experience on emotional self-reports and psychophysiological responses to dissonance. *Psychophysiology, 48*(3), 337–349. doi:10.1111/j.1469-8986.2010.01075.x

Demorest, S. M., & Morrison, S. J. (2000). Does music make you smarter? This discussion explores some of the research studies that have proposed connections between musical involvement and general intelligence. *Music Educators Journal, 87*(2), 33–58. doi:10.2307/3399646

DeNora, T. (2003). Music sociology: Getting the music into the action. *British Journal of Music Education, 20*(2), 165–177. doi:10.1017/S0265051703005369

Deutsch, D. (2010). The paradox of pitch circularity. *Acoustics Today, 7,* 8–15. https://acousticstoday.org/wp-content/uploads/2019/09/THE-PARADOX-OF-PITCH-CIRCULARITY-Diana-Deutsch.pdf

Deutsch, D. (2013). Grouping mechanisms in music. In D. Deutsch (Ed.), *The psychology of music* (3rd ed., pp. 183–248). San Diego, CA: Academic Press.

Deutsch, D. (2019). *Musical illusions and phantom words.* New York, NY: Oxford University Press.

Dhule, S. S., Sunita, B. N., & Gawali, S. R. (2013). Pulmonary function tests in wind instrument players. *International Journal of Science and Research, 2*(5), 384–386.

Di Stadio, A., Dipietro, L., Ricci, G., Della Volpe, A., Minni, A., Greco, A., de Vincentiis, M., & Ralli, M. (2018). Hearing loss, tinnitus, hyperacusis, and diplacusis in professional musicians: A systematic review. *International Journal of Environmental Research and Public Health, 15*(10). https://doi.org/10.3390/ijerph15102120

Diaz, F. M. (2018). Relationships among meditation, perfectionism, mindfulness, and performance anxiety among collegiate music students. *Journal of Research in Music Education, 66*(2), 150–167. doi:10.1177/0022429418765447

Diaz, F. M., & Silveira, J. M. (2012). Dimensions of flow in academic and social activities among summer music camp participants. *International Journal of Music Education, 31*(3), 310–320. doi:10.1177/0255761411434455

Diaz, F. M., Silveira, J. M., & Strand, K. (2020). A neurophenomenological investigation of mindfulness among collegiate musicians. *Journal of Research in Music Education, 68*(3), 351–374. doi:10.1177/0022429420921184

Dibben, N., & Haake, A. B. (2013). Music and the construction of space in office-based work settings. In G. Born (Ed.), *Music, sound and space: Transformations of public and private experience* (pp. 151–168). Cambridge, UK: Cambridge University Press.

Dibben, N., & Williamson, V. J. (2007). An exploratory survey of in-vehicle music listening. *Psychology of Music, 35*(4), 571–589. doi:10.1177/0305735607079725

Dietrich, A. (2014). The mythconception of the mad genius. *Frontiers in Psychology, 5,* article 79. https://doi.org/10.3389/fpsyg.2014.00079

Dilworth, J. (2004). Artistic expression as interpretation. *British Journal of Aesthetics*, *44*(1), 10–28. https://doi.org/10.1093/bjaesthetics/44.1.10

Dobos, B., Piko, B. F., & Kenny, D. T. (2019). Music performance anxiety and its relationship with social phobia and dimensions of perfectionism. *Research Studies in Music Education*, *41*(3), 310–326. doi:10.1177/1321103X18804295

Dobson, M. C. (2010). New audiences for classical music: The experiences of non-attenders at live orchestral concerts. *Journal of New Music Research*, *39*(2), 111–124. doi:10.1080/09298215.2010.489643

Dobson, M. C. (2011). Insecurity, professional sociability, and alcohol: Young freelance musicians' perspectives on work and life in the music profession. *Psychology of Music*, *39*(2), 240–260. doi:10.1177/0305735610373562

Doffman, M. (2012). Jammin' an ending: Creativity, knowledge, and conduct among jazz musicians. *Twentieth Century Music*, *8*(2), 203–225. doi:10.1017/S1478572212000084

Doğantan-Dack, M. (2014). Philosophical reflections on expressive music performance. In D. Fabian, R. Timmers, & E. Schubert (Eds.), *Expressiveness in music performance: Empirical approaches across styles and cultures* (pp. 3–21). Oxford, UK: Oxford University Press.

Draves, T. J. (2008). Music achievement, self-esteem, and aptitude in a college songwriting class. *Bulletin of the Council for Research in Music Education*, *178*, 35–46. https://www.jstor.org/stable/40319337

Duby, M. (2020). Minds, music, and motion: Ecologies of ensemble performance. *Music and Practice*, *6*. doi:10.32063/0607

Duke, R. A., & Davis, C. M. (2006). Procedural memory consolidation in the performance of brief keyboard sequences. *Journal of Research in Music Education*, *54*(2), 111–124.

Duke, R. A., & Simmons, A. L. (2006). The nature of expertise: Narrative descriptions of 19 common elements observed in the lessons of three renowned artist-teachers. *Bulletin of the Council for Research in Music Education*, *170*, 7–19. https://www.jstor.org/stable/40319345

Duke, R. A., Simmons, A. L., & Cash, C. D. (2009). It's not how much; it's how: Characteristics of practice behavior and retention of performance skills. *Journal of Research in Music Education*, *56*(4), 310–321. doi:10.1177/0022429408328

Dunn, P. G., de Ruyter, B., & Bouwhuis, D. G. (2012). Toward a better understanding of the relation between music preference, listening behavior, and personality. *Psychology of Music*, *40*(4), 411–428. doi:10.1177/0305735610388897

Dweck, C. S. (2006). *Mindset: The new psychology of success*. New York, NY: Penguin Random House.

Dyndahl, P., & Nielsen, S. G. (2014). Shifting authenticities in Scandinavian music education. *Music Education Research*, *16*(1), 105–118. doi:10.1080/14613808.2013.847075

Eccles, J. S., & Wigfield, A. (2020). From expectancy-value theory to situated expectancy-value theory: A developmental, social cognitive, and sociocultural perspective on motivation. *Contemporary Educational Psychology*, *61*. https://doi.org/10.1016/j.cedpsych.2020.101859

Edison, T. A. (1878). The phonograph and its future. *North American Review*, *126*(262), 527–536.

Eerola, T., Jakubowski, K., Moran, N., Keller, P. E., & Clayton, M. (2018). Shared periodic performer movements coordinate interactions in duo improvisations. *Royal Society Open Science*, *5*, 171520. https://doi.org/10.1098/rsos.171520

Eerola, T., & Vuoskoski, J. K. (2011). A comparison of the discrete and dimensional models of emotion in music. *Psychology of Music, 39*(1), 18–49. doi:10.1177/0305735610362821

Elder, D. (1982). *Pianists at play: Interviews, master lessons, and technical regimes.* Evanston, IL: Instrumentalist Company.

Elliott, D., & Silverman, M. (2017). Identities and musics: Reclaiming personhood. In R. MacDonald, D. J. Hargreaves, & D. Miell (Eds.), *Handbook of musical identities* (pp. 27–45). Oxford, UK: Oxford University Press.

Ericsson, K. A., & Harwell, K. W. (2019). Deliberate practice and proposed limits on the effects of practice on the acquisition of expert performance: Why the original definition matters and recommendations for future research. *Frontiers in Psychology, 10,* article 2396. https://doi.org/10.3389/fpsyg.2019.02396

Ericsson, K. A., Krampe, R. T., & Tesch-Romer, C. (1993). The role of deliberate practice in the acquisition of expert performance. *Psychological Review, 100*(3), 363–406. doi:10.1037//0033-295X.100.3.363

Ericsson, K. A., & Moxley, J. H. (2013). Working memory that mediates experts' performance: Why it is qualitatively different from traditional working memory. In T. P. Alloway & R. G. Alloway (Eds.), *Working memory: The connected intelligence* (pp. 109–136). New York, NY: Psychology Press.

Ericsson, K. A., & Pool, R. (2016). *Peak: Secrets from the new science of expertise.* New York, NY: Houghton Mifflin & Harcourt.

Evans, P. (2015). Self-determination theory: An approach to motivation in music education. *Musicae Scientiae, 19*(1), 65–83. doi:10.1177/1029864914568044

Evans, P. (2016). Motivation. In G. E. McPherson (Ed.), *The child as musician: A handbook of musical development* (2nd ed., pp. 325–339). Oxford, UK: Oxford University Press.

Evans, P., & Bonneville-Roussy, A. (2015). Self-determined motivation for practice in university music students. *Psychology of Music, 44*(5) 1095–1110. doi:10.1177/0305735615610926

Evans, P., & Liu, M. Y. (2019). Psychological needs and motivational outcomes in a high school orchestra program. *Journal of Research in Music Education, 67,* 83–105. https://doi.org/10.1177/0022429418812769

Evans, P., & McPherson, G. E. (2015). Identity and practice: The motivational benefits of a long-term musical identity. *Psychology of Music, 43*(3), 407–422. https://doi-org.libproxy.unl.edu/10.1177/0305735613514471

Evans, P., McPherson, G. E., & Davidson, J. W. (2012). The role of psychological needs in ceasing music and music learning activities. *Psychology of Music, 41*(5), 600–619. doi:10.1177/0305735612441736f

Fachner, J. (2006). Music and altered states of consciousness: An overview. In D. Aldridge & J. Fachner (Eds.), *Music and altered states: Consciousness, transcendence, therapy and addiction* (pp. 15–37). London, UK: Jessica Kingsley.

Fancourt, D. (2016). An introduction to the psychoneuroimmunology of music: History, future collaboration and a research agenda. *Psychology of Music, 44*(2), 168–182. doi:10.1177/0305735614558901

Farnsworth-Grodd, V. A., & Cameron, L. (2013). Mindfulness and the self-regulation of music performance anxiety. In A. Williamon & W. Goebl (Eds.), *Proceedings of the International Symposium on Performance Science 2013* (pp. 317–322). Brussels, Belgium: Association Européenne des Conservatoires. http://researchonline.rcm.ac.uk/339/1/isps2013_proceedings.pdf

Feichas, H. (2010). Bridging the gap: Informal learning practices as a pedagogy of integration. *British Journal of Music Education, 27*, 47–58. doi:10.1017/S0265051709990192

Fernholz, I., Mumm, J. L. M., Plag, J., Noeres, K., Rotter, G., Willich, S. N., Ströhle, A., Berghöfer, A., & Schmidt, A. (2019). Performance anxiety in professional musicians: A systematic review on prevalence, risk factors and clinical treatment effects. *Psychological Medicine, 49*(14), 2287–2306. doi.org/10.1017/S0033291719001910

Fine, P., Rosner, B., & Berry, A. (2006). The effect of pattern recognition and tonal predictability on sight-singing ability. *Psychology of Music, 34*(4), 431–447. doi:10.1177/0305735606067152

Fischinger, T., Kaufmann, M., & Scholtz, W. (2020). If it's Mozart, it must be good? The influence of textual information and age on musical appreciation. *Psychology of Music, 48*(4), 579–597. doi:10.1177/0305735618812216

Fitts, P. M., & Posner, M. I. (1967). *Human performance.* Belmont, CA: Brooks/Cole.

Flath, C. M., Friesike, S., Wirth, M., & Thiesse, F. (2017). Copy, transform, combine: Exploring the remix as a form of innovation. *Journal of Information Technology, 32*(4), 306–325. doi:10.1057/s41265-017-0043-9

Flegal, K. E., & Anderson, M. C. (2008). Overthinking skilled motor performance: Or why those who teach can't do. *Psychonomic Bulletin & Review, 15*, 927–932. doi:10.3758/PBR.15.5.927

Flett, G. L., Hewitt, P. L., & Heisel, M. J. (2014). The destructiveness of perfectionism revisited: Implications for the assessment of suicide risk and the prevention of suicide. *Review of General Psychology, 18*(3), 156–172. http://dx.doi.org/10.1037/gpr0000011

Folkestad, G. (2012). Digital tools and discourse in music: The ecology of composition. In D. J. Hargreaves, D. E. Miell, & R. A. R. MacDonald (Eds.), *Musical imaginations: Multidisciplinary perspectives on creativity, performance, and perception* (pp. 193–205). Oxford, UK: Oxford University Press.

Forbes, M. (2021). Giving voice to jazz singers' experiences of flow in improvisation. *Psychology of Music. 49*(4), 789–803. doi:10.1177/0305735619899137

Forbes, M. (2020). "We're pushing back": Group singing, social identity, and caring for a spouse with Parkinson's. *Psychology of Music.* Advance online publication. doi:10.1177/0305735620944230

Ford, J. L., Vosloo, J., & Arvinen-Barrow, M. (2020). "Pouring everything that you are": Musicians' experiences of optimal performances. *British Journal of Music Education, 37*(2), 141–153. doi:10.1017/S0265051720000078

Ford, L., & Davidson, J. W. (2003). An investigation of members' roles in wind quintets. *Psychology of Music, 31*, 53–74. https://doi.org/10.1177/0305735603031001323

Forman, M. (2002). Soundtrack to a crisis: Music, context, discourse. *Television & New Media, 3*(2), 191–204. https://doi.org/10.1177/152747640200300211

Forrester, M. A., & Borthwick-Hunter, E. (2015). Understanding the development of musicality: Contributions from longitudinal studies. *Psychomusicology: Music, Mind, and Brain, 25*(1), 93–102.

Forsyth, A. J., Lennox, J. C., & Emslie, C. (2016). "That's cool, you're a musician and you drink": Exploring entertainers' accounts of their unique workplace relationship with alcohol. *International Journal of Drug Policy, 36*, 85–94. http://dx.doi.org/10.1016/j.drugpo.2016.07.001

Freer, E., & Evans, P. (2018). Psychological needs satisfaction and value in students' intentions to study music in high school. *Psychology of Music, 46*(6), 881–895. doi:10.1177/0305735617731613

Fritz, B. S., & Avsec, A. (2007). The experience of flow and subjective well-being of music students. *Horizons of Psychology, 16*(2), 5–17.

Fuentes, C., Hagberg, J., & Kjellberg, H. (2019). Soundtracking: Music listening practices in the digital age. *European Journal of Marketing, 53*(3), 483–503. https://doi.org/ 10.1108/EJM-10-2017-0753

Furuya, S., & Altenmüller, E. (2013). Flexibility of movement organization in piano performance. *Frontiers in Human Neuroscience, 7*, article 173. https://www.frontiersin. org/articles/10.3389/fnhum.2013.00173/full

Furuya, S., & Altenmüller, E. (2015). Acquisition and reacquisition of motor coordination in musicians. *Annals of the New York Academy of Sciences, 1337*, 118–124. doi:10.1111/ nyas.12659

Gabor, E. (2011). Turning points in the development of classical musicians. *Journal of Ethnographic & Qualitative Research, 5*, 138–156.

Gaboury, V., Lavoie, N., & Lessard, A. (2020). A combined music and writing program helps second graders learn to spell. *International Journal of Music Education, 38*(4), 513–524. doi:10.1177/0255761420950982

Gabrielsson, A. (2010). Strong experiences with music. In P. N. Juslin & J. A. Sloboda (Eds.), *Handbook of music and emotion: Theory, research, applications* (pp. 547–604). Oxford, UK: Oxford University Press.

Gabrielsson. (2016). The relationship between musical structure and perceived expression. In S. Hallam, I. Cross, & M. Thaut (Eds.), *The Oxford handbook of music psychology* (2nd ed., pp. 215–232). Oxford, UK: Oxford University Press.

Gabrielsson, A., & Lindström, E. (2010). The role of structure in the musical expression of emotions. In P. N. Juslin & J. A. Sloboda (Eds.), *Handbook of music and emotion: Theory, research, applications* (pp. 367–399). Oxford, UK: Oxford University Press.

Gabrielsson, A., Whaley, J., & Sloboda, J. (2016). Peak experiences in music. In S. Hallam, I. Cross, & M. Thaut (Eds.), *The Oxford handbook of music psychology* (2nd ed., pp. 745–758). Oxford, UK: Oxford University Press.

Gagné, F. (2013). The DMGT: Changes within, beneath, and beyond. *Talent Development & Excellence, 5*(2), 5–19.

Galeyev, B. M. (2007). The nature and functions of synesthesia in music. *Leonardo, 40*(3), 285–288. https://doi.org/10.1162/leon.2007.40.3.285

Gallate, J., Wong, C., Ellwood, S., Roring, R. W., & Snyder, A. (2012). Creative people use nonconscious processes to their advantage. *Creativity Research Journal, 24*(2–3), 146– 151. doi:10.1080/10400419.2012.677282

Gardner, H. (2011). *Creating minds* (2nd ed.). New York, NY: Basic Books.

Gardner, H., & Weinstein, E. (2018). Creativity: The view from Big C and the introduction of tiny C. In R. J. Sternberg & J. C. Kaufman (Eds.), *The nature of human creativity* (pp. 94–109). Cambridge, UK: Cambridge University Press.

Garofalo, R. (2010). Politics, mediation, social context, and public use. In P. N. Juslin & J. A. Sloboda (Eds.), *Handbook of music and emotion: Theory, research, applications* (pp. 725–754). Oxford, UK: Oxford University Press.

Garofalo, R. (2012). Pop goes to war, 2001–2004: US popular music after 9/11. In J. Ritter & J. M. Daughtry (Eds.), *Music in the post-9/11 world* (pp. 3–26). New York, NY: Routledge.

Gaunt, H., Creech, A., Long, M., & Hallam, S. (2012). Supporting conservatoire students towards professional integration: One-to-one tuition and the potential of mentoring. *Music Education Research, 14*(1), 25–43. doi:10.1080/14613808.2012.657166

Gawboy, A. M., & Townsend, J. (2012). Scriabin and the possible. *Music Theory Online, 18*(2). https://mtosmt.org/issues/mto.12.18.2/mto.12.18.2.gawboy_townsend.php

George, A. M., Brown, P. M., Scholz, B., Scott-Parker, B., & Rickwood, D. (2018). "I need to skip a song because it sucks": Exploring mobile phone use while driving among young adults. *Transportation Research Part F: Traffic Psychology and Behaviour, 58*, 382–391. https://doi.org/10.1016/j.trf.2018.06.014

Georgievski, M. J., & Stephan, U. (2016). Advancing the psychology of entrepreneurship: A review of the psychological literature and an introduction. *Applied Psychology, 65*(3), 437–468. https://doi.org/10.1111/apps.12073

Geringer, J. M., Madsen, C. K., & Gregory, D. (2004). A fifteen-year history of the Continuous Response Digital Interface: Issues relating to validity and reliability. *Bulletin of the Council for Research in Music Education, 160*, 1–15. https://www.jstor.org/stable/40319214

Gerlich, R. N., Browning, L., & Westermann, L. (2010). I've got the music in me: A study of peak musical memory age and the implications for future advertising. *Journal of College Teaching & Learning, 7*(2), 610–669. https://doi.org/10.19030/tlc.v7i2.90

Giebelhausen, R., & Kruse, A. J. (2018). "A smile on everybody's face": A multiple case study of community ukulele groups. *International Journal of Music Education, 36*(3), 347–365. doi:10.1177/0255761417744371

Giesbrecht, M., & Andrews, B. W. (2015). Towards understanding of contemporary music composition. In S. Schonmann (Ed.), *International yearbook for research in arts education* (Vol. 3, pp. 38–42). Münster, Germany: Waxmann.

Gilbert, E. (2002, June). Play it like your hair's on fire. *GQ, 72*(6), 248–255, 268–270.

Gilboa, A., & Tal-Shmotkin, M. (2010). String quartets as self-managed teams: An interdisciplinary perspective. *Psychology of Music, 40*(1), 19–41. doi:10.1177/0305735610377593

Gillespie, W., & Myors, B. (2000). Personality of rock musicians. *Psychology of Music, 28*, 154–165. https://doi.org/10.1177/0305735600282004

Ginsborg, J. (2004). Strategies for memorizing music. In A. Williamon (Ed.), *Enhancing musical performance* (pp. 123–142). Oxford, UK: Oxford University Press.

Ginsborg, J., Kreutz, G., Thomas, M., & Williamon, A. (2009). Healthy behaviours in music and non-music performance students. *Health Education, 109*(3), 242–258. https://doi.org/10.1108/09654280910955575

Gioia, T. (2006). *Work songs.* Durham, NC: Duke University Press.

Gioia, T. (2016). *How to listen to jazz.* New York, NY: Basic Books.

Gjermunds, N., Brechan, I., Johnsen, S. Å. K., & Watten, R. G. (2020). Personality traits in musicians. *Current Issues in Personality Psychology, 8*(2), 100–107. https://doi.org/10.5114/cipp.2020.97314

Gladwell, M. (2008). *Outliers: The story of success.* New York, NY: Little, Brown and Company.

Gläveanu, V. P. (2013). Rewriting the language of creativity: The five A's framework. *Review of General Psychology, 17*(1), 69–81. doi:10.1037/a0029528

Glennie, E. (2003, February). *How to truly listen* [Video]. TED. https://www.ted.com/talks/evelyn_glennie_how_to_truly_listen

Glowinski, D., Badino, L., Ausilio, A., Camurri, A., & Fadiga, L. (2012, October). Analysis of leadership in a string quartet. In *Third International Workshop on Social Behaviour in Music at ACM ICMI 2012* (pp. 763–774). Santa Monica, CA: ACM ICMI. https://doi.org/10.1145/2388676.2388805

Gobet, F. (1998). Memory for the meaningless: How chunks help. In *Proceedings of the 20th Meeting of the Cognitive Science Society* (pp. 398–403). Mahwah, NJ: Erlbaum.

Gobet, F., & Simon, H. (1998). Expert chess memory: Revisiting the chunking hypothesis. *Memory, 6*(3), 225–255. doi:10.1080/741942359

Goebl, W., & Palmer, C. (2009). Synchronization of timing and motion among performing musicians. *Music Perception, 26*(5), 427–438. doi:10.1525/MP.2009.26.5.427

Goehr, L. (2007). *The imaginary museum of musical works: An essay in the philosophy of music* (rev. ed.). New York, NY: Oxford University Press.

Goldin, C., & Rouse, C. (2000). Orchestrating impartiality: The impact of "blind" auditions on female musicians. *American Economic Review, 90*(4), 715–741. doi:10.1257/aer.90.4.715

Good, A., Reed, M. J., & Russo, F. A. (2014). Compensatory plasticity in the deaf brain: Effects on perception of music. *Brain Sciences, 4*(4), 560–574. doi:10.3390/brainsci4040560

Goodman, E. (2002). Ensemble performance. In J. Rink (Ed.), *Musical performance: A guide to understanding* (pp. 153–167). Cambridge, UK: Cambridge University Press.

Goolsby, T. W. (1994). Profiles of processing: Eye movements during sightreading. *Music Perception, 12*, 97–123. https://doi.org/10.2307/40285757

Gordon, E. E. (1986a). *Intermediate measures of music audiation.* Chicago, IL: GIA

Gordon, E. E. (1986b). *Primary measures of music audiation.* Chicago, IL: GIA

Gordon, E. E. (1989). *Advanced measures of music audiation.* Chicago, IL: GIA.

Gordon, E. E. (1999). All about audiation and music aptitudes. *Music Educators Journal, 86*(2), 41–44. doi:10.2307/3399589

Gordon, E. E. (2003). *Learning sequences in music: Skill, content, and patterns. A music learning theory.* Chicago, IL: GIA.

Goudreau, G., Weber-Pillwax, C., Cote-Meek, S., Madill, H., & Wilson, S. (2008). Hand drumming: Health-promoting experiences of Aboriginal women from a northern Ontario urban community. *International Journal of Indigenous Health, 4*(1), 72–83.

Greasley, A., Lamont, A., & Sloboda, J. (2013). Exploring musical preferences: An in-depth qualitative study of adults' liking for music in their personal collections. *Qualitative Research in Psychology, 10*(4), 402–427. doi:10.1080/14780887.2011.647259

Greasley, A. E., Fulford, R. J., Pickard, M., & Hamilton, N. (2020). Help Musicians UK hearing survey: Musicians' hearing and hearing protection. *Psychology of Music, 48*(4), 529–546. doi:10.1177/0305735618812238

Greasley, A. E., & Lamont, A. (2011). Exploring engagement with music in everyday life using experience sampling methodology. *Musicae Scientiae, 15*(1), 45–71.

Greb, F., Schlotz, W., & Steffens, J. (2018). Personal and situational influences on the functions of music listening. *Psychology of Music, 46*(6), 763–794. doi:10.1177/0305735617724883

Green, B., & Gallwey, W. T. (2015). *The inner game of music.* London, UK: Pan Macmillan.

Green, L. (2002). *How popular musicians learn: A way ahead for music education.* Aldershot, UK: Ashgate.

Green, L. (2014). Teenagers, musical identity and classical music: The classroom as a catalyst. In L. Green (Ed.), *Music education as critical theory and practice* (pp. 277–290). London: Routledge.

Greenberg, D. M., Müllensiefen, D., Lamb, M. E., & Rentfrow, P. J. (2015). Personality predicts musical sophistication. *Journal of Research in Personality, 58*, 154–158. http://dx.doi.org/10.1016/j.jrp.2015.06.002

Greenspon, T. S. (2014). Is there an antidote to perfectionism? *Psychology in the Schools*, *51*(9), 986–998. doi:10.1002/pits.21797

Gregg, M. J., Clark, T. W., & Hall, C. R. (2008). Seeing the sound: An exploration of the use of mental imagery by classical musicians. *Musicae Scientiae*, *12*(2), 231–247. https://doi.org/10.1177/102986490801200203

Griffiths, N. K. (2010). "Posh music should equal posh dress": An investigation into the concert dress and physical appearance of female soloists. *Psychology of Music*, *38*(2), 159–177.

Grimmer, S. (2011). Continuity and change: The guru-shishya relationship in Karnatic classical music training. In L. Green (Ed.), *Learning, teaching, and musical identity: Voices across cultures* (pp. 91–108). Bloomington, IN: Indiana University Press.

Grings, A. F. S., & Hentschke, L. (2017). Attributional theory in investigating public music performance in higher music education. *International Journal of Music Education*, *35*(1), 31–46. doi:10.1177/0255761415619393

Gritten, A. (2017). Developing trust in others; or, how to empathise like a performer. In E. King & C. Waddington (Eds.), *Music and empathy* (pp. 248–266). Abingdon, UK: Routledge.

Gruszka, A., & Tang, M. (2017). The 4P's creativity model and its application in different fields. In C. H. Werner & M. Tang (Eds.), *Handbook of the management of creativity and innovation* (pp. 51–71). London, UK: World Scientific.

Gruzelier, J. H., & Egner, T. (2004). Physiological self-regulation: Biofeedback and neurofeedback. In A. Willamon (Ed.), *Musical excellence: Strategies and techniques to enhance performance* (pp. 197–220). Oxford, UK: Oxford University Press.

Güsewell, A., & Ruch, W. (2015). Character strengths profiles of musicians and non-musicians. *Journal of Arts and Humanities*, *4*(6), 1–17. https://theartsjournal.org/index.php/site/article/view/734

Haake, A. B. (2011). Individual music listening in workplace settings: An exploratory survey of offices in the UK. *Musicae Scientiae*, *15*(1), 107–129. doi:10.1177/1029864911398065

Haddon, E. (2011). Multiple teachers: Multiple gains? *British Journal of Music Education*, *28*(1), 69–85. doi:10.1017/S0265051710000422

Hajdu, D. (2011, May 23). Forever young? In some ways, yes. *New York Times*. https://www.nytimes.com/2011/05/24/opinion/24hajdu.html

Hallam, S. (2010). Transitions and the development of expertise. *Psychology Teaching Review*, *16*(2), 3–32.

Hallam, S. (2011). What predicts level of expertise attained, quality of performance, and future musical aspirations in young instrumental players? *Psychology of Music*, *41*(3), 267–291. doi:10.1177/0305735611425902

Hallam, S. (2016). Musicality. In G. E. McPherson (Ed.), *The child as musician: A handbook of musical development* (2nd ed., pp. 67–80). Oxford, UK: Oxford University Press.

Hallam, S., & Bautista, A. (2018). Processes of instrumental learning: The development of musical expertise. In G. E. McPherson & G. F. Welch (Eds.), *Vocal, instrumental, and ensemble learning and teaching: An Oxford handbook of music education* (Vol. 3, pp. 108–125). New York, NY: Oxford University Press.

Hallam, S., & Burns, S. (2018). *Progression in instrumental music making for learners from disadvantaged communities: A literature review.* Leeds, UK: Opera North/Arts Council England.

Hallam, S., Creech, A., Papageorgi, I., Gomes, T., Rinta, T., Varvarigou, M., & Lanipekun, J. (2016). Changes in motivation as expertise develops: Relationships with musical aspirations. *Musicae Scientiae*, *20*(4), 528–550. doi:10.1177/1029864916634420

Hallam, S., & MacDonald, R. (2016). The effects of music in community and educational settings. In S. Hallam, I. Cross, & M. Thaut (Eds.), *The Oxford handbook of music psychology* (2nd ed., pp. 775–788). Oxford, UK: Oxford University Press.

Hallett, R., & Lamont, A. (2015). How do gym members engage with music during exercise? *Qualitative Research in Sport, Exercise and Health*, *7*(3), 411–427. doi:10.1080/2159676X.2014.949835

Hallett, R., & Lamont, A. (2017). Music use in exercise: A questionnaire study. *Media Psychology*, *20*(4), 658–684. doi:10.1080/15213269.2016.1247716

Hansen, D. J., Lumpkin, G. T., & Hills, G. E. (2011). A multidimensional examination of a creativity-based opportunity recognition model. *International Journal of Entrepreneurial Behaviour and Research*, *17*(5), 515–533. doi:10.1108/13552551111158835

Hanser, S. B. (2010). Music, health, and well-being. In P. N. Juslin & J. A. Sloboda (Eds.), *Handbook of music and emotion: Theory, research, applications* (pp. 849–877). Oxford, UK: Oxford University Press.

Hanser, W. E., ter Bogt, T. F., Van den Tol, A. J., Mark, R. E., & Vingerhoets, A. J. (2016). Consolation through music: A survey study. *Musicae Scientiae*, *20*(1), 122–137. doi:10.1177/1029864915620264

Hao, N. (2010). The effects of domain knowledge and instructional manipulation on creative idea generation. *Journal of Creative Behavior*, *44*(4), 237–257.

Hargreaves, D., & Lamont, A. (2017). Wellbeing and health. In *The psychology of musical development* (pp. 245–277). Cambridge, UK: Cambridge University Press.

Hargreaves, D. J., & Bonneville-Roussy, A. (2018) What is "open-earedness," and how can it be measured? *Musicae Scientiae*, *22*(2), 161–174. doi:10.1177/1029864917697783

Hargreaves, D. J., Hargreaves, J. J., & North, A. C. (2012). Imagination and creativity in music listening. In D. Hargreaves, D. Miell, & R. A. R. MacDonald (Eds.), *Musical imaginations: Multidisciplinary perspectives on creativity, performance, and perception* (pp. 156–172). Oxford, UK: Oxford University Press.

Hargreaves, D. J., & North, A. C. (2010). Experimental aesthetics and liking for music. In P. N. Justin & J. A. Sloboda (Eds.), *Handbook of music and emotion: Theory, research, applications* (pp. 515–546). Oxford, UK: Oxford University Press.

Hargreaves, D. J., North, A. C., & Tarrant, M. (2016). How and why do musical preferences change in childhood and adolescence? In G. E. McPherson (Ed.), *The child as musician: A handbook of musical development* (pp. 303–322). Oxford, UK: Oxford University Press.

Harrison, K. (2019). The social potential of music for addiction recovery. *Music & Science*. doi:10.1177/2059204319842058

Hash, P. M. (2012). An analysis of the ratings and interrater reliability of high school band contests. *Journal of Research in Music Education*, *60*(1), 81–100. doi:10.1177/0022429411434932

Hatfield, J. L. (2016). Performing at the top of one's musical game. *Frontiers in Psychology*, *7*, article 1356. https://doi.org/10.3389/fpsyg.2016.01356

Hatfield, J. L., Halvari, H., & Lemyre, P. (2017). Instrumental practice in the contemporary music academy: A three-phase cycle of Self-Regulated Learning in music students. *Music Scientiae*, *21*, 316–337. doi:10.1177/1029864916658342

Hays, T., & Minichiello, V. (2005). The meaning of music in the lives of older people: A qualitative study. *Psychology of Music, 33*(4), 437–451. doi:10.1177/0305735605056160

Hebert, D. G., & Kertz-Welzel, A. (Eds.). (2016). *Patriotism and nationalism in music education.* Abingdon, UK: Routledge.

Heidemann, K. (2016). A system for describing vocal timbre in popular song. *Music Theory Online: A Journal of the Society for Music Theory, 22*(1). http://www.mtosmt.org/issues/mto.16.22.1/mto.16.22.1.heidemann.html

Helmefalk, M., & Hultén, B. (2017). Multi-sensory congruent cues in designing retail store atmosphere: Effects on shoppers' emotions and purchase behavior. *Journal of Retailing and Consumer Services, 38*, 1–11. http://dx.doi.org/10.1016/j.jretconser.2017.04.007

Henninger, J. C. (2018). The nature of expertise in instrumental music settings: A comparative analysis of common elements observed in band rehearsals and applied lessons. *Journal of Band Research, 53*(2), 48–72.

Herbrand, M. K., & Silverman, M. J. (2020). A randomized pilot study of patient-preferred live music addressing fatigue, energy, and pain in adults on a medical oncology/hematology unit. *Psychology of Music* Advance online publication. doi:10.1177/0305735620967723

Herget, A., Breves, P., & Schramm, H. (2020). The influence of different levels of musical fit on the efficiency of audio-visual advertising. *Musicae Scientiae.* Advance online publication. https://doi.org/10.1177/1029864920904095

Herholz, S. C., Boh, B., & Pantev, C. (2011). Musical training modulates encoding of higher-order regularities in the auditory cortex. *European Journal of Neuroscience, 34*(3), 524–529. doi:10.1111/j.1460-9568.2011.07775.x

Herholz, S. C., Halpern, A. R., & Zatorre, R. J. (2012). Neuronal correlates of perception, imagery, and memory for familiar tunes. *Journal of Cognitive Neuroscience, 24*(6), 1382–1397. https://doi.org/10.1162/jocn_a_00216

Herholz, S. C., & Zatorre, R. J. (2012). Musical training as a framework for brain plasticity: Behavior, function, and structure. *Neuron, 76*(3), 486–502. http://dx.doi.org/10.1016/j.neuron.2012.10.011

Héroux, I. (2016). Understanding the creative process in the shaping of an interpretation by expert musicians: Two case studies. *Musicae Scientiae, 20*(3), 304–324. doi:10.1177/1029864916634422

Héroux, I. (2018). Creative processes in the shaping of a musical interpretation: A study of nine professional musicians. *Frontiers in Psychology, 9*, article 665. https://doi.org/10.3389/fpsyg.2018.00665

Hess, J. (2018). Detroit youth speak back: Rewriting deficit perspectives through songwriting. *Bulletin of the Council for Research in Music Education, 216*, 7–30. https://doi.org/10.5406/bulcouresmusedu.216.0007

Hevner, K. (1935). The affective character of the major and minor modes in music. *American Journal of Psychology, 47*, 103–118.

Hevner, K. (1936). Experimental studies of the elements of expression in music. *American Journal of Psychology, 48*, 246–268.

Hewitt, A., & Allan, A (2013). Advanced youth music ensembles: Experiences of, and reasons for, participation. *International Journal of Music Education, 31*(3), 257–575. doi:10.1177/0255761411434494

Heye, A., & Lamont, A. (2010). Mobile listening situations in everyday life: The use of MP3 players while travelling. *Musicae Scientiae, 14*(1), 95–120. https://doi.org/10.1177/102986491001400104f

Heyman, L., Perkins, R., & Araújo, L. (2019). Examining the health and wellbeing experiences of singers in popular music. *Journal of Popular Music Education, 3*, 173–201. https://doi.org/10.1386/jpme.3.2.173_1

Hibbett, R. (2005). What is indie rock? *Popular Music and Society, 28*(1), 55–77. doi:10.1080/03007760420000300972

Hickey, M. (2009). Can improvisation be "taught"?: A call for free improvisation in our schools. *International journal of music education, 27*(4), 285–299. doi:10.1177/0255761409345442

Hill, B. M., & Monroy-Hernández, A. (2012). The remixing dilemma: The trade-off between generativity and originality. *American Behavioral Scientist, 57*(5), 643–663. doi:10.1177/0002764212469359

Hill, J. (2017). Incorporating improvisation into classical music performance. In J. Rink, H. Gaunt, & A. Williamon (Eds.), *Musicians in the making: Pathways to creative performance* (pp. 222–240). Oxford, UK: Oxford University Press.

Hill, J. (2018). *Becoming creative: Insights from musicians in a diverse world.* New York, NY: Oxford University Press.

Hill, S. C. (2019). "Give me actual music stuff!": The nature of feedback in a collegiate songwriting class. *Research Studies in Music Education, 41*(2), 135–153. https://doi.org/10.1177/1321103X19826385

Hodges, D. A. (2016). Bodily responses to music. In S. Hallam, I. Cross, & M. Thaut (Eds.), *Oxford handbook of music psychology* (2nd ed., pp. 183–196). Oxford, UK: Oxford University Press.

Hoffman, A. R. (2015). "Blessed": Musical talent, smartness, & figured identities. *Equity & Excellence in Education, 48*(4), 606–620.

Hoffman, S. L., & Hanrahan, S. J. (2012). Mental skills for musicians: Managing music performance anxiety and enhancing performance. *Sport, Exercise, and Performance Psychology, 1*(1), 17–28. doi:10.1037/a0025409

Holmes, J. A. (2017). Expert listening beyond the limits of hearing: Music and deafness. *Journal of the American Musicological Society, 70*(1), 171–220. https://doi.org/10.1525/jams.2017.70.1.171

Holmes, P. (2005). Imagination in practice: A study of the integrated roles of interpretation, imagery and technique in the learning and memorisation processes of two experienced solo performers. *British Journal of Music Education, 22*(3), 217–235. doi:10.1017/S0265051705006613

Holtz, P. (2009). What's your music? Subjective theories of music-creating artists. *Musicae Scientiae, 13*(2), 207–230. https://doi.org/10.1177/102986490901300202

Honing, H. (2010). Lure(d) into listening: The potential of cognition-based music information retrieval. *Empirical Musicology Review, 5*(4), 146–151. https://doi.org/10.18061/1811/48549

Horan, R. (2009). The neuropsychological connection between creativity and meditation. *Creativity Research Journal, 21*(2–3), 199–222. doi:10.1080/10400410902858691

Horden, P. (Ed.). (2017). *Music as medicine: The history of music therapy since antiquity.* Abingdon, UK: Routledge.

Hu, X., Chen, J., & Wang, Y. (2021). University students' use of music for learning and well-being: A qualitative study and design implications. *Information Processing and Management, 58*(1). https://doi.org/10.1016/j.ipm.2020.102409

Hughes, E. (2010). Musical memory in piano playing and piano study. *Musical Quarterly, 1*(4), 592–603. https://www.jstor.org/stable/738068

Hunter, M. (2005). "To play as if from the soul of the composer": The idea of the performer in early Romantic aesthetics. *Journal of the American Musicological Society*, *58*(2), 357–398. https://doi.org/10.1525/jams.2005.58.2.357

Huron, D. (2006). *Sweet anticipation: Music and the psychology of expectation*. Cambridge, MA: MIT Press.

Huron, D. (2011). Why is sad music pleasurable? A possible role for prolactin. *Musicae Scientiae*, *15*(2), 146–158. doi:10.1177/1029864911401171

Huron, D., & Margulis, E. H. (2010). Musical expectancy and thrills. In P. N. Juslin & J. A. Sloboda (Eds.), *Handbook of music and emotion: Theory, research, applications* (pp. 575–604). Oxford, UK: Oxford University Press.

Hyry-Beihammer, E. K. (2011). Master-apprentice relation in music teaching. From a secret garden to a transparent modelling. *Nordic Research in Music Education Yearbook*, *12*, 161–178. http://hdl.handle.net/11250/172285

Isbell, D., & Stanley, A. M. (2011). Keeping instruments out of the attic: The concert band experiences of the non-music major. *Music Education Research International*, *5*, 22–33.

Iuşcă, D. G. (2020). "Seeing is believing": The importance of visual factors in music performance assessment. *Review of Artistic Education*, *20*(1), 355–360. doi:10.2478/rae-2020-0039

Jellison, J. A. (2016). Inclusive music classrooms: A universal approach. In G. E. McPherson (Ed.), *The child as musician: A handbook of musical development* (2nd ed., pp. 31–51). Oxford, UK: Oxford University Press.

Johansson, K. (2012). Organ improvisation: Edition, expansion, and instant composition. In D. J. Hargreaves, D. E. Miell, & R. A. R. MacDonald (Eds.), *Musical imaginations: Multidisciplinary perspectives on creativity, performance, and perception* (pp. 220–232). Oxford, UK: Oxford University Press.

Johnson, C. M. (2000). Effect instruction in appropriate rubato usage on the onset timings of musicians in performances of Bach. *Journal of Research in Music Education*, *48*, 78–84. https://doi.org/10.2307/3345458

Johnson, D., Allison, C., & Baron-Cohen, S. (2013). The prevalence of synesthesia: The consistency revolution. In J. Simner & E. Hubbard (Eds.), *Oxford handbook of synesthesia* (pp. 3–22). Oxford, UK: Oxford University Press.

Johnson, M. (2009). *Pop music theory: Harmony, form, and composition*. Boston, MA: Cinemasonique Music and MonoMyth Media.

Johnson, N., Shiju, A. M., Parmar, A., & Prabhu, P. (2020). Evaluation of auditory stream segregation in musicians and nonmusicians. *International Archives of Otorhinolaryngology*, *25*(1), e77–e80. doi:10.1055/s-0040-1709116f

Johnson-Laird, P. N. (2002). How jazz musicians improvise. *Music Perception*, *19*(3), 415–442. https://doi.org/10.1525/mp.2002.19.3.415

Jones, M. R. (2010). Attending to sound patterns and the role of entrainment. In A. C. Nobre & J. T. Coull (Eds.), *Attention and time* (pp. 317–330). Oxford, UK: Oxford University Press.

Jones, P. M. (2009). Lifewide as well as lifelong: Broadening primary and secondary school music education's service to students' musical needs. *International Journal of Community Music*, *2*(2–3), 201–214. doi:10.1386/ijcm.2.2&3.201/1

Jorgensen, E. R. (2020). To love or not to love (Western classical music): That is the question (for music educators). *Philosophy of Music Education Review*, *28*(2), 128–144. doi:10.2979/philmusieducrevi.28.2.02

Juchniewicz, J., Kelly, S. N., & Acklin, A. I. (2014). Rehearsal characteristics of "superior" band directors. *Update: Applications of Research in Music Education, 32*(2), 35–43. doi:10.1177/8755123314521221

Juncos, D. G., & Markman, E. J. (2016). Acceptance and Commitment Therapy for the treatment of music performance anxiety: A single subject design with a university student. *Psychology of Music, 44*(5), 935–952. doi:10.1177/0305735615596236

Juslin, P. 'N. (2013). What does music express? Basic emotions and beyond. *Frontiers in Psychology, 4*, article 596. https://doi.org/10.3389/fpsyg.2013.00596

Juslin, P. N. (2019). *Musical emotions explained: Unlocking the secrets of musical affect.* Oxford, UK: Oxford University Press.

Juslin, P. N., Friberg, A., Schoonderwaldt, E., & Karlsson, J. (2004). Feedback learning of musical expressivity. In A. Williamon (Ed.), *Musical excellence: Strategies and techniques for enhancing performance* (pp. 247–270). New York, NY: Oxford University Press.

Juslin, P. N., Karlsson, J., Lindström, E., Friberg, A., & Schoonderwaldt, E. (2006). Play it again with feeling: Computer feedback in musical communication of emotions. *Journal of Experimental Psychology: Applied, 12*(2), 79–95. https://doi.org/10.1037/1076-898X.12.2.79

Juslin, P. N., & Laukka, P. (2000). Improving emotional communication in music through cognitive feedback. *Musicae Scientiae, 4*, 151–183. https://doi.org/10.1177/102986490000400202

Juslin, P. N., & Laukka, P. (2003). Communication of emotions in vocal expression and music performance: Different channels, same code? *Psychological Bulletin, 129*(5), 770–814. https://doi.org/10.1037/0033-2909.129.5.770

Juslin, P. N., Liljeström, S., Västfjäll, D., Barradas, G., & Silva, A. (2008). An experience sampling study of emotional reactions to music: Listener, music, and situation. *Emotion, 8*(5), 668–683. doi:10.1037/a0013505

Juslin, P. N., & Lindström, E. (2016). Emotion in music performance. In S. Hallam, I. Cross, & M. Thaut (Eds.), *The Oxford handbook of music psychology* (2nd ed., pp. 597–614). Oxford, UK: Oxford University Press.

Juslin, P. N., & Scherer, K. R. (2005). Vocal expression of affect. In J. A. Harrigan, R. Rosenthal, & K. R. Scherer (Eds.), *The new handbook of methods in nonverbal behavior research* (pp. 65–136). New York, NY: Oxford University Press.

Juslin, P. N., & Sloboda, J. A. (2010). The past present, and future of music and emotion research. In P. N. Justin & J. A. Sloboda (Eds.), *Handbook of music and emotion: Theory, research, applications* (pp. 933–955). Oxford, UK: Oxford University Press.

Juslin, P. N., & Timmers, R. (2010). Expression and communication of emotion in music performance. In P. N. Justin & J. A. Sloboda (Eds.), *Handbook of music and emotion: Theory, research, applications* (pp. 453–489). Oxford, UK: Oxford University Press.

Juslin, P. N., & Västfjäll, D. (2008). Emotional responses to music: The need to consider underlying mechanisms. *Behavioral and Brain Sciences, 31*, 559–575. doi:10.1017/S0140525X08005293

Kaleńska-Rodzaj, J. (2020). Pre-performance emotions and music performance anxiety beliefs in young musicians. *Research Studies in Music Education, 42*(1), 77–93. doi:10.1177/1321103X19830098.

Kamin, S., Richards, H., & Collins, D. (2007). Influences on the talent development process of non-classical musicians: Psychological, social and environmental influences. *Music Education Research, 9*(3), 449–468. doi:10.1080/14613800701587860

Kapsetaki, M. E., & Easmon, C. (2019). Eating disorders in musicians: A survey investigating self-reported eating disorders of musicians. *Eating and Weight Disorders-Studies on Anorexia, Bulimia and Obesity, 24*(3), 541–549. doi:10.1007/s40519-017-0414-9

Karageorghis, C. I. (2020). Music-related interventions in the exercise domain: A theory-based approach. In G. Tenenbaum & R. C. Eklund (Eds.), *Handbook of sport psychology* (4th ed., pp. 929–949). Hoboken, NJ: Wiley.

Karageorghis, C. I., & Priest, D. (2012). Music in the exercise domain: A review and synthesis (Part I). *International Review of Sport and Exercise Psychology, 5*(1), 44–66. http://dx.doi.org/10.1080/1750984X.2011.631026

Karlsson, J., & Juslin, P. N. (2008). Musical expression: An observational study of instrumental teaching. *Psychology of Music, 36*(3), 309–334. doi:10.1177/0305735607086040

Karma, K. (2007). Musical aptitude definition and measure validation: Ecological validity can endanger the construct validity of musical aptitude tests. *Psychomusicology: A Journal of Research in Music Cognition, 19*(2), 79–90.

Kaspersen, M., & Götestam, K. G. (2002). A survey of performance anxiety among Norwegian music students. *European Journal of Psychiatry, 16*, 69–80.

Katz, S. L. (2009). *Dichotomous forces of inspiration in the creative process: A study of within-domain versus beyond-domain music composers* (Publication No. 3357299) [Doctoral dissertation, Harvard University]. ProQuest Dissertations & Theses A&I.

Katz, S. L., & Gardner, H. (2012). Musical materials or metaphorical models? A psychological investigation of what inspires composers. In D. J. Hargreaves, D. E. Miell, & R. A. R. MacDonald (Eds.), *Musical imaginations: Multidisciplinary perspectives on creativity, performance, and perception* (pp. 107–123). Oxford, UK: Oxford University Press.

Kaufman, J. C., & Beghetto, R. A. (2009). Beyond big and little: The Four C Model of creativity. *Review of General Psychology, 13*(1), 1–12. doi:10.1037/a0013688

Kaufman, S. B. (2013). Opening up openness to experience: A four-factor model and relations to creative achievement in the arts and sciences. *Journal of Creative Behavior, 47*(4), 233–255. doi:10.1002/jocb.33

Kaufman, S. B., & Gregoire, C. (2015). *Wired to create: Unraveling the mysteries of the creative mind.* New York, NY: Pedigree.

Kaur, J., & Singh, S. (2016). Neuromusculoskeletal problems of upper extremities in musicians-a literature review. *International Journal of Therapies and Rehabilitation Research, 5*(2), 14–18. doi:10.5455/ijtrr.000000120

Keeler, J. R., Roth, E. A., Neuser, B. L., Spitsbergen, J. M., Waters, D. J. M., & Vianney, J. M. (2015). The neurochemistry and social flow of singing: Bonding and oxytocin. *Frontiers in Human Neuroscience, 9*, article 518. https://doi.org/10.3389/fnhum.2015.00518

Keen, I. (2020). Agency, history and tradition in the construction of "Classical" music: The debate over "authentic performance." In C. Pinney & N. Thomas (Eds.), *Beyond aesthetics: Art and the technologies of enchantment* (pp. 31–56). Abingdon, UK: Routledge.

Keller, P. (2014). Ensemble performance. In D. Fabian, R. Timmers, & E. Schubert (Eds.), *Expressiveness in music performance: Empirical approaches across styles and cultures* (pp. 260–282). Oxford, UK: Oxford University Press.

Keller, P. E. (2007). Musical ensemble synchronisation. In E. Schubert, K. Buckley, R. Eliott, B. Koboroff, J. Chen, & C. Stevens (Eds.), *Proceedings of the International Conference on Music Communication Science* (pp. 80–83). Sydney, Australia.

Keller, P. E. (2008). Joint action in music performance. In F. Morganti, F. A. Carassa, & G. Riva (Eds.), *Enacting intersubjectivity: A cognitive and social perspective on the study of interactions* (pp. 205–221). Amsterdam, The Netherlands: IOS Press.

Keller, P. E., & Appel, M. (2010). Individual differences, auditory imagery, and the coordination of body movements and sounds in musical ensembles. *Music Perception, 28*(1), 27–46. doi:10.1525/mp.2010.28.1.27

Kelly, S. N. (2002). A sociological basis for music education. *International Journal of Music Education, 39*(1), 40–49. https://doi.org/10.1177/025576140203900105

Kenny, D. T. (2011). *The psychology of music performance anxiety.* Oxford, UK: Oxford University Press.

Kenny, D. T., & Ackermann, B. J. (2016). Optimizing physical and psychological health in performing musicians. In S. Hallam, I. Cross, & M. Thaut (Eds.), *The Oxford handbook of music psychology* (2nd ed., pp. 633–647). Oxford, UK: Oxford University Press.

Kenny, D. T., Davis, P., & Oates, J. (2004). Music performance anxiety and occupational stress amongst opera chorus artists and their relationship with state and trait anxiety and perfectionism. *Journal of Anxiety Disorders, 18*, 757–777. doi:10.1016/j.janxdis.2003.09.004

Kenny, D. T., Driscoll, T., & Ackermann, B. (2014). Psychological well-being in professional orchestral musicians in Australia: A descriptive population study. *Psychology of Music, 42*(2), 210–232. doi:10.1177/0305735612463950

Kenny, D. T., Fortune, J. M., & Ackermann, B. (2013). Predictors of music performance anxiety during skilled performance in tertiary flute players. *Psychology of Music, 41*(3), 306–328. doi:10.1177/0305735611425904

Kenny, D. T., & Osborne, M. S. (2006). Music performance anxiety: New insights from young musicians. *Advances in Cognitive Psychology, 2*(2–3), 103–112. doi:10.2478/v10053-008-0049-5

Kent, G. (2007). Unpeaceful music. In O. Urbain (Ed.), *Music and conflict transformation: Harmonies and dissonances in geopolitics* (pp. 112–119). New York, NY: I.B. Tauris.

Kertz-Welzel, A. (2020). "Kim had the same idea as Haydn": International perspectives on classical music and music education. *Philosophy of Music Education Review, 28*(2), 239–256. doi:10.2979/philmusieducrevi.28.2.08

Khalfa, S., Roy, M., Rainville, P., Dalla Bella, S., & Peretz, I. (2008). Role of tempo entrainment in psychophysiological differentiation of happy and sad music? *International Journal of Psychophysiology, 68*(1), 17–26. https://doi.org/10.1016/j.ijpsycho.2007.12.001

Kim, B. S. K., & Alamilla, S. G. (2017). Acculturation and enculturation: A review of theory and research. In A. M. Czopp & A. W. Blume (Eds.), *Social issues in living color: Challenges and solutions from the perspective of ethnic minority psychology: Societal and global issues* (Vol. 2, pp. 25–52). Santa Barbara, CA: Praeger/ABC-CLIO.

Kim, Y. (2008). The effect of improvisation-assisted desensitization, and music-assisted progressive muscle relaxation and imagery on reducing pianists' music performance anxiety. *Journal of Music Therapy, 45*(2), 165–191. doi:10.1093/jmt/45.2.165

King, E. (2013). Social familiarity: Styles of interaction in chamber ensemble rehearsal. In E. King & H. M. Prior (Eds.), *Music and familiarity: Listening, musicology and performance* (pp. 253–270). Abingdon, UK: Routledge.

King, E., & Gritten, A. (2017). Dialogue and beyond. In J. Rink, H. Gaunt, & A. Williamon (Eds.), *Musicians in the making: Pathways to creative performance* (pp. 306–321). Oxford, UK: Oxford University Press.

King, E. C. (2006). The roles of student musicians in quartet rehearsals. *Psychology of Music, 34*(2), 262–282. doi:01.0077/1315735616160855

Kingsbury, H. (2010). *Music, talent, & performance: A conservatory culture system* (2nd ed.). Philadelphia, PA: Temple University Press.

Kingsford-Smith, A., & Evans, P. (2021). A longitudinal study of psychological needs satisfaction, value, achievement, and elective music intentions. *Psychology of Music, 49*(3), 382–398. doi:10.1177/0305735619868285

Kinney, D. W. (2009). Internal consistency of performance evaluations as a function of music expertise and excerpt familiarity. *Journal of Research in Music Education, 56*(4), 322–337. 10.1177/0022429408328934

Klein, S. D., Bayard, C., & Wolf, U. (2014). The Alexandre Technique and musicians: A systematic review of controlled trials. *Complementary and Alternative Medicine, 14*, article 414. https://doi.org/10.1186/1472-6882-14-414

Kleinsmith, A. L., Friedman, R. S., & Neill, W. T. (2016). Exploring the impact of final ritardandi on evaluative responses to cadential closure. *Psychomusicology: Music, Mind, and Brain, 26*(4), 346–357. http://dx.doi.org/10.1037/pmu0000159

Knobel, M., & Lankshear, C. (2008). Remix: The art and craft of endless hybridization. *Journal of Adult & Adolescent Literacy, 52*(1), 22–33. doi:10.1598/JAAL.52.1.3

Knudsen, J. S. (2017). Music in the aftermath of the 2011 Utøya massacre. In F. Holt & A. Kärjä (Eds.), *The Oxford handbook of popular music in the Nordic countries* (pp. 257–276). New York: Oxford University Press.

Kodály, Z. (1974). *The selected writings of Zoltán Kodály*. London, UK: Boosey & Hawkes.

Koelsch, S., Vuust, P., & Friston, K. (2019). Predictive processes and the peculiar case of music. *Trends in Cognitive Sciences, 23*(1), 63–77. https://doi.org/10.1016/j.tics.2018.10.006

Kokotsaki, D., & Davidson, J. W. (2003). Investigating musical performance anxiety among music college singing students: A quantitative analysis. *Music Education Research, 5*(1), 45–59. doi:10.1080/14613800307103

Kolb, B. (2018). Brain plasticity and experience. In R. Gibb & B. Kolb (Eds.), *The neurobiology of brain and behavioral development* (pp. 341–389). London, UK: Academic Press.

Konečni, V. J. (2012). Composers' creative process: The role of life-events, emotion and reason. In D. J. Hargreaves, D. E. Miell, & R. A. R. MacDonald (Eds.), *Musical imaginations: Multidisciplinary perspectives on creativity, performance, and perception* (pp. 141–155). Oxford, UK: Oxford University Press.

Konrad, U. (2006). Compositional method. In C. Eisen & S. P. Keefe (Eds.), *The Cambridge Mozart encyclopedia*. Cambridge, UK: Cambridge University Press.

Kontukoski, M., Paakki, M., Thureson, J., Uimonen, H., & Hopia, A. (2016). Imagined salad and steak restaurants: Consumers' colour, music and emotion associations with different dishes. *International Journal of Gastronomy and Food Science, 4*, 1–11. http://dx.doi.org/10.1016/j.ijgfs.2016.04.001

Kopiez, R., & Lee, J. I. (2008). Towards a general model of skills involved in sight reading music. *Music Education Research, 10*(1), 41–62. doi:10.1080/14613800701871363

Kopiez, R., & Lehmann, M. (2008). The "open-earedness" hypothesis and the development of age-related aesthetic reactions to music in elementary school children. *British Journal of Music Education, 25*(2), 121–138. doi:10.1017/S0265051708007882

Kopiez, R., Wolf, A., & Platz, F. (2017). Small influence of performing from memory on audience evaluation. *Empirical Musicology Review, 12*(1–2), 2–14. http://dx.doi.org/10.18061/emr.v12i1-2.5553

Korczynski, M. (2003). Music at work: Toward a historical overview. *Folk Music Journal, 8*(3), 314–334. https://www.jstor.org/stable/4522689

Kozbelt, A. (2008). One-hit wonders in classical music: Evidence and (partial) explanations for an early career peak, *Creativity Research Journal, 20*(2), 179–195. doi:10.1080/10400410802059952

Kozbelt, A. (2012). Process, self-evaluation, and lifespan creativity trajectories in eminent composers. In D. Collins (Ed.), *The act of musical composition: Studies in the creative process* (pp. 27–51). Surrey, UK: Ashgate.

Kozbelt, A., Beghetto, R. A., & Runco, M. A. (2010). Theories of creativity. In J. C. Kaufman & R. J. Sternberg (Eds.), *The Cambridge handbook of creativity* (pp. 20–47). Cambridge, UK: Cambridge University Press.

Krahé, C., Hahn, U., & Whitney, K. (2015). Is seeing (musical) believing? The eye versus the ear in emotional responses to music. *Psychology of Music, 43*(1), 140–148. doi:10.1177/0305735613498920

Kraus, N., & Chandrasekaran, B. (2010). Music training for the development of auditory skills. *Nature Reviews Neuroscience, 11*, 599–605. doi:10.1038/nrn2882

Krause, A., North, A., & Hewitt, L. (2014). Music selection behaviors in everyday listening. *Journal of Broadcasting & Electronic Media, 58*(2), 306–323. doi:10.1177/0305735613496860

Krause, A. E., North, A. C., & Hewitt, L. Y. (2016). The role of location in everyday experiences of music. *Psychology of Popular Media Culture, 5*(3), 232–257. http://dx.doi.org/10.1037/ppm0000059

Kreutz, G. (2014). Does singing facilitate social bonding. *Music & Medicine, 6*(2), 51–60. http://dx.doi.org/10.47513/mmd.v6i2.180

Lacaille, N., Koestner, R., & Gaudreau, P. (2007). On the value of intrinsic rather than traditional achievement goals for performing artists: A short-term prospective study. *International Journal of Music Education, 25*(3), 245–257. doi:10.1177/0255761407083578

Lacaille, N., Whipple, N., & Koestner, R. (2005). Reevaluating the benefits of performance goals: The relation of goal type to optimal performance for musicians and athletes. *Medical Problems of Performing Artists, 20*, 11–16.

Lamont, A. (2011a). The beat goes on: Music education, identity and lifelong learning. *Music Education Research, 13*(4), 369–388. doi:10.1080/14613808.2011.638505

Lamont, A. (2011b). University students' strong experiences of music: Pleasure, engagement, and meaning. *Musicae Scientiae, 15*, 229–249. doi:10.1177/1029864911403368

Lamont, A. (2012). Emotion, engagement and meaning in strong experiences of music performance. *Psychology of Music, 40*(5), 574–594. doi:10.1177/0305735612448510

Lamont, A. (2017). Musical identity, interest, and involvement. In R. A. R. MacDonald, D. J. Hargreaves, & D. Miell (Eds.), *Handbook of musical identities* (pp. 176–196). Oxford, UK: Oxford University Press.

Lamont, A., Greasley, A., & Sloboda, J. (2016). Choosing to hear music: Motivation, process, and effect. In S. Hallam, I. Cross, & M. Thaut (Eds.), *The Oxford handbook of music psychology* (2nd ed., pp. 711–724). Oxford, UK: Oxford University Press.

Lamont, A., & Hargreaves, D. (2019). Musical preference and social identity in adolescence. In K. McFerran, P. Derrington, & S. Saarikallio (Eds.), *Handbook of music, adolescents, and wellbeing* (pp. 109–118). Oxford, UK: Oxford University Press.

Landay, K., & Harms, P. D. (2019). Whistle while you work? A review of the effects of music in the workplace. *Human Resource Management Review, 29*(3), 371–385. https://doi.org/10.1016/j.hrmr.2018.06.003

Lane, D. M., & Chang, Y. A. (2018). Chess knowledge predicts chess memory even after controlling for chess experience: Evidence for the role of high-level processes. *Memory & Cognition, 46*(3), 337–348. https://doi.org/10.3758/s13421-017-0768-2

Langner, J., Kopiez, R., Stoffel, C., & Wilz, M. (2000). Realtime analysis of dynamic shaping. In C. Woods, G. Luck, F. Brochard, F. Seddon, & J. Sloboda (Eds.), *Proceedings of the Sixth International Conference on Music Perception and Cognition*. Staffordshire, UK: Keele University.

Latimer, M. E., Jr., Bergee, M. J., & Cohen, M. L. (2010). Reliability and perceived pedagogical utility of a weighted music performance assessment rubric. *Journal of Research in Music Education, 58*(2), 168–183. doi:10.1177/0022429410369836

Laukka, P. (2004). Instrumental music teachers' views on expressivity: A report from music conservatoires. *Music Education Research, 6*(1), 45–56. https://doi.org/10.1080/1461380032000182821

Laukka, P., Eerola, T., Thingujam, N. S., Yamasaki, T., & Beller, G. (2013). Universal and culture-specific factors in the recognition and performance of musical affect expressions. *Emotion, 13*, 434–449. doi:10.1037/a0031388

Laukka, P., & Quick, L. (2013). Emotional and motivational uses of music in sports and exercise: A questionnaire study among athletes. *Psychology of Music, 41*(2), 198–215. doi:10.1177/0305735611422507

Laurila, K., & Willingham, L. (2017). Drum circles and community music: Reconciling the difference. *International Journal of Community Music, 10*(2), 139–156. doi:10.1386/ijcm.10.2.139_1

Law, L. N. C., & Zentner, M. (2012). Assessing musical abilities objectively: Construction and validation of the Profile of Music Perception Skills. *PLoS ONE, 7*(12), e52508. https://doi.org/10.1371/journal.pone.0052508

Lazarus, A. A., & Abramovitz, A. A. (2004). A multimodal behavioral approach to performance anxiety. *Journal of Clinical Psychology, 60*(8), 831–840. doi:10.1002/jclp.20041

Lebowitz, E. R., Leckman, J. F., Silverman, W. K., & Feldman, R. (2016). Cross-generational influences on childhood anxiety disorders: Pathways and mechanisms. *Journal of Neural Transmission, 123*(9), 1053–1067. doi:10.1007/s00702-016-1565-y

Lecanuet, J. P., & Schaal, B. (2002). Sensory performances in the human foetus: A brief summary of research. *Intellectica, 1*(34), 29–56. https://doi.org/10.3406/intel.2002.1072

Lee, J. D., Roberts, S. C., Hoffman, J. D., & Angell, L. S. (2012). Scrolling and driving: How an MP3 player and its aftermarket controller affect driving performance and visual behavior. *Human Factors, 54*(2), 250–263. https://doi.org/10.1177/0018720811429562

Lee, J. I. (2006). The role of inner hearing in sight-reading music as an example of intermodal perception. *Musikpsychologie, 18*, 35–52.

Lehman, P. R. (2007). Getting down to basics: Keynote address. In T. S. Brophy (Ed.), *Assessment in music education: Integrating curriculum, theory, and practice: Proceedings of the 2007 Symposium on Assessment in Music Education* (pp. 17–28). Chicago, IL: GIA Publications.

Lehmann, A. C., & Davidson, J. W. (2006). Taking an acquired skills perspective on music performance. In R. Colwell (Ed.), *MENC handbook of musical cognition and development* (pp. 225–259). New York, NY: Oxford University Press.

Lehmann, A. C., & Ericsson, K. A. (1998). The historical development of domains of expertise: Performance standards and innovations in music. In A. Steptoe (Ed.), *Genius and the mind: Studies of creativity and temperament in the historical record* (pp. 64–97). Oxford, UK: Oxford University Press.

Lehmann, A. C., Gruber, H., & Kopiez, R. (2018). Expertise in music. In K. A. Ericsson, R. R. Hoffman, A. Kozbelt, & A. M. Williams (Eds.), *Cambridge handbook of expertise and expert performance* (2nd ed., pp. 535–549). Cambridge, UK: Cambridge University Press.

Lehmann, A. C., & Jørgensen, H. (2018). Practice. In G. E. McPherson & G. F. Welch (Eds.), *Vocal, instrumental, and ensemble learning and teaching: An Oxford handbook of music education* (Vol. 3, pp. 126–144). New York, NY: Oxford University Press.

Leman, M., Desmelt, F., Styns, F., van Noorden, L., & Moelants, D. (2008). Sharing musical expression through embodied listening: A case study based on Chinese gun music. *Music Perception, 26*(3), 263–278. doi:10.1525/MP.2009.26.3.263

Leung, B. W., & McPherson, G. W. (2011). Case studies of factors affecting the motivation of musical high achievers to learn music in Hong Kong. *Music Education Research, 13*(1), 69–91. doi:10.1080/14613808.2011.553278

Levitin, D. (2006). *This is your brain on music: The science of a human obsession.* New York, NY: Dutton.

Levitin, D. J., & Rogers, S. E. (2005). Absolute pitch: Perception, coding, and controversies. *Trends in Cognitive Sciences, 9*(1), 26–33. doi:10.1016/j.tics.2004.11

Lim, M. C. (2014). In pursuit of harmony: The social and organisational factors in a professional vocal ensemble. *Psychology of Music, 42*(3), 307–324. doi:10.1177/0305735612469674

Limb, C. J., & Braun, A. R. (2008). Neural substrates of spontaneous musical performance: An fMRI study of jazz improvisation. *PLoS ONE, 3*(2), e1679. doi:10.1371/journal.pone.0001679

Lin, P., Chang, J., Zemon, V., & Midlarsky, E. (2007). Silent illumination: A study on Chan (Zen) meditation, anxiety, and musical performance quality. *Psychology of Music, 36*(2), 139–155. doi:10.1177/0305735607080840

Lindblom, A. (2017). "It gives them a place to be proud"—Music and social inclusion. Two diverse cases of young First Nations people diagnosed with autism in British Columbia, Canada. *Psychology of Music, 45*(2), 268–282. doi:10.1177/0305735616659553

Lindström, E., Juslin, P. N., Bresin, R., & Williamon, A. (2003). "Expressivity comes from within your soul": A questionnaire study of music students' perspectives on expressivity. *Research Studies in Music Education, 20,* 23–47. https://doi.org/10.1177/1321103X030200010201

Linnenbrink-Garcia, L., Maehr, M. L. Y., & Pintrich, P. R. (2011). Motivation and achievement. In R. Colwell & P. R. Webster (Eds.), *MENC handbook of research on music learning: Volume 1: Strategies* (pp. 216–264). New York, NY: Oxford University Press.

Lisboa, T., Williamon, A., Zicari, M., & Eiholzer, H. (2005). Mastery through imitation: A preliminary study. *Musicae Scientiae, 19*(1), 75–110. doi:10.1177/102986490500900103

Liston, M., Frost, A. A. M., & Mohr, P. B. (2003). The prediction of musical performance anxiety. *Medical Problems of Performing Artists, 18*(3), 120–125.

Loimusalo, N. J., & Huovinen, E. (2018). Memorizing silently to perform tonal and nontonal notated music: A mixed-methods study with pianists. *Psychomusicology: Music, Mind, and Brain, 28*(4), 222. http://dx.doi.org/10.1037/pmu0000227

Loimusalo, N., Huovinen, E., & Puurtinen, M. (2019). Successful approaches to mental practice: A case study of four pianists. *Music Performance Research, 9,* 101–127. http://urn.fi/URN:NBN:fi:jyu-201904252286

López-Íñiguez, G., & Bennett, D. (2020). A lifespan perspective on multi-professional musicians: Does music education prepare classical musicians for their careers? *Music Education Research, 22*(1), 1–14. doi:10.1080/14613808.2019.1703925

Lothwesen, K. S. (2020). The profile of music as a creative domain in people's conceptions: Expanding Runco & Bahleda's 1986 study on implicit theories of creativity in conceptual replication. *Musicae Scientiae, 24*(3), 277–298. doi:10.1177/1029864918798417

Lotto, A., & Holt, L. (2011). Psychology of auditory perception. *Wiley Interdisciplinary Reviews: Cognitive Science, 2*(5), 479–489. doi:10.1002/wcs.123

Lotze, M., Scheler, G., Tan, H. R., Braun, C., & Birbaumer, N. (2003). The musician's brain: Functional imaging of amateurs and professionals during performance and imagery. *Neuroimage, 20*, 1817–1829. doi:10.1016/j.neuroimage.2003.07.018

Louven, C. (2016). Hargreaves' "open-earedness": A critical discussion and new approach on the concept of musical tolerance and curiosity. *Musicae Scientiae, 20*, 235–247. doi:10.1177/1029864916633264

Lu, X., Yi, F., & Hu, L. (2020). Music-induced analgesia: An adjunct to pain management. *Psychology of Music.* Advance online publication. doi:10.1177/0305735620928585

Lubart, T., & Guignard, J. (2004). The generality-specificity of creativity: A multi-variant approach. In R. J. Sternberg, E. L. Grigorenko, & J. L. Singer (Eds.), *Creativity: From potential to realization* (pp. 43–56). Washington, DC: American Psychological Association.

Lucey, B. (2013, November 5). *Shattering the myths of Wolfgang Amadeus Mozart.* Newspaper Alum. https://www.newspaperalum.com/2013/11/shattering-the-myths-of-wolfgang-amadeus-mozart.html

Ludden, D. (2015, July 31). Is music a universe language? [Blog post]. https://www.psychologytoday.com/us/blog/talking-apes/201507/is-music-universal-language/

Lumpkin, G. T., Hills, G. E., & Shrader, R. C. (2004). Opportunity recognition. In H. P. Welsch (Ed.), *Entrepreneurship: The way ahead* (pp. 73–90). New York, NY: Routledge.

Lussy, M. (1874). *Traité de l'expression musicale: Accents, nuances et mouvements dans la musique vocal et instrumentale.* Paris, France: Berger-Levrault & Heugel.

Lussy, M. (1883). *Le Rythme musicale: Son origine, sa unction et son accentuation.* Paris, France: Heugel.

Lynar, E., Cvejic, E., Schubert, E., & Vollmer-Conna, U. (2017). The joy of heartfelt music: An examination of emotional and physiological responses. *International Journal of Psychophysiology, 120*, 118–125. http://dx.doi.org/10.1016/j.ijpsycho.2017.07.012

MacGregor, E. H. (2020). Participatory performance in the secondary music classroom and the paradox of belonging. *Music Education Research, 22*(2), 229–241. https://doi.org/10.1080/14613808.2020.1737927

Mach, E. (1980). *Great pianists speak for themselves.* New York, NY: Dodd, Mead.

MacIntyre, P. D., Schnare, B., & Ross, J. (2017). Self-determination theory and motivation for music. *Psychology of Music, 46*(5), 699–715. doi:10.1177/0305735617721637

MacLeod, R. B., & Nápoles, J. (2015). The influences of teacher delivery and student progress on experienced teachers' perceptions of teaching effectiveness. *Journal of Music Teacher Education, 24*(3), 24–36. doi:10.1177/1057083714527111

MacNamara, A., Holmes, P., & Collins, D. (2006). The pathway to excellence: The role of psychological characteristics in negotiating the challenges of musical development. *British Journal of Music Education, 23*(3), 285–302. doi:10.1017/S0265051706007066

Macnamara, B. N., Hambrick, D. Z., & Oswald, F. L. (2014). Deliberate practice and performance in music, games, sports, education, and professions: A meta-analysis. *Psychological Science, 25,* 1608–1618. doi:10.1177/0956797614535810

Madison, G., Holmquist, J., & Vestin, M. (2018). Musical improvisation skill in a prospective partner is associated with mate value and preferences, consistent with sexual selection and parental investment theory: Implications for the origin of music. *Evolution and Human Behavior, 39*(1), 120–129. https://doi.org/10.1016/j.evolhumbehav.2017.10.005

Mainwaring, J. (1941). The meaning of musicianship: A problem in the teaching of music. *British Journal of Educational Psychology, 11*(3), 205–214.

Mainwaring, J. (1951). *Teaching music in schools.* London, UK: Paxton.

Mamlok, D. (2017). Active listening, music education, and society. In G. W. Noblit (Ed.), *Oxford research encyclopedia of education.* Oxford University Press. https://doi.org/10.1093/acrefore/9780190264093.013.186

Manfredo, J. (2008). Factors influencing curricular content for undergraduate instrumental conducting courses. *Bulletin of the Council for Research in Music Education, 175,* 43–57. https://www.jstor.org/stable/40319412

Manning, F. C., & Schutz, M. (2016). Trained to keep a beat: Movement-related enhancements to timing perception in percussionists and non-percussionists. *Psychological Research, 80,* 532–542. doi:10.1007/s00426-015-0678-5

Margulis, E. H. (2005). A model of melodic expectation. *Music Perception, 22*(4), 663–714. https://doi.org/10.1525/mp.2005.22.4.663

Margulis, E. H. (2014). *On repeat: How music plays the mind.* New York, NY: Oxford University Press.

Marsh, K., & Young, S. (2016). Musical play. In G. E. McPherson (Ed.), *The child as musician: A handbook of musical development* (2nd ed., pp. 462–484). Oxford, UK: Oxford University Press.

Marshall, E. A., & Butler, K. (2015). School-to-work transitions in emerging adulthood. In J. J. Arnett (Ed.), *The Oxford handbook of emerging adulthood* (pp. 316–333). New York, NY: Oxford University Press.

Martin-Gagnon, G., & Creech, A. (2019). Cool jazz: Music performance anxiety in jazz performance students. *Music Education Research, 21*(4), 414–425. doi:10.1080/14613808.2019.1605346

Martin-Saavedra, J. S., Vergara-Mendez, L. D., Pradilla, I., Vélez-van-Meerbeke, A., & Talero-Gutiérrez, C. (2018). Standardizing music characteristics for the management of pain: A systematic review and meta-analysis of clinical trials. *Complementary Therapies in Medicine, 41,* 81–89. https://doi.org/10.1016/j.ctim.2018.07.008

Martin-Saavedra, J. S., Vergara-Mendez, L. D., & Talero-Gutiérrez, C. (2018). Music is an effective intervention for the management of pain: An umbrella review. *Complementary Therapies in Clinical Practice, 32,* 103–114. https://doi.org/10.1016/j.ctcp.2018.06.003

Maruyama, K., & Hosokawa, S. (2006). Yearning for *eleki*: On Ventures tribute bands in Japan. In S. Homan (Ed.), *Access all eras: Tribute bands and global pop cultures* (pp. 151–165). New York, NY: Open University Press.

Marvin, E. W., VanderStel, J., & Siu, J. C. (2020). In their own words: Analyzing the extents and origins of absolute pitch. *Psychology of Music, 48*(6), 8080823. doi:10.1177/0305735619832959

Mas-Herrero, E., Singer, N., Ferreri, L., McPhee, M., Zatorre, R., & Ripolles, P. (2020). Rock'n'roll but not sex or drugs: Music is negatively correlated to depressive symptoms during the COVID-19 pandemic via reward-related mechanisms. *PsyArXiv*. https:// doi.org/10.31234/osf.io/x5upn

Massie-Laberge, C., Cossette, I., & Wanderley, M. M. (2019). Kinematic analysis of pianists' expressive performances of romantic excepts: Applications for enhanced pedagogical approaches. *Frontiers in Psychology, 9*, article 2725. https://doi.org/10.3389/ fpsyg.2018.02725

Matei, R., Broad, S., Goldbart, J., & Ginsborg, J. (2018). Health education for musicians. *Frontiers in Psychology, 9*, article 1137. https://doi.org/10.3389/fpsyg.2018.01137

Matei, R., & Ginsborg, J. (2017). Music performance anxiety in classical musicians— what we know about what works. *BJPsych International, 14*(2), 33–35. doi:10.1192/ s2056474000001744

McClellan, E. (2014). Undergraduate music education major identity formation in the university music department. *Action, Criticism & Theory for Music Education, 13*(1), 279–309. http://act.maydaygroup.org/articles/McClellan13_1.pdf

McClellan, E. (2017). A social-cognitive theoretical framework for examining music teacher identity. *Action, Criticism, and Theory for Music Education, 16*(2), 65–101. doi:10.22176/act16.2.65.

McGillen, C., & McMillan, R. (2005). Engaging with adolescent musicians: Lessons in song writing, cooperation and the power of original music. *Research Studies in Music Education, 25*(1), 1–20. https://doi.org/10.1177/1321103X050250010401

McGinnis, A. M., & Milling, L. S. (2005). Psychological treatment of musical performance anxiety: Current status and future directions. *Psychotherapy: Theory, Research, Practice, Training, 42*(3), 357–373. doi:10.1037/0033-3204.42.3.357

McIntosh, J. (2018). Child musicians and dancers performing in sync: Teaching, learning, and rehearsing collectively in Bali. In S. A. Reily & K. Brucher (Eds.), *The Routledge companion to the study of local musicking* (pp. 213–224). New York, NY: Routledge.

McMullen, E., & Saffran, J. R. (2004). Music and language: A developmental comparison. *Music Perception, 21*(3), 289–311. https://doi.org/10.1525/mp.2004.21.3.289

McPhee, E. A. (2011). Finding the muse: Teaching musical expression to adolescents in the one-to-one studio environment. *International Journal of Music Education, 29*(4), 333–346. doi:10.1177/0255761411421084

McPherson, G. E. (2005). From child to musician: Skill development during the beginning stages of learning an instrument. *Psychology of Music, 33*(1), 5–35. doi:10.1177/ 0305735605048012

McPherson, G. E. (2009). The role of parents in children's musical development. *Psychology of Music, 37*(1), 91–110. doi:10.1177/0305735607086049

McPherson, G. E., Bailey, M., & Sinclair, K. E. (1997). Path analysis of a theoretical model to describe the relationship among five types of musical performance. *Journal of Research in Music Education, 45*, 103–129. https://doi.org/10.2307/3345469

McPherson, G. E., Davidson, J. W., & Faulkner, R. (2012). *Music in our lives*. Oxford, UK: Oxford University Press.

McPherson, G. E., & Gabrielsson, A. (2002). From sound to sign. In R. Parncutt & G. E. McPherson (Eds.), *The science and psychology of music performance: Creative strategies for teaching and learning* (pp. 99–115). New York, NY: Oxford University Press.

McPherson, G. E., & Hendricks, K. S. (2010). Students' motivation to study music: The United States of America. *Research Studies in Music Education, 32*, 201–213. doi:10.1177/1321103X10384200

McPherson, G. E., & McCormick, J. (2006). Self-efficacy and music performance. *Psychology of Music, 34*(3), 322–336. doi:10.1177/0305735606064841

McPherson, G. E., Osborne, M. S., Evans, P., & Miksza, P. (2019). Applying self-regulated learning microanalysis to study musicians' practice. *Psychology of Music, 47*(1), 18–32. doi:10.1177/0305735617731614

McPherson, G. E., & Williamon, A. (2016). Building gifts into musical talents. In G. E. McPherson (Ed.), *The child as musician: A handbook of musical development* (2nd ed., pp. 340–359). Oxford, UK: Oxford University Press.

McPherson, G. E., & Zimmerman, B. J. (2011). Self-regulation of musical learning: A social cognitive perspective on developing performance skills. In R. Colwell & P. Webster (Eds.), *MENC handbook of research on music learning, Volume 2: Applications* (pp. 130–175). New York, NY: Oxford University Press.

Meissner, H. (2017). Instrumental teachers' instructional strategies for facilitating children's learning of expressive music performance: An exploratory study. *International Journal of Music Education, 35*(1), 118–135. doi:10.1177/0255761416643850

Meissner, H., & Timmers, R. (2020). Young musicians' learning of expressive performance: The importance of dialogic teaching and modeling. *Frontiers in Education, 5,* article 11. https://doi.org/10.3389/feduc.2020.00011

Merriam, A. P. (1964). *The anthropology of music.* Chicago, IL: Northwestern University Press.

Merrotsy, P. (2013). A note on Big-C creativity and little-c creativity. *Creativity Research Journal, 25*(4), 474–476. doi:10.1080/10400419.2013.843921

Merter, S. (2017). Synesthetic approach in the design process for enhanced creativity and multisensory experiences. *Design Journal, 20*(Supp 1), S4519–S4528. doi:10.1080/14606925.2017.1352948

Miksza, P. (2005). The effect of mental practice on the performance achievement of high school trombonists. *Contributions to Music Education, 35,* 75–93.

Miksza, P. (2007). Effective practice: An investigation of observed practice behaviors, self-reported practice habits, and the performance achievement of high school wind players. *Journal of Research in Music Education, 55*(4), 359–375. doi:10.1177/0022429408317513

Miksza, P. (2011). A review of research on practicing: Summary and synthesis of the extant research with implications for a new theoretical orientation. *Bulletin of the Council for Research in Music Education, 190,* 51–92. doi:10.5406/bulcouresmusedu.190.0051uc

Miksza, P. (2015). The effect of self-regulation instruction on the performance achievement, musical self-efficacy, and practicing of advanced wind players. *Psychology of Music, 43*(2), 219–243. doi:10.1177/0305735613500832

Miksza, P., Blackwell, J., & Roseth, N. E. (2018). Self-regulated music practice: Microanalysis as a data collection technique and inspiration for pedagogical intervention. *Journal of Research in Music Education, 66*(3), 295–319. doi:10.1177/0022429418788557

Miksza, P., Tan, L., & Dye, C. (2012). Achievement motivation for band: A cross-cultural examination of the 2 × 2 achievement goal motivation framework. *Psychology of Music, 44,* 1372–1388. doi:10.1177/0305735616628659

Miksza, P., Watson, K., & Calhoun, I. (2018). The effect of mental practice on melodic jazz improvisation achievement. *Psychomusicology: Music, Mind, and Brain, 28*(1), 40. http://dx.doi.org/10.1037/pmu0000206

Mikutta, C. A., Maissen, G., Altorfer, A., Strik, W., & König, T. (2014). Professional musicians listen differently to music. *Neuroscience, 268*, 102–111. http://dx.doi.org/10.1016/j.neuroscience.2014.03.007

Miller, K. E., & Quigley, B. M. (2012). Sensation-seeking, performance genres and substance use among musicians. *Psychology of Music, 40*(4), 389–410. doi:10.1177/0305735610387776

Miller, L. K. (2014). On the nature and origin of musical savants. In *Musical savants: Exceptional skill in the mentally retarded* (pp. 177–207). New York, NY: Psychology Press.

Millet, B., Ahn, S., & Chattah, J. (2019). The impact of music on vehicular performance: A meta-analysis. *Transportation Research Part F: Traffic Psychology and Behaviour, 60*, 743–760. https://doi.org/10.1016/j.trf.2018.10.007

Mills, J. (2006). Performing and teaching: The beliefs and experience of music students as instrumental Teachers, *Psychology of Music, 34*(3), 372–390.

Mills, J., & McPherson, G. E. (2016). Musical literacy: Reading traditional clef notation. In G. E. McPherson (Ed.), *The child as musician: A handbook of musical development* (2nd ed., pp. 177–191). Oxford, UK: Oxford University Press.

Mindell, J. A., & Williamson, A. A. (2018). Benefits of a bedtime routine in young children: Sleep, development, and beyond. *Sleep Medicine Reviews, 40*, 93–108. https://doi.org/10.1016/j.smrv.2017.10.007

Miranda, D. (2020). The emotional bond between neuroticism and music. *Psychomusicology: Music, Mind, and Brain, 30*(2), 53–63. http://dx.doi.org/10.1037/pmu0000250

Miranda, D., Gaudreau, P., & Morizot, J. (2010). Blue notes: Coping by music listening predicts neuroticism changes in adolescence. *Psychology of Aesthetics, Creativity, and the Arts, 4*(4), 247. doi:10.1037/a0019496

Mishra, J. (2014). Improving sightreading accuracy: A meta-analysis. *Psychology of Music, 42*(2), 131–156. doi:10.1177/0305735612463770

Mitchell, H., & Benedict, R. (2017). The moot audition: Preparing music performers as expert listeners. *Research Studies in Music Education, 39*(2), 195–208. doi:10.1177/1321103X17709631

Mitchell, L., & MacDonald, R. (2012). Music and pain: Evidence from experimental perspectives. In R. A. R. MacDonald, G. Kreutz, & L. Mitchell (Eds.), *Music, health and well-being* (pp. 230–238). Oxford, UK: Oxford University.

Moelants, D. (2012). Conveying syncopation in music performance. In E. Cambouropoulos, C. Tsougras, P. Mavromatis, & K. Pastiadis (Eds.), *Proceedings of the 12th International Conference on Music Perception and Cognition and the 8th Triennial Conference of the European Society for the Cognitive Sciences of Music* (pp. 686–691). Thessaloniki, Greece: Aristotle University of Thessaloniki.

Montuori, A. (2020). Diversity. In *Encyclopedia of creativity* (3rd ed., pp. 368–376). Amsterdam, The Netherlands: Elsevier. https://doi.org/10.1016/B978-0-12-809324-5.23866-2

Moore, D. G., Burland, K., & Davidson, J. W. (2003). The social context of musical success: A developmental account. *British Journal of Psychology, 94*, 529–549.

Mornell, A., Osborne, M. S., & McPherson, G. E. (2020). Evaluating practice strategies, behavior and learning progress in elite performers: An exploratory study. *Musicae Scientiae, 24*(1), 130–135. doi:10.1177/1029864918771731

Mornell, A., & Wulf, G. (2019). Adopting an external focus of attention enhances musical performance. *Journal of Research in Music Education*, *66*(4), 375–391. doi:10.1177/0022429418801573

Morrison, S., & Selvey, J. (2014). The effect of conductor expressivity on choral ensemble evaluation. *Bulletin of the Council for Research in Music Education*, 199, 7–18. https://www.jstor.org/stable/10.5406/bulcouresmusedu.199.0007

Mosing, M. A., Madison, G., Pedersen, N. L., Kuja-Halkola, R., & Ullén, F. (2014). Practice does not make perfect: No causal effect of music practice on music ability. *Psychological Science*, *25*(9), 1795–1803. doi:10.1177/0956797614541990

Mudede, C. (2013, March 27). The language of hiphop hands. The Stranger. https://www.thestranger.com/seattle/the-language-of-hiphop-hands/Content?oid=16346921

Münte, T. F., Altenmüller, E., & Jäncke, L. (2002). The musician's brain as a model of neuroplasticity. *Nature Reviews Neuroscience*, *3*(6), 473–478. https://doi.org/10.1038/nrn843

Musco, A. M. (2009). Effects of learning melodies by ear on performance skills and student attitudes. *Contributions to Music Education*, *36*(2), 79–95. https://www.jstor.org/stable/24127180

Musco, A. M. (2010). Playing by ear: Is expert opinion supported by research? *Bulletin of the Council for Research in Music Education*, 184, 49–63. https://www.jstor.org/stable/27861482

Myers, D. E. (2008). Lifespan engagement and the question of relevance: Challenges for music education research in the twenty-first century. *Music Education Research*, *10*(1), 1–14. doi:10.1080/14613800701871330

Myers, S. A., & Anderson, C. M. (2008). *The fundamentals of small group communication*. Los Angeles, CA: Sage.

Myint, E. E. P., & Pwint, M. (2010, July). An approach for multi-label music mood classification. In *Proceedings of the 2010 2nd International Conference on Signal Processing Systems* (Vol. 1, pp. 290–294). Piscataway, NJ: Institute of Electrical and Electronics Engineers.

Nagel, J. J. (2010). Treatment of music performance anxiety via psychological approaches: A review of selected CBT and psychodynamic literature. *Medical Problems of Performing Artists*, *25*(4), 141–148.

Nager, W., Kohlmetz, C., Altenmüller, E., Rodriguez-Fornells, A., & Münte, T. (2003). The fate of sounds in conductors' brains: An ERP study. *Cognitive Brain Research*, *17*, 83–93. doi:10.1016/s0926-6410(03)00083-1

Nakamura, J., & Csikszentmihalyi, M. (2014). The concept of flow. In M. Csikszentmihalyi (Ed.), *Flow and the foundations of positive psychology* (pp. 239–263). Dordrecht, The Netherlands: Springer.

Nan, Y., Sun, Y., & Peretz, I. (2010). Congenital amusia in speakers of a tone language: Association with lexical tone agnosia. *Brain*, *133*(9), 2635–2642. doi:10.1093/brain/awq178

Nanayakkara, S. C., Taylor, E., Wyse, L., & Ong, S. H. (2009). An enhanced musical experience for the deaf: Design and evaluation of a music display and a haptic chair. In S. Greenberg, S. E. Hudson, K. Hinckley, M. R. Morris, & D. R. Olsen Jr. (Eds.), *Proceedings of the SIGCHI Conference on Human Factors in Computing Systems* (pp. 337–346). New York, NY: Association for Computing Machinery.

Nanayakkara, S. C., Wyse, L., Ong, S. H., & Taylor, E. A. (2013). Enhancing musical experience for the hearing-impaired using visual and haptic displays. *Human–Computer Interaction*, *28*(2), 115–160. doi:10.1080/07370024.2012.697006

Napoles, J., & MacLeod, R. B. (2013). The influences of teacher delivery and student progress on preservice teachers' perceptions of teaching effectiveness. *Journal of Research in Music Education*, *61*(3), 249–261. doi:10.1177/0022429413497234

Narducci, D. M. (2020). Musculoskeletal and associated conditions in the instrumental musician. In S. Lee, M. L. Morris, & S. V. Nicosia (Eds.), *Perspectives in performing arts medicine practice* (pp. 197–239). Cham, Switzerland; Springer.

Negus, K., Street, J., & Behr, A. (2017). Copying, copyright and originality: Imitation, transformation and popular musicians. *European Journal of Cultural Studies*, *20*(4), 363–380. doi:10.1177/1367549417718206

Newberger, J. (2020). Music in times of upheaval. *Psychoanalytic Social Work*, *27*(1), 31–41. doi:10.1080/15228878.2019.1656651

Nielsen Music. (2020). *Year-end music report: U.S. 2019.* https://static.billboard.com/files/pdfs/NIELSEN_2019_YEARENDreportUS.pdf

Nielsen, S. (2001). Self-regulating learning strategies in instrumental music practice. *Music Education Research*, *3*(2), 155–167. doi:10.1080/14613800120089223

Nielsen, S. G. (2015). Learning pre-played solos: Self-regulated learning strategies in jazz/improvised music. *Research Studies in Music Education*, *37*(2), 233–246. doi:10.1177/1321103X15615661

Niermann, H. C. M., Figner, B., & Roelofs, K. (2017). Individual differences in defensive stress-responses: The potential relevance for psychopathology. *Current Opinion in Behavioral Sciences*, *14*, 94–101. https://doi.org/10.1016/j.cobeha.2017.01.002

Nilsson, U. (2008). The anxiety- and pain-reducing effects of music interventions: A systematic review. *AORN Journal*, *87*, 780–807.

Niven, K., & Miles, E. (2013). Affect arousal. In M. D. Gellman & J. R. Turner (Eds.), *Encyclopedia of behavioral medicine* (pp. 50–52). New York, NY: Springer. https://doi.org/10.1007/978-1-4419-1005-9_1089

Njoora, T. K. (2015). More than just good feelings: Advocacy for music among mainstream subjects. *Muziki*, *12*(1), 23–40. doi:10.1080/18125980.2015.1031367

Noice, H., Jeffrey, J., Noice, T., & Chaffin, R. (2008). Memorization by a jazz musician: A case study. *Psychology of Music*, *36*(1), 63–79. doi:10.1177/0305735607080834

Norris, C. E., & Borst, J. D. (2007). An examination of the reliabilities of two choral festival adjudication forms. *Journal of Research in Music Education*, *55*(3), 237–251. https://doi.org/10.1177/002242940705500305

North, A. C., & Hargreaves, D. J. (2010). Music and marketing. In P. N. Juslin & J. A. Sloboda (Eds.), *Handbook of music and emotion: Theory, research, applications* (pp. 909–930). Oxford, UK: Oxford University Press.

North, A. C., & Hargreaves, D. J. (2012). Pop music subcultures and wellbeing. In R. A. R. MacDonald, G. Kreutz, & L. Mitchell (Eds.), *Music, health and well-being* (pp. 502–512). Oxford, UK: Oxford University.

North, A. C., Hargreaves, D. J., & Hargreaves, J. J. (2004). Uses of music in everyday life. *Music Perception*, *22*, 41–77. https://doi.org/10.1525/mp.2004.22.1.41

Nozaradan, S., Schwartze, M., Obermeier, C., & Kotz, S. A. (2017). Specific contributions of basal ganglia and cerebellum to the neural tracking of rhythm. *Cortex*, *95*, 156–168. http://dx.doi.org/10.1016/j.cortex.2017.08.015

Oare, S. (2012). Decisions made in the practice room: A qualitative study of middle school students' thought processes while practicing. *Update: Applications of Research in Music Education, 30*(2), 63–70. doi:10.1177/8755123312437051

O'Bryan, J. (2015). "We ARE our instrument!": Forming a singer identity. *Research Studies in Music Education, 37*(1), 123–137. doi:10.1177/1321103X15592831

Ockelford, A., & Welch, G. F. (2018). Mapping musical development in learners with the most complex needs: The Sounds of Intent project. In G. F. Welch & G. E. McPherson (Eds.), *Special needs, community music, and adult learning: An Oxford handbook of music education* (Vol. 4, pp. 7–27). New York, NY: Oxford University Press.

O'Connor, J. (2012). Is it good to be gifted: The social construction of the gifted child. *Children & Society, 26*, 293–303. doi:10.1111/j.1099-0860.2010.00341.x

Oechslin, M. S., Gschwind, M., & James, C. E. (2018). Tracking training-related plasticity by combining fMRI and DTI: The right hemisphere ventral stream mediates musical syntax processing. *Cerebral Cortex, 28*(4), 1209–1218. doi:10.1093/cercor/bhx033

Ohriner, M. S. (2012). Grouping hierarchy and trajectories of pacing in performances of Chopin's mazurkas. *Music Theory Online: A Journal of the Society for Music Theory, 18*(1). http://www.mtosmt.org/issues/mto.12.18.1/mto.12.18.1.ohriner.php

O'Neill, S., & Sloboda, J. (2017). Responding to performers. In J. Rink, H. Gaunt, & A. Williamon (Eds.), *Musicians in the making: Pathways to creative performance* (pp. 322–340). Oxford, UK: Oxford University Press.

O'Neill, S. A. (2011). Developing a young musician's growth mindset: The role of motivation, self-theories, and resiliency. In I. Deliège & J. W. Davidson (Eds.), *Music and the mind: Essays in honour of John Sloboda* (pp. 31–46). Oxford, UK: Oxford University Press.

Onyebadi, U. (Ed.). (2017). *Music as a platform for political communication*. Hershey, PA: IGI Global.

Osborne, M. S. (2016). Building performance confidence. In G. E. McPherson (Ed.), *The child as musician: A handbook of musical development* (2nd ed., pp. 422–440). Oxford, UK: Oxford University Press.

Osborne, M. S., Greene, D. J., & Immel, D. T. (2014). Managing performance anxiety and improving mental skills in conservatoire students through performance psychology training: A pilot study. *Psychology of Well-Being: Theory, Research and Practice, 4*, article 18. doi:10.1186/s13612-014-0018-3

Osborne, M. S., & Kenny, D. T. (2005). Development and validation of a music performance anxiety inventory for gifted adolescent musicians. *Journal of Anxiety Disorders, 19*(7), 725–751. doi:10.1016/j.janxdis.2004.09.002

Osborne, M. S., & Kenny, D. T. (2008). The role of sensitizing experiences in music performance anxiety in adolescent musicians. *Psychology of Music, 36*(4), 447–462. doi:10.1177/0305735607086051

Osborne, M. S., & McPherson, G. E. (2019). Precompetitive appraisal, performance anxiety and confidence in conservatorium musicians: A case for coping. *Psychology of Music, 47*(3), 451–462. doi:10.1177/0305735618755000

Osborne, M. S., McPherson, G. E., Miksza, P., & Evans, P. (2020). Using a microanalysis intervention to examine shifts in musicians' self-regulated learning. *Psychology of Music*. doi:10.1177/0305735620915265

Oviedo-Trespalacios, O., Williamson, A., & King, M. (2019). User preferences and design recommendations for voluntary smartphone applications to prevent distracted driving. *Transportation Research Part F: Traffic Psychology and Behaviour, 64*, 47–57. https://doi.org/10.1016/j.trf.2019.04.018

Packer, C., & Packer, D. (2005). Beta-blockers, stage fright, and vibrato: A case report. *Medical Problems of Performing Artists, 20*(3), 126–130.

Papageorgi, I. (2020). Prevalence and predictors of music performance anxiety in adolescent learners: Contributions of individual, task-related and environmental factors. *Musicae Scientiae.* Advance online publication. doi:10.1177/1029864920923128

Papageorgi, I., Creech, A., Haddon, E., Morton, F., De Bezenac, C., Himonides, E., Potter, J., Duffy, C., Whyton, T., & Welch, G. (2009). Investigating musical performance: Perceptions and prediction of expertise in advanced musical learners. *Psychology of Music, 38*(1), 31–66. doi:10.1177/0305735609336044

Papageorgi, I., Creech, A., & Welch, G. (2011). Perceived performance anxiety in advanced musicians specializing in different musical genres. *Psychology of Music, 41*(1), 18–41. doi:10.1177/0305735611408995

Paparo, S. A. (2013). The *Accafellows*: Exploring the music making and culture of a collegiate a cappella ensemble. *Music Education Research, 15*(1), 19–38. doi:10.1080/14613808.2012.712508

Parker, E. C. (2010). Exploring student experiences of belonging within an urban high school choral ensemble: An action research study. *Music Education Research, 12*(4), 339–352. doi:10.1080/14613808.2010.519379

Parker, E. C. (2016). The experience of creating community: An intrinsic case study of four Midwestern public school choral teachers. *Journal of Research in Music Education, 64*, 220–237. doi:10.1177/0022429416648292

Parker, E. C. (2018). A grounded theory of adolescent high school women's choir singers' process of social identity development. *Journal of Research in Music Education, 65*(4), 439–460. doi:10.1177/0022429417743478

Parker, E. C. (2020). *Adolescents on music: Why music matters to young people in our lives.* New York, NY: Oxford University Press.

Parncutt, R. (2016a). Prenatal development and the phylogeny and ontogeny of musical behavior. In S. Hallam, I. Cross, & M. Thaut (Eds.), *The Oxford handbook of music psychology* (2nd ed., pp. 371–386). Oxford, UK: Oxford University Press.

Parncutt, R. (2016b). Prenatal development. In G. E . McPherson (Ed.), *The child as musician: A handbook of musical development* (pp. 3–30). Oxford, UK: Oxford University Press.

Parncutt, R., & Levitin, D. J. (2001). Absolute pitch. In S. Sadie (Ed.), *The new Grove dictionary of music and musicians* (2nd ed., pp. 27–29). London, UK: Macmillan.

Parry, C. B. W. (2004). Managing the physical demands of musical performance. In A. Williamon (Ed.), *Musical excellence: Strategies and techniques to enhance performance* (pp. 41–60). Oxford, UK: Oxford University Press.

Parsons, J. E., & Simmons, A. L. (2020). Focus of attention verbalizations in beginning band: A multiple case study. *Journal of Research in Music Education, 69*(2), 152–166. doi:10.1177/ 0022429420973638.

Patel, A. D., & Demorest, S. M. (2013). Comparative music cognition: Cross-species and cross-cultural studies. In D. Deutsch (Ed.), *The psychology of music* (3rd ed., pp. 647–681). San Diego, CA: Academic Press.

Patston, T. (2014). Teaching stage fright?—Implications for music educators. *British Journal of Music Education, 31*(1), 85–98. doi:10.1017/S0265051713000144

Patston, T., & Loughlan, T. (2014). Playing with performance: The use and abuse of beta-blockers in the performing arts. *Victorian Journal of Music Education, 1*, 3–10.

Patston, T., & Osborne, M. S. (2016). The developmental features of music performance anxiety and perfectionism in school age music students. *Performance Enhancement & Health, 4*(1–2), 42–49. http://dx.doi.org/10.1016/j.peh.2015.09.003

Pawłusz, E. (2018). Can musicians build the nation? Popular music and identity in Estonia. In A. Polese, J. Morris, E. Pawlusz, & O. Seliverstova (Eds.), *Identity and nation building in everyday post-socialist life* (pp. 34–51). Abingdon, UK: Routledge.

Pearce, E., Launay, J., van Duijn, M., Rotkirch, A., David-Barrett, T., & Dunbar, R. I. (2016). Singing together or apart: The effect of competitive and cooperative singing on social bonding within and between sub-groups of a university Fraternity. *Psychology of music, 44*(6), 1255–1273. doi:10.1177/0305735616636208

Peltola, H. R., & Eerola, T. (2016). Fifty shades of blue: Classification of music-evoked sadness. *Musicae Scientiae, 20*(1), 84–102. doi:10.1177/1029864915611206

Pembrook, R., & Craig, C. (2002). Teaching as a profession: Two variations on a theme. In R. Colwell & C. Richardson (Eds.), *The new handbook of research on music teaching and learning* (pp. 786–817). New York, NY: Oxford University Press.

Peretz, I., & Zatorre, R. J. (2005). Brain organization for music processing. *Annual Review of Psychology, 56*, 89–114. doi:10.1146/annurev.psych.56.091103.070225

Perkins, R., & Williamon, A. (2014). Learning to make music in older adulthood: A mixed-methods exploration of impacts on well-being. *Psychology of Music, 42*(5), 550–567. doi:10.1177/0305735613483668

Pflederer, M. (1964). The responses of children to musical tasks embodying Piaget's principles of conservation. *Journal of Research in Music Education, 12*, 251–268.

Pfordresher, P. Q. (2019). *Sound and action in music performance.* London, UK: Academic Press.

Philippe, R. A., Kosirnik, C., Vuichoud, N., Clark, T., Williamon, A., & McPherson, G. E. (2020). Conservatory musicians' temporal organization and self-regulation processes in preparing for a music exam. *Frontiers in Psychology, 11*, article 89. https://doi.org/10.3389/fpsyg.2020.00089

Piaget, J. (1958). *The child's construction of reality.* London, UK: Routledge.

Pietschnig, J., Voracek, M., & Formann, A. K. (2010). Mozart effect–Shmozart effect: A meta-analysis. *Intelligence, 38*(3), 314–323. doi:10.1016/j.intell.2010.03.001

Pike, P. (2015). The ninth semester: Preparing undergraduates to function as professional musicians in the 21st century. *College Music Symposium, 55.* https://www.jstor.org/stable/26574399

Pinho, A. L., de Manzano, Ö., Fransson, P., Eriksson, H., & Ullén, F. (2014). Connecting to create: Expertise in musical improvisation Is associated with increased functional connectivity between premotor and prefrontal areas. *Journal of Neuroscience, 34*(18), 6156–6163. doi:10.1523/JNEUROSCI.4769-13.2014

Pipe, L. (2019). "I see you, baby . . . ": Expressive gesture and nonverbal communication in popular music performance education. In B. Powell, G. D. Smith, & Z. Moir (Eds.), *The Bloomsbury handbook of popular music education* (pp. 321–336). London, UK: Bloomsbury Academic.

Pitts, S. (2005). *Valuing musical participation.* Aldershot, UK: Ashgate.

Pitts, S. E. (2007). Music beyond school: Learning through participation. In L. Bresler (Ed.), *International handbook of research in arts education* (pp. 759–772). Dordrecht, The Netherlands: Springer.

Pitts, S. E., & Robinson, K. (2016). Dropping in and dropping out: Experiences of sustaining and ceasing amateur participation in classical music. *British Journal of Music Education, 33*(3), 327–346. doi:10.1017/S0265051716000152.

Platz, F., & Kopiez, R. (2013). When the first impression counts: Music performers, audience and the evaluation of stage entrance behaviour. *Musicae Scientiae, 17*(2), 167–197. doi:10.1177/1029864913486369

Platz, F., Kopiez, R., Lehmann, A. C., & Wolf, A. (2014). The influence of deliberate practice on musical achievement: A meta-analysis. *Frontiers in Psychology, 7*, article 646. https://doi.org/10.3389/fpsyg.2014.00646

Poggi, I., & Ansani, A. (2018, June). The lexicon of the conductor's gaze. In *Proceedings of the 5th International Conference on Movement and Computing* (pp. 1–8). New York, NY: Association for Computing Machinery. https://dl.acm.org/doi/pdf/10.1145/3212721.3212811

Poggi, I., D'Errico, F., & Ansani, A. (2020). The conductor's intensity gestures. *Psychology of Music*. Advance online publication.

Pohjannoro, U. (2014). Inspiration and decision-making: A case study of a composer's intuitive and reflective thought. *Musicae Scientiae, 18*(2), 166–188. doi:10.1177/1029864914520848

Posner, J., Russell, J. A., & Peterson, B. S. (2005). The circumplex model of affect: An integrative approach to affective neuroscience, cognitive development, and psychopathology. *Development and Psychopathology, 17*(3), 715–734. doi:10.1017/S0954579405050340

Pressing, J. (2001). Improvisation: Methods and models. In J. Sloboda (Ed.), *Generative processes in music: The psychology of performance, improvisation, and composition* (pp. 129–178). Oxford, UK: Oxford University Press.

Price, H. E., & Byo, J. L. (2002). Rehearsing and conducting. In R. Parncutt & G. E. McPherson (Eds.), *The science and psychology of music performance: Creative strategies for teaching and learning* (pp. 335–351). New York, NY: Oxford University Press.

Price, H. E., Mann, A., & Morrison, S. J. (2016). Effect of conductor expressivity on ensemble evaluations by nonmusic majors. *International Journal of Music Education, 34*(2), 135–142. doi:10.1177/0255761415617925

Prichard, C., Korczynski, M., & Elmes, M. (2007). Music at work: An introduction. *Group & Organization Management, 32*(1), 4–21. doi:10.1177/1059601106294485

Provasi, J., Anderson, D. I., & Barbu-Roth, M. (2014). Rhythm perception, production, and synchronization during the perinatal period. *Frontiers in Psychology, 5*, article 1048. https://doi.org/10.3389/fpsyg.2014.01048

Rae, G., & McCambridge, K. (2004). Correlates of performance anxiety in practical music exams. *Psychology of Music, 32*(4), 432–439. doi:01.0077/1315735614146011

Ragert, M., Fairhurst, M. T., & Keller, P. E. (2014). Segregation and integration of auditory streams when listening to multi-part music. *PloS ONE, 9*(1), e84085. doi:10.1371/journal.pone.0084085

Ragert, P., Schmidt, A., Altenmüller, E., & Dinse, H. R. (2004). Superior tactile performance and learning in professional pianists: Evidence for meta-plasticity in musicians. *European Journal of Neuroscience, 19*(2), 473–478. https://doi.org/10.1111/j.0953-816X.2003.03142.x

Ragert, M., Schroeder, T., & Keller, P. (2013). Knowing too little or too much: The effects of familiarity with a co-performer's part on interpersonal coordination in musical ensembles. *Frontiers in Psychology, 4*, article 368. https://doi.org/10.3389/fpsyg.2013.00368

Raines, R. (2015). *Composition in the digital world: Conversations with 21st-century American composers.* New York, NY: Oxford University Press.

Ramsey, G. P. (2000). The muze 'n the hood: Musical practice and film in the age of hip hop. *Institute for Studies in American Music Newsletter, 29*(2), 1–2, 12.

Rankin, S. (2018). *Writing sounds in Carolingian Europe: The invention of musical notation.* Cambridge, UK: Cambridge University Press.

Rauscher, F. H., & Hinton, S. C. (2003). Type of music training selectively influences perceptual processing. In R. Kopiez, A. Lehmann, I. Wolther, & C. Wolf (Eds.), *Proceedings of the Fifth Triennial Conference of the European Society for the Cognitive Sciences of Music.* Hannover, Germany: University of Music and Drama.

Rauscher, F. H., Shaw, G. L., & Ky, C. N. (1993). Music and spatial task performance. *Nature, 365*(6447), 611. https://link.springer.com/content/pdf/10.1038/365611a0.pdf

Rawlings, J. R., & Young, J. (2020). Relational aggression and youth empowerment within a high school instrumental music program. *Psychology of Music.* doi:10.1177/0305735620923140

Reese, J. A. (2019). Uke, flow and rock'n'roll. *International Journal of Community Music, 12*(2), 207–227. doi:10.1386/ijcm.12.2.207_1

Rentfrow, P. J., & Gosling, S. D. (2003). The do re mi's of everyday life: The structure and personality correlates of music preferences. *Journal of Personality and Social Psychology, 84*(6), 1236. doi:10.1037/0022-3514.84.6.1236

Renwick, J. M., & McPherson, G. E. (2002). Interest and choice: Student-selected repertoire and its effect on practising behaviour. *British Journal of Music Education, 19*(2), 173–188. doi:10.1017/S0265051702000256

Repp, B. H. (2005). Sensorimotor synchronization: A review of the tapping literature. *Psychonomic Bulletin & Review, 12*(6), 969–992. https://doi.org/10.3758/BF03206433

Richard-Lalonde, M., Gélinas, C., Boitor, M., Gosselin, E., Feeley, N., Cossette, S., & Chlan, L. L. (2020). The effect of music on pain in the adult intensive care unit: A systematic review of randomized controlled trials. *Journal of Pain and Symptom Management, 59*(6), 1304–1319. https://doi.org/10.1016/j.jpainsymman.2019.12.359

Rickels, D. A., Brewer, W. D., Councill, K. H., Fredrickson, W. E., Hairston, M., Perry, D. L., Porter, A. M., & Schmidt, M. (2013). Career influences of music education audition candidates. *Journal of Research in Music Education, 61*(1), 115–134. doi:10.1177/0022429412474896

Rickels, D. A., Hoffman, E. C., III, & Fredrickson, W. E. (2019). A comparative analysis of influences on choosing a music teaching occupation. *Journal of Research in Music Education, 67*(3), 286–303. doi:10.1177/0022429419849937

Ring, C., & Kavussanu, M. (2018). The impact of achievement goals on cheating in sport. *Psychology of Sport and Exercise, 35*, 98–103. https://doi.org/10.1016/j.psychsport.2017.11.016

Roberts, M. (2012, October 17). Creativity "closely entwined with mental illness." *BBC News Online.* http://www.bbc.co.uk/news/health-19959565

Robinson, S. M. (2013). *Chamber music in alternative venues in the 21st century U.S.: Investigating the effect of new venues on concert culture, programming and the business of classical music* [Unpublished doctoral dissertation]. University of South Carolina.

Robson, K. E., & Kenny, D. T. (2017). Music performance anxiety in ensemble rehearsals and concerts: A comparison of music and non-music major undergraduate musicians. *Psychology of Music, 45*(6), 868–885. doi:10.1177/0305735617693472

Roels, H. (2016). Comparing the main compositional activities in a study of eight composers. *Musicae Scientiae, 20*(3), 413–435. doi:10.1177/1029864915624737

Roesler, R., & McGaugh, J. L. (2010). Memory consolidation. In G. F. Koob, M. L. Moal, & R. F. Thompson (Eds.), *Encyclopedia of behavioral neuroscience* (pp. 206–214). London, UK: Academic Press.

Rogers, G. L. (2007). Popular music in the classroom (letter to the editor). *Music Educators Journal, 93*(5), 7.

Rohwer, D., & Polk, J. (2006). Practice behaviors of eighth-grade instrumental musicians. *Journal of Research in Music Education, 54*(4), 350–362. https://doi.org/10.1177/002242940605400407

Rose, D., Bartoli, A. J., & Heaton, P. (2019). Formal-informal musical learning, sex and musicians' personalities. *Personality and Individual Differences, 142*, 207–213. https://doi.org/10.1016/j.paid.2018.07.015

Rosenbaum, A. J., Vanderzanden, J., Morse, A. S., & Uhl, R. L. (2012). Injuries complicating musical practice and performance: The hand surgeon's approach to the musician-patient. *Journal of Hand Surgery, 37*(6), 1269–1272. doi:10.1016/j.jhsa.2012.01.018

Rosenkranz, K., Williamon, A., & Rothwell, J. C. (2007). Motorcortical excitability and synaptic plasticity is enhanced in professional musicians. *Journal of Neuroscience, 27*(19), 5200–5206. doi:10.1523/JNEUROSCI.0836-07.2007

Rostvall, A., & West, T. (2003). Analysis of interaction and learning in instrumental teaching. *Music Education Research, 5*(3), 213–226. doi:10.1080/1461380032000126319

Roy, L., & Zhang, Y. (2019). The health of a musician: Identifying musicians' unstated/unrecognized health information needs. In S. Kurbanoğlu et al. (Eds.), *Information literacy in everyday life: 6th European Conference, ECIL 2018* (pp. 115–123). Cham, Switzerland: Springer. https://doi.org/10.1007/978-3-030-13472-3_11fc

Ruddock, E. (2012). "Sort of in your blood": Inherent musicality survives cultural judgment. *Research Studies in Music Education, 34*, 207–221. doi:10.1177/1321103x12461747

Runco, M. A. (2008). Creativity and education. *New Horizons in Education, 56*, 107–115.

Rusinek, G. (2008). Disaffected learners and school music culture: An opportunity for inclusion. *Research Studies in Music Education, 30*, 9–23. doi:10.1177/1321103x08089887

Ryan, C., & Costa-Giomi, E. (2004). Attractiveness bias in the evaluation of young pianists' performances. *Journal of Research in Music Education, 52*(2), 141–154. https://doi.org/10.2307/3345436

Ryan, R. M., & Deci, E. L. (2002). Overview of self-determination theory: An organismic dialectical perspective. In E. L. Deci & R. M. Ryan (Eds.), *Handbook of self-determination research* (pp. 3–33). Rochester, NY: University of Rochester Press.

Saarikallio, S., Alluri, V., Maksimainen, J., & Toiviainen, P. (2021). Emotions of music listening in Finland and in India: Comparison of an individualistic and a collectivistic culture. *Psychology of Music, 49*(4), 989–1005. doi:10.1177/0305735620917730.

Saarikallio, S., Nieminen, S., & Brattico, E. (2013). Affective reactions to musical stimuli reflect emotional use of music in everyday life. *Musicae Scientiae, 17*(1), 27–39. doi:10.1177/1029864912462381

Sachs, H. (1982). *Virtuoso*. London, UK: Thames & Hudson.

Sadie, S. (2006). *Mozart: The early years, 1756–1781*. Oxford, UK: Oxford University Press.

Salganik, M. J., Dodds, P. S., & Watts, D. J. (2006). Experimental study of inequality and unpredictability in an artificial cultural market. *Science, 311*(5762), 854–856. doi:10.1126/science.1121066

Salimpoor, V. N., Zald, D. H., Zatorre, R. J., Dagher, A., & McIntosh, A. R. (2015). Predictions and the brain: How musical sounds become rewarding. *Trends in Cognitive Sciences, 19*(2), 86–91. http://dx.doi.org/10.1016/j.tics.2014.12.001

Salmon, M., Doery, K., Dance, P., Chapman, J., Gilbert, R., Williams, R., & Lovett, R. (2019). Defining the indefinable: Descriptors of Aboriginal and Torres Strait Islander peoples' cultures and their links to health and wellbeing (2nd ed.). Carlton South VIC, Australia: Lowitja Institute. https://openresearch-repository.anu.edu.au/handle/1885/148406

Sawyer, R. K. (2003). *Group creativity: Music, theater, collaboration.* Mahwah, NJ: Lawrence Erlbaum Associates.

Scanlon, M. B. (1942). Lowell Mason's philosophy of music education. *Music Educators Journal, 28*(3), 24–25, 70.

Scarborough, R. C. (2017). Making it in a cover music scene: Negotiating artistic identities in a "Kmart-level market." *Sociological Inquiry, 87*(1), 153–178. https://doi.org/10.1111/soin.12153

Schäfer, T. (2016). The goals and effects of music listening and their relationship to the strength of music preference. *PLoS ONE, 11*(3), e0151634. doi:10.1371/journal.pone.0151634

Schäfer, T., Sedlmeier, P., Städtler, C., & Huron, D. (2013). The psychological functions of music listening. *Frontiers in Psychology, 4,* article 511. https://doi.org/10.3389/fpsyg.2013.00511

Schellenberg, E. G. (2012). Cognitive performance after music listening: A review of the Mozart effect. In R. A. R. MacDonald, G. Kreutz, & L. Mitchell (Eds.), *Music, health and well-being* (pp. 324–338). Oxford, UK: Oxford University Press.

Schellenberg, E. G. (2016). Music and nonmusical abilities. In G. E. McPherson (Ed.), *The child as musician: A handbook of musical development* (pp. 149–176). Oxford, UK: Oxford University Press.

Schiavio, A., Biasutti, M., van der Schyff, D., & Parncutt, R. (2020). A matter of presence: A qualitative study on teaching individual and collective music classes. *Musicae Scientiae, 24*(3), 356–376. doi:10.1177/1029864918808833

Schiavio, A., Moran, N., van der Schyff, D., Biasutti, M., & Parncutt, R. (2020). Processes and experiences of creative cognition in seven Western classical composers. *Musicae Scientiae.* Advance online publication. doi:10.1177/1029864920943931

Schippers, H. (2006). "As if a little bird is sitting on your finger . . .": Metaphor as a key instrument in training professional musicians. *International Journal of Music Education, 24*(3), 209–217. doi:10.1177/0255761406069640

Schlesinger, J. (2009). Creative mythconceptions: A closer look at the evidence for the "mad genius" hypothesis. *Psychology of Aesthetics, Creativity, and the Arts, 3*(2), 62–72. doi:10.1037/a0013975

Schmidt, N. B., Richey, J. A., Zvolensky, M. J., & Maner, J. K. (2008). Exploring human freeze responses to a threat stressor. *Journal of Behavior Therapy and Experimental Psychiatry, 39*(3), 292–304. doi:10.1016/j.jbtep.2007.08.002

Schmuckler, M. A. (2016). Tonality and contour in melodic processing. In S. Hallam, I. Cross, & M. Thaut (Eds.), *The Oxford handbook of music psychology* (2nd ed., pp. 143–165). Oxford, UK: Oxford University Press.

Schubert, E. (2003). Update of the Hevner adjective checklist. *Perceptual and Motor Skills, 96*, 1117–1122. https://doi.org/10.2466/pms.2003.96.3c.1117

Schubert, E. (2004). Modeling perceived emotion with continuous musical features. *Music Perception, 21*(4), 561–585. https://doi.org/10.1525/mp.2004.21.4.561

Schubert, E. (2010). Continuous self-report methods. In P. N. Juslin & J. A. Sloboda (Eds.), *Handbook of music and emotion: Theory, research, applications* (pp. 223–253). Oxford, UK: Oxford University Press.

Schubert, E. (2012). Spreading activation and dissociation: A cognitive mechanism for creative processing in music. In D. J. Hargreaves, D. E. Miell, & R. A. R. MacDonald (Eds.), *Musical imaginations: Multidisciplinary perspectives on creativity, performance, and perception* (pp. 124–140). Oxford, UK: Oxford University Press.

Seashore, C. E. (1960). *Seashore measures of musical talents* (rev. ed.). New York, NY: Psychological Corporation.

Seashore, C. E. (1967). *Psychology of music.* New York, NY: Dover.

Seddon, F. A. (2005). Modes of communication during jazz improvisation. *British Journal of Music Education, 22*(1), 47–61. doi:10.1017/S0265051704005984

Seeger, A. (2018). Music of struggle and protest in the 20th century. In R. Bader (Ed.), *Springer handbook of systematic musicology* (pp. 1029–1042). Berlin, Germany: Springer.

Segovia, A. (1976). *Andrés Segovia: An autobiography of the years 1893–1920* (W. F. O'Brien, Trans.). New York, NY: Macmillan.

Seligman, M. (2008). Positive health. *Applied Psychology, 57*, 3–18.

Seligman, M. E. P. (2011). *Flourish: A visionary new understanding of happiness and well-being.* New York, NY: Free Press.

Seung, Y., Kyong, J., Woo, S., Lee, B., & Lee, K. (2005). Brain activation during music listening in individuals with or without prior music training. *Neuroscience Research, 52*(4), 323–329. https://doi.org/10.1016/j.neures.2005.04.011

Shanahan, D., Neubarth, K., & Conklin, D. (2016). *Mining musical traits of social functions in Native American music.* In J. Devaney, M. I. Mandel, D. Turnbull, & G. Tzanetakis (Eds.), *Proceedings of the 17th International Society for Music Information Retrieval Conference* (pp. 681–687). New York, NY: International Society for Music Information Retrieval. http://archives.ismir.net/ismir2016/paper/000167.pdf

Shaw, R. D. (2017). I can hardly wait to see what I am going to do today: Lesson planning perspectives of experienced band teachers. *Contributions to Music Education, 42*, 129–152. https://www.jstor.org/stable/10.2307/26367440

Sheldon, D. A. (2004). Listeners' identification of musical expression through figurative language and musical terminology. *Journal of Research in Music Education, 52*, 357–368. https://doi.org/10.1177/002242940405200407

Sheldon, D. A., & Brittin, R. V. (2012). A comparison of pre- and post-student teachers' perceptions of instrumental music educators' verbal and vocal teaching strategies. In *Proceedings of the 24th ISME Research Commission Seminar* (pp. 188–197). Thessaloniki, Greece: International Society for Music Education. https://www.isme.org/sites/default/files/documents/proceedings/2012_Research_proceedings_optimised.pdf

Shouldice, H. N. (2014). Elementary students' definitions and self-perceptions of being a "good musician." *Music Education Research, 16*(3), 330–345. doi:10.1080/14613808.2014.909396

Shouldice, H. N. (2020). An investigation of musical ability beliefs and self-concept among fourth-grade students in the United States. *International Journal of Music Education, 38*(4), 525–536. doi:10.1177/0255761420914667

Sievers, B., Polansky, L., Casey, M., & Wheatley, T. (2013). Music and movement share a dynamic structure that supports universal expressions of emotion. *Proceedings of the National Academy of Sciences of the United States of America, 110*(1), 70–75. doi:10.1073/pnas.1209023110

Silverman, M. (2008). A performer's creative processes: Implications for teaching and learning musical interpretation. *Music Education Research, 10*(2), 249–269. doi:10.1080/14613800802079114

Silvey, B. A. (2011). Effects of score study on novices' conducting and rehearsing: A preliminary investigation. *Bulletin of the Council for Research in Music Education, 187,* 33–48. http://www.jstor.org/stable/41162322

Silvey, B. A. (2014). Strategies for improving rehearsal technique: Using research findings to promote better rehearsals. *Update: Applications of Research in Music Education, 32*(2), 11–17. doi:10.1177/8755123313502348

Simmonds-Moore, C. A., Alvarado, C. S., & Zingrone, N. L. (2019). A survey exploring synesthetic experiences: Exceptional experiences, schizotypy, and psychological well-being. *Psychology of Consciousness: Theory, Research, and Practice, 6*(1), 99–121. http://dx.doi.org/10.1037/cns0000165

Simmons, A. L. (2012). Distributed practice and procedural memory consolidation in musicians skill learning. *Journal of Research in Music Education, 59*(4), 357–368. doi:10.1177/0022429411424798

Simner, J., Mulvenna, C., Sagiv, N., Tsakanikos, E., Witherby, S. A., Fraser, C., Scott, K., & Ward, J. (2006). Synaesthesia: The prevalence of atypical cross-modal experiences. *Perception, 35*(8), 1024–1033. doi:10.1068/p5469

Simoens, V. L., & Tervaniemi, M. (2013). Musician–instrument relationship as a candidate index for professional well-being in musicians. *Psychology of Aesthetics, Creativity, and the Arts, 7*(2), 171. doi:10.1037/a0030164

Simones, L., Rodger, M., & Schroeder, F. (2017). Seeing how it sounds: Observation, imitation, and improved learning in piano playing. *Cognition and Instruction, 35*(2), 125–140. doi:10.1080/07370008.2017.1282483

Simonton, D. K. (1995). Exceptional personal influence: An integrative paradigm. *Creativity Research Journal, 8*(4), 371–373.

Simonton, D. K. (2000). Creative development as acquired expertise: Theoretical issues and an empirical test. *Developmental Review, 20*(2), 283–318. doi:10.1006/drev.1999.0504

Simonton, D. K. (2005). Are genius and madness related? Contemporary answers to an ancient problem. *Psychiatric Times, 22*(7). https://www.psychiatrictimes.com/view/are-genius-and-madness-related-contemporary-answers-ancient-question

Simonton, D. K. (2009). Genius, creativity and leadership. In T. Rickards, M. A. Runco, & S. Moger (Eds.), *The Routledge companion to creativity* (pp. 247–255). New York, NY: Routledge.

Simonton, D. K. (2010). Creativity in highly eminent individuals. In J. C. Kaufman & R. J. Sternberg (Eds.), *The Cambridge handbook of creativity* (pp. 174–188). Cambridge, UK: Cambridge University Press.

Simonton, D. K. (2014). More method in the mad-genius controversy: A historiometric study of 204 historic creators. *Psychology of Aesthetics, Creativity, and the Arts, 8*(1), 53–61. https://doi.org/10.1037/a0035367

Sinclair, G., & Dolan, P. (2015). Heavy metal figurations: Music consumption, subcultural control and civilizing processes. *Marketing Theory, 15*(3), 423–441. doi:10.1177/1470593115569015

Sindberg, L. (2012). *Just good teaching: Comprehensive musicianship through performance (CMP) in theory and practice.* Lanham, MD: Rowman & Littlefield.

Skånland, M. S. (2011). Use of mp3-players as a coping resource. *Music and Arts in Action, 3*(2), 15–33. http://hdl.handle.net/10036/3964

Skånland, M. S. (2013). Everyday music listening and affect regulation: The role of MP3 players. *International Journal of Qualitative Studies on Health and Well-Being, 8*(1), article 20595. doi:10.3402/qhw.v8i0.20595d

Sloboda, J. A. (1983). The communication of musical metre in piano performance. *Quarterly Journal of Experimental Psychology, 35,* 377–396.

Sloboda, J. A. (1985). *The musical mind: The cognitive psychology of music.* Oxford, UK: Clarendon.

Sloboda, J. A. (2000). Individual differences in music performance. *Trends in Cognitive Sciences, 4*(10), 397–403.

Sloboda, J. A. (2000). Individual differences in music performance. *Trends in Cognitive Sciences, 4,* 397–403. https://doi.org/10.1016/S1364-6613(00)01531-X

Sloboda, J. (2005a). Are some children more gifted for music than others? In *Exploring the musical mind* (pp. 297–316). Oxford, UK: Oxford University Press.

Sloboda, J. (2005b). Empirical studies of emotional response to music. In *Exploring the musical mind* (pp. 203–212). Oxford, UK: Oxford University Press.

Sloboda, J. (2005c). Everyday uses of music listening: A preliminary study. In *Exploring the musical mind* (pp. 319–331). Oxford, UK: Oxford University Press.

Sloboda, J. (2005d). Music as a language. In *Exploring the musical mind* (pp. 175–189). Oxford, UK: Oxford University Press.

Sloboda, J. (2005e). Musical expertise. In *Exploring the musical mind* (pp. 244–263). Oxford, UK: Oxford University Press.

Sloboda, J. (2005f). The psychology of music reading. In *Exploring the musical mind* (pp. 3–26). Oxford, UK: Oxford University Press.

Sloboda, J. A. (2010). Music in everyday life: The role of emotions. In P. N. Juslin & J. A. Sloboda (Eds.), *Handbook of music and emotion: Theory, research, applications* (pp. 493–514). Oxford, UK: Oxford University Press.

Sloboda, J. A. (2014). The acquisition of musical performance expertise: Deconstructing the "talent" account of individual differences in musical expressivity. In K. A. Ericsson (Ed.), *The road to excellence* (pp. 107–126). New York, NY: Psychology Press.

Sloboda, J. A., Davidson, J. W., Howe, M. J., & Moore, D. G. (1996). The role of practice in the development of performing musicians. *British Journal of Psychology, 87*(2), 287–309. https://doi.org/10.1111/j.2044-8295.1996.tb02591.x

Sloboda, J. A., & Lehmann, A. C. (2001). Performance correlates of perceived emotionality in different interpretations of a Chopin piano prelude. *Music Perception, 19,* 87–120. https://www.jstor.org/stable/10.1525/mp.2001.19.1.87

Small, C. (2011). *Music of the common tongue* (rev. ed.). Middletown, CT: Wesleyan University Press.

Smilde, R. (2009). Musicians as lifelong learners. In P. Alheit & H. von Felden (Eds.), *Lebenslanges Lernen und erziehungswissenschaftliche Biographieforschung*. Wiesbaden, Germany: VS Verlag für Sozialwissenschaften. https://doi.org/10.1007/978-3-531-91520-3_10

Smith, B. P. (2005). Goal orientation, implicit theory of ability, and collegiate instrumental music practice. *Psychology of Music, 33*(1), 36–57. doi:10.1177/0305735605048013

Smith, J. (2014). Entrepreneurial music education. In M. Kaschub & J. Smith (Eds.), *Promising practices in 21st century music teacher education* (pp. 61–78). New York, NY: Oxford University Press.

Spahn, C. (2015). Treatment and prevention of music performance anxiety. In E. Altenmüller, S. Finger, & F. Boller (Eds.), *Music, neurology, and neuroscience: Evolution, the musical brain, medical conditions, and therapies* (pp. 129–140). Amsterdam, The Netherlands: Elsevier. https://doi.org/10.1016/bs.pbr.2014.11.024

Spahn, C., Strukely, S., & Lehmann, A. (2004). Health conditions, attitudes toward study, and attitudes toward health at the beginning of university study: Music students in comparison with other student populations. *Medical Problems of Performing Musicians, 19*, 26–33. https://doi.org/10.21091/mppa.2004.1005

Spahn, C., Walther, J. C., & Nusseck, M. (2016). The effectiveness of a multimodal concept of audition training for music students in coping with music performance anxiety. *Psychology of Music, 44*(4), 893–909. doi:10.1177/0305735615597484

Spence, C., Puccinelli, N. M., Grewal, D., & Roggeveen, A. L. (2014). Store atmospherics: A multisensory perspective. *Psychology & Marketing, 31*(7), 472–488. https://doi.org/10.1002/mar.20709

Staecker, H., & Thompson, J. (2013). Central auditory system, anatomy. In S. E. Kountakis (Ed.), *Encyclopedia of otolaryngology, head and neck surgery* (pp. 376–383). Berlin, Germany: Springer-Verlag. https://doi.org/10.1007/978-3-642-23499-6_536

Stavrou, N. A. M., Psychountaki, M., Georgiadis, E., Karteroliotis, K., & Zervas, Y. (2015). Flow theory—goal orientation theory: Positive experience is related to athlete's goal orientation. *Frontiers in Psychology, 6*, article 1499. https://doi.org/10.3389/fpsyg.2015.01499

Sternberg, R. J. (2005). Creativity or creativities? *International Journal of Human-Computer Studies, 63*(4–5), 370–382. doi:10.1016/j.ijhcs.2005.04.003

Sternberg, R. J. (2018). The triangle of creativity. In R. J. Sternberg & J. C. Kaufman (Eds.), *The nature of human creativity* (pp. 318–344). Cambridge, UK: Cambridge University Press.

Steyn, B. J. M., Steyn, M. H., Maree, D. J. F., & Panebianco-Warrens, C. (2016). Psychological skills and mindfulness training effects on the psychological wellbeing of undergraduate music students: An exploratory study. *Journal of Psychology in Africa, 26*(2), 167–171. http://dx.doi.org/10.1080/14330237.2016.1163906

Stoeber, J., & Eismann, U. (2007). Perfectionism in young musicians: Relations with motivation, effort, achievement, and distress. *Personality and Individual Differences, 43*(8), 2182–2192. doi:10.1016/j.paid.2007.06.036

Stoeber, J., Madigan, D. J., Damian, L. E., Esposito, R. M., & Lombardo, C. (2016). Perfectionism and eating disorder symptoms in female university students: The central role of perfectionistic self-presentation. *Eating and Weight Disorders, 22*, 641–648. doi:10.1007/s40519-016-0297-1

Studer, R., Danuser, B., Hildebrandt, H., Arial, M., & Gomez, P. (2011). Hyperventilation complaints in music performance anxiety among classical music students. *Journal of Psychosomatic Research, 70*(6), 557–564. Doi:10.1016/j.jpsychores.2010.11.004

Sturman, J. (Ed.). (2019). *The SAGE international encyclopedia of music and culture.* Thousand Oaks, CA: Sage.

Sundberg, J., Friberg, A., & Bresin, R. (2003) Attempts to reproduce a pianist's expressive timing with Director Musices performance rules. *Journal of New Music Research, 32*(3), 317–325. https://doi.org/10.1076/jnmr.32.3.317.16867

Suzuki, S. (1966). *Nurtured by love: The classic approach to talent education* (W. Suzuki, Trans.). Fort Lauderdale, FL: Exposition-Phoenix Press.

Swaminathan, S., & Schellenberg, E. G. (2018). Musical competence is predicted by music training, cognitive abilities, and personality. *Scientific Reports, 8*(1), 1–7. doi:10.1038/s41598-018-27571-2

Swanwick, K. (2003). *Musical knowledge: Intuition, analysis, and music education.* London, UK: Taylor & Francis e-Library. https://doi.org/10.4324/9780203424575

Swanwick, K. & Tillman, J. (2016). The sequence of musical development: A study of children's composition. In *A developing discourse: The selected works of Keith Swanwick* (pp. 68–98). London, UK: Routledge.

Syed, M. (2010). *Bounce: Mozart, Federer, Picasso, Beckham and the science of success.* New York, NY: HarperCollins.

Syed, M. (2015). Emerging adulthood: Developmental stage, theory, or nonsense? In J. J. Arnett (Ed.)., *The Oxford handbook of emerging adulthood* (pp. 11–25). New York, NY: Oxford University Press.

Talamini, F., Altoè, G., Carretti, B., & Grassi, M. (2017). Musicians have better memory than nonmusicians: A meta-analysis. *PLoS ONE, 12*(10), e0186773. https://doi.org/10.1371/journal.pone.0186773

Talent. (2021). *Oxford English Dictionary.* https://www.oed.com/view/Entry/197208?

Tamir, I. (2021). "I am grateful that god hates the reds": Persistent values and changing trends in Israel football chants. *Sport in Society, 24*(2), 222–234. https://doi.org/10.1080/17430437.2019.1627331

Tan, L. (2017). Concept teaching in instrumental music education: A literature review. *Update: Applications of Research in Music Education, 35*(2), 38–45. doi:10.1177/8755123315604455

Taylor, J. (2012). Taking it in the ear: On musico-sexual synergies and the (queer) possibility that music is sex. *Continuum, 26*(4), 603–614. doi:10.1080/10304312.2012.698039

Temperley, D., & Tan, D. (2013). Emotional connotations of diatonic modes. *Music Perception: An Interdisciplinary Journal, 30*(3), 237–257. doi:10.1525/MP.2012.30.3.237

Thakur, D., Martens, M. A., Smith, D. S., & Roth, E. (2018). Williams syndrome and music: A systematic integrative review. *Frontiers in Psychology, 9,* article 2203. https://doi.org/10.3389/fpsyg.2018.02203

Thaut, M. H., & Hodges, M. (Eds.). (2019). *The Oxford handbook of music and the brain.* Oxford, UK: Oxford University Press.

Theorell, T., Kowalski, J., Theorell, A. M. L., & Horwitz, E. B. (2020). Choir singers without rehearsals and concerts? A questionnaire study on perceived losses from restricting choral singing during the Covid-19 pandemic. *Journal of Voice.* Advance online publication. https://doi.org/10.1016/j.jvoice.2020.11.006

Thomas, J. P., & Nettelbeck, T. (2014). Performance anxiety in adolescent musicians. *Psychology of Music, 42*(4), 624–634. doi:10.1177/0305735613485151

Thompson, W., Graham, P., & Russo, F. (2005). Seeing music performance: Visual influences on perception and experience. *Semiotica, 2005*(156), 203–227. doi:10.1515/semi.2005.2005.156.203

Thompson, W. F., Russo, F. A., & Livingston, S. R. (2010). Facial expressions of singers influence perceived pitch relations. *Psychonomic Bulletin & Review, 17*(3), 317–322. doi:10.3758/PBR.17.3.317

Thompson, W. F., Russo, F. A., & Quinto, L. (2008). Audio-visual integration of emotional cues in song. *Cognition and Emotion, 22*(8), 1457–1470. doi:10.1080/02699930701813974

Thurber, M. R., Bodenhamer-Davis, E., Johnson, M., Chesky, K., & Chandler, C. K. (2010). Effects of heart rate variability coherence biofeedback training and emotional management techniques to decrease music performance anxiety. *Biofeedback, 38*(1), 28–39.

Time Magazine. (1976, October 4). Ozmosis in Central Park. *Time, 108*(14), 68.

Topolinski, S., & Strack, F. (2008). Where there's a will—there's no intuition. The unintentional basis of semantic coherence judgments. *Journal of Memory and Language, 58*(4), 1032–1048. doi:10.1016/j.jml.2008.01.002

Traasdahl, S. (2017). *"Big music doesn't need huge halls": Investigating the audience experience of classical music concerts in alternative music venues* [Unpublished master's thesis]. University of Oslo.

Trehub, S. E. (2017). The maternal voice as a special signal for infants. In M. Filippa, P. Kuhn, & B. Westrup (Eds.), *Early vocal contact and preterm infant brain development* (pp. 39–54). Cham, Switzerland: Springer.

Trehub, S. E., & Degé, F. (2016). Reflections on infants as musical connoisseurs. In G. E. McPherson (Ed.), *The child as musician: A handbook of musical development* (2nd ed., pp. 361–372). Oxford, UK: Oxford University Press.

Trehub, S. E., & Hannon, E. E. (2006). Infant music perception: Domain-general or domain-specific mechanisms? *Cognition, 100*(1), 73–99. doi:10.1016/j.cognition.2005.11.006

Trehub, S. E., Hannon, E. E., & Schachner, A. (2010). Perspectives on music and affect in the early years. In P. N. Juslin & J. A. Sloboda (Eds.), *Handbook of music and emotion: Theory, research, applications* (pp. 645–668). Oxford, UK: Oxford University Press.

Tsay, C. (2013). Sight over sound in the judgment of music performance. *Proceedings of the National Academy of Sciences of the United States of America, 110*(36), 14580–14585. https://doi.org/10.1073/pnas.1221454110

Turino, T. (2008). *Music as social life: The politics of participation.* Chicago, IL: University of Chicago Press.

Tversky, A., & Kahneman, D. (1973). Availability: A heuristic for judging frequency and probability. *Cognitive Psychology, 5*(2), 207–232. https://doi-org.libproxy.unl.edu/10.1016/0010-0285(73)90033-9

Upitis, R. (2018). Stages of notational development. In *This too is music* (pp. 117–147). New York: Oxford University Press.

Vaag, J., Sund, E. R., & Bjerkeset, O. (2018). Five-factor personality profiles among Norwegian musicians compared to the general workforce. *Musicae Scientiae, 22*(3), 434–445. doi:10.1177/1029864917709519

Valentine, E. (2002). The fear of performance. In J. Rink (Ed.), *Musical performance: A guide to understanding* (pp. 168–182). Cambridge, UK: Cambridge University Press.

Valentine, E. (2004). Alexander technique. In A. Williamon (Ed.), *Musical excellence* (pp. 179–195). Oxford, UK: Oxford University Press.

Valenzuela, R., Codina, N., & Pestana, J. V. (2018). Self-determination theory applied to flow in conservatoire music practice: The roles of perceived autonomy and competence, and autonomous and controlled motivation. *Psychology of Music, 46,* 33–48.

Valera, W., Abrami, P. C., & Upitis, R. (2016). Self-regulation and music learning: A systematic review. *Psychology of Music, 44*(1), 55–74. doi:10.1177/0305735614554639

Vaquero, L., Hartmann, K., Ripollés, P., Rojo, N., Sierpowska, J., Francois, C., Càmara, E., van Vugt, F. T., Mohammadi, B., Samii, A., Münte, T. F., Rodríguez-Fornells, A., & Altenmüller, E. (2016). Structural neuroplasticity in expert pianists depends on the age of musical training onset. *NeuroImage, 126,* 106–119. doi:10.1016/j.neuroimage.2015.11.008

Vervainioti, A., & Alexopoulos, E. C. (2015). Job-related stressors of classical instrumental musicians: A systematic qualitative review. *Medical Problems of Performing Artists, 30*(4), 197–202. https://doi.org/10.21091/mppa.2015.4037

Vetter, D. E. (2008, January 31). How do the hammer, anvil and stirrup bones amplify sound into the inner ear? *Scientific American.* https://www.scientificamerican.com/article/experts-how-do-the-hammer-anvil-a/

Vines, B. W., Krumhansl, C. L., Wanderley, M. M., Dalca, I. M., & Levitin, D. J. (2011). Music to my eyes: Cross-modal interactions in the perception of emotions in musical performance. *Cognition, 118,* 157–170. doi:10.1016/j.cognition.2010.11.010

Violisist.com. (2017, November 17). *Discussion forum—Beta blockers and performance anxiety.* https://www.violinist.com/discussion/thread.cfm?page=761

Volk, T. (1993). Factors influencing music educators in the "rote-tote" controversy, 1865–1900. *Bulletin of Historical Research in Music Education, 15*(1), 31–43. https://www.jstor.org/stable/40214824

Vuoskoski, J. K., Thompson, M. R., Clarke, E. F., & Spence, C. (2014). Crossmodal interactions in the perception of expressivity in musical performance. *Attention, Perception, & Psychophysics, 76,* 591–604. doi:10.3758/s13414-013-0582-2

Vuvan, D. T., Nunes-Silva, M., & Peretz, I. (2015). Meta-analytic evidence for the nonmodularity of pitch processing in congenital amusia. *Cortex, 69,* 186–200.

Waddell, G., & Williamon, A. (2017). Eye of the beholder: Stage entrance behavior and facial expression affect continuous quality ratings in music performance. *Frontiers in Psychology, 8,* article 513. https://doi.org/10.3389/fpsyg.2017.00513

Waddington, C. (2017). When it clicks: Co-performer empathy in ensemble playing. In E. King & C. Waddington (Eds.), *Music and empathy* (pp. 230–247). Abingdon, UK: Routledge.

Waggoner, D. T. (2011). Effects of listening conditions, error types, and ensemble textures on error detection skills. *Journal of Research in Music Education, 59*(1), 56–71. doi:10.1177/0022429410396094

Waldron, J. (2009). Exploring a virtual music "community of practice": Informal music learning on the Internet. *Journal of Music, Technology and Education, 2,* 97–112. doi:10.1386/jmte.2.2-3.97_1

Waldron, J. (2018). Questioning 20th century assumptions about 21st century music practices. *Action, Criticism, & Theory for Music Education, 17*(1), 97–113. doi:10.22176/act17.1.97

Wallas, G. (1926). *The art of thought.* New York, NY: Harcourt, Brace and Company.

Wallentin, M., Nielsen, A. H., Friis-Olivarius, M., Vuust, C., & Vuust, P. (2010). The Musical Ear Test, a new reliable test for measuring musical competence. *Learning and Individual Differences, 20,* 188–196. doi:10.1016/j.lindif.2010.02.004

Walton, A. E., Richardson, M. J., Langland-Hassan, P., & Chemero, P. (2015). Improvisation and the self-organization of multiple musical bodies. *Frontiers in Psychology, 6,* article 313. https://doi.org/10.3389/fpsyg.2015.00313

Wan, C. Y., & Huon, G. F. (2005). Performance degradation under pressure in music: An examination of attentional processes. *Psychology of Music, 33*(2), 155–172. doi:10.1177/0305735605050649

Wang, W. C., Brashier, N. M., Wing, E. A., Marsh, E. J., & Cabeza, R. (2016). On known unknowns: Fluency and the neural mechanisms of illusory truth. *Journal of Cognitive Neuroscience, 28*(5), 739–746. https://doi-org.libproxy.unl.edu/10.1162/jocn_a_00923

Wapnick, J., Campbell, L., Siddell-Strebel, J., & Darrow, A. (2009). Effects of non-musical attributes and excerpt duration on ratings of high-level piano performances. *Musicae Scientiae, 13*(1), 35–54. doi:10.1177/1029864909013001002

Warnet, V. (2020). Verbal behaviors of instrumental music teachers in secondary classrooms: A review of literature. *Update: Applications of Research in Music Education, 39*(1), 8–16. doi:10.1177/8755123320924827.

Waxman, J. (2012). *Prefacing music in the concert hall: Program books, composer commentaries, and the conflict over musical meaning* (Publication No. 3546489) [Doctoral dissertation, New York University]. ProQuest Dissertations Publishing.

Weidner, B. N. (2020). A grounded theory of musical independence in the concert band. *Journal of Research in Music Education, 68*(1), 53–77. doi:10.1177/0022429419897616

Weiner, B. (2004). Attribution theory revised: Transforming cultural plurality into theoretical unity. In D. McInerney & S. Etten (Eds.), *Big theories revised* (pp. 13–29). Charlotte, NC: Information Age.

Weisberg, R. W. (2006). *Creativity: Understanding innovation in problem solving, science, invention, and the arts.* Hoboken, NJ: John Wiley.

Wesolowski, B. C. (2016). Assessing jazz big band performance: The development, validation, and application of a facet-factorial rating scale. *Psychology of Music, 44*(3), 324–339. doi:10.1177/0305735614567700

West, R. (2004). Drugs and musical performance. In A. Williamon (Ed.), *Musical excellence: Strategies and techniques to enhance performance* (pp. 271–290). Oxford, UK: Oxford University Press.

Whipple, C. M., Gfeller, K., Driscoll, V., Oleson, J., & McGregor, K. (2015). Do communication disorders extend to musical messages? An answer from children with hearing loss or autism spectrum disorders. *Journal of Music Therapy, 52*(1), 78–116. doi:10.1093/jmt/thu039

Wiggins, J. (2016). Musical agency. In G. E. McPherson (Ed.), *The child as musician: A handbook of musical development* (2nd ed., pp. 102–121). Oxford, UK: Oxford University Press.

Wiggins, J., & Medvinsky, M. (2013). Scaffolding student composers. In M. Kaschub & J. Smith (Eds.), *Composing our future: Preparing music educators to teach composition* (pp. 109–125). New York, NY: Oxford University Press.

Wigram, T. (2006). Musical creativity in children with cognitive and social impairment. In I. Deliège & G. Wiggins (Eds.), *Musical creativity: Multidisciplinary research in theory and practice* (pp. 221–237). Hove, UK: Psychology Press.

Williamon, A. (1999). The value of performing from memory. *Psychology of Music, 27*(1), 84–95. https://doi.org/10.1177/0305735699271008

Williamon, A. (Ed.). (2004). *Musical excellence: Strategies and techniques to enhance performance.* Oxford, UK: Oxford University Press.

Williamon, A. (2014). Implications for education. In D. Fabian, R. Timmers, & E. Schubert (Eds.), *Expressiveness in music performance: Empirical approaches across styles and cultures* (pp. 348–351). Oxford, UK: Oxford University Press.

Williamon, A., Clark, T., & Küssner, M. (2017). Learning in the spotlight. In J. Rink, H. Gaunt, & A. Williamon (Eds.), *Musicians in the making: Pathways to creative performance* (pp. 206–221). Oxford, UK: Oxford University Press.

Williamon, A., & Davidson, J. W. (2002). Exploring co-performer communication. *Musicae Scientiae, 6,* 53–72. https://doi.org/10.1177/102986490200600103

Williamon, A., Wasley, D., Burt-Perkins, R., Ginsborg, J., & Hildebrandt, W. (2009). Profiling musicians' health, wellbeing, and performance. In A Williamon, S. Pretty, & Buck (Eds.), *Proceedings of the International Symposium on Performance Science 2009* (pp. 85–90). Utrecht, The Netherlands: European Association of Conservatoires. http://performancescience.org/wp-content/uploads/2018/08/isps2009_proceedings.pdf

Williams, E., Dingle, G. A., Calligeros, R., Sharman, L., & Jetten, J. (2020). Enhancing mental health recovery by joining arts-based groups: A role for the social cure approach. *Arts & Health, 12*(2), 169–181. doi:10.1080/17533015.2019.1624584

Williams, L. R. (2008). Effect of music complexity on nonmusicians' focus of attention to melody or harmony. *Update: Applications of Research in Music Education, 26*(2), 27–32. doi:10.1177/8755123308317952

Williamson, V. (2014). *You are the music: How music reveals what it means to be human.* London, UK: Icon Books.

Wilson, G. D. (2002). *Psychology for performing artists: Butterflies and bouquets.* London, UK: Whurr.

Wilson, G. D., & Roland, D. (2002). Performance anxiety. In R. Parncutt & G. E. McPherson (Eds.), *The science and psychology of music performance: Creative strategies for teaching and learning* (pp. 47–61). New York, NY: Oxford University Press.

Wing, H. D. (1981). *Standardised tests of musical intelligence.* Windsor, UK: National Foundation for Educational Research.

Wise, K., James, M., & Rink, J. (2017). Performers in the practice room. In J. Rink, H. Gaunt, & A. Williamon (Eds.), *Musicians in the making: Pathways to creative performance* (pp. 143–163). Oxford, UK: Oxford University Press.

Wolfe, J. (2019). An investigation into the nature and function of metaphor in advanced music instruction. *Research Studies in Music Education, 41*(3), 280–292. doi:10.1177/1321103X18773113

Wong, P. C., Ciocca, V., Chan, A. H., Ha, L. Y., Tan, L.-H., & Peretz, I. (2012). Effects of culture on musical pitch perception. *PLoS ONE, 7*(4), e33424. https://doi.org/10.1371/journal.pone.0033424

Woody, R. H. (1999). The relationship between advanced musicians' explicit planning and their expressive performance of dynamic variations in an aural modeling task. *Journal of Research in Music Education, 47,* 331–342. https://doi.org/10.2307/3345488

Woody, R. H. (2000). Learning expressivity in music performance: An exploratory study. *Research Studies in Music Education, 14,* 14–23. https://doi.org/10.1177/1321103X0001400102

Woody, R. H. (2001). Learning from the experts: Applying research in expert performance to music education. *Update: Applications of Research in Music Education, 19*(2), 9–14.

Woody, R. H. (2002a). Emotion, imagery and metaphor in the acquisition of musical performance skill. *Music Education Research, 4*(2), 213–224. doi:10.1080/1461380022000011920

Woody, R. H. (2002b). The relationship between musicians' expectations and their perception of expressive features in an aural model. *Research Studies in Music Education, 18*, 53–61.

Woody, R. H. (2003). Explaining expressive performance: Component cognitive skills in an aural modeling task. *Journal of Research in Music Education, 51*, 51–63.

Woody, R. H. (2006a). Musician's cognitive processing of imagery-based instructions for expressive performance. *Journal of Research in Music Education, 54*(2), 125–137. https://doi.org/10.1177/002242940605400204

Woody, R. H. (2006b). The effect of various instructional conditions on expressive music performance. *Journal of Research in Music Education, 54*(1), 21–36. https://doi.org/10.1177/002242940605400103

Woody, R. H. (2012). Playing by ear: Foundation or frill? *Music Educators Journal, 99*(2), 82–88. doi:10.1177/0027432112459199

Woody, R. H. (2019). *Becoming a real musician: Inspiration and guidance for teachers and parents of musical kids.* Lanham, MD: Rowman & Littlefield.

Woody, R. H. (2020a). Musicians' use of harmonic cognitive strategies when playing by ear. *Psychology of Music, 48*(5), 674–692. doi:10.1177/0305735618816365

Woody, R. H. (2020b). Music education students' intrinsic and extrinsic motivation: A quantitative analysis of personal narratives. *Psychology of Music.* Advance online publication. doi:10.1177/0305735620944224

Woody, R. H., & Adams, M. C. (2019). Vernacular and popular music. In C. Conway, K. Pellegrino, A. M. Stanley, & C. West (Eds.), *Oxford handbook of preservice music teacher education in the United States* (pp. 893–902). New York, NY: Oxford University Press.

Woody, R. H., Fraser, A., Nannen, B., & Yukevich, P. (2019). Musical identities of older adults are not easily changed: An exploratory study. *Music Education Research, 21*(3), 315–330. https://doi.org/10.1080/14613808.2019.1598346

Woody, R. H., & Lehmann, A. C. (2010). Student musicians' ear playing ability as a function of vernacular music experiences. *Journal of Research in Music Education, 58*(2), 101–115. doi:10.1177/0022429410370785

Woody, R. H., Lui, X., Rom, B., Smith, B., & Wassemiller, J. (2021). Musical engagement and identity: Exploring youth experiences, tastes, and beliefs. *Music Education Research, 23*(4), 430–442. doi: 10.1080/14613808.2021.1949272

Woody, R. H., & McPherson, G. E. (2010). Emotion and motivation in the lives of performers. In P. N. Juslin & J. A. Sloboda (Eds.), *Handbook of music and emotion: Theory, research, applications* (pp. 401–424). Oxford, UK: Oxford University Press.

Woody, R. H., & Parker, E. C. (2012). Encouraging participatory musicianship among university students. *Research Studies in Music Education, 34*(2), 130–146.

Wristen, B. G. (2013). Depression and anxiety in university music students. *Update: Applications of Research in Music Education, 31*(2), 20–27. doi:10.1177/8755123312473613

Young, V., Burwell, K., & Pickup, D. (2003). Areas of study and teaching strategies in instrumental teaching: A case study research project. *Music Education Research, 5*, 139–155. doi:10.1080/1461380032000085522

Zakaria, J. B., Musib, H. B., & Shariff, S. M. (2013). Overcoming performance anxiety among music undergraduates. *Procedia—Social and Behavioral Sciences, 90*, 226–234. doi:10.1016/j.sbspro.2013.07.086

Zelenak, M. S. (2015). Measuring the sources of self-efficacy among secondary school music students. *Journal of Research in Music Education, 62*(4), 389–404. doi:10.1177/0022429414555018

Zembylas, T., & Niederauer, M. (2018). *Composing processes and artistic agency: Tacit knowledge in composing.* Abingdon, UK: Routledge.

Zendel, B. R., & Alain, C. (2009). Concurrent sound segregation is enhanced in musicians. *Journal of Cognitive Neuroscience, 21*(8), 1488–1498. https://doi.org/10.1162/jocn.2009.21140

Zentner, M., Grandjean, D., & Scherer, K. R. (2008). Emotions evoked by the sound of music: Characterization, classification, and measurement. *Emotion, 8*(4), 494–521. doi:10.1037/1528-3542.8.4.494

Zhang, J. D., Susino, M., McPherson, G. E., & Schubert, E. (2020). The definition of a musician in music psychology: A literature review and the six-year rule. *Psychology of Music, 48*(3), 389–409. doi:10.1177/0305735618804038

Zhang, L., & Sternberg, R. J. (2009). Intellectual styles and creativity. In T. Rickards, M. A. Runco, & S. Moger (Eds.), *The Routledge companion to creativity* (pp. 256–266). New York, NY: Routledge.

Zimmerman, B. J. (1998). Developing self-fulfilling cycles of academic regulation: An analysis of exemplary models In D. H. Schunk & B. J. Zimmerman (Eds.), *Self-regulated learning. From teaching to self-reflective practice* (pp. 1–20). London, UK: Guilford Press.

Zorzal, R. C. (2020). Emotion-related words and emotional analogies as teaching strategies for expressivity. *Research Studies in Music Education.* Advance online publication. https://doi.org/10.1177/1321103X19899169

Index

For the benefit of digital users, indexed terms that span two pages (e.g., 52–53) may, on occasion, appear on only one of those pages.

Tables and figures are indicated by *t* and *f* following the page number

absolute pitch, 33
acculturation, 10–11
acquired skill. *See* skill acquisition
adolescence, 23, 38–39, 169, 259–60, 275
adrenaline, 171, 176–77
Alexander Technique, 176
altered states, 147–48
amusement park model, 143
amusia, 31
anticipation, 160, 160*f*, 210. *See also*
    expectancy/expectation
anxiety, 52–53, 111, 169–92
aptitude, 24–26
arch structure, 126
Armstrong, Louis, 30, 144
arousal, 171–73, 172*f*, 182–83, 255–
    56, 286–87
artistry, 7, 11–12, 19–20, 22, 41–42, 63–64,
    111–12, 116, 117, 125–26, 128–
    29, 135
atonal, 97, 110–11
attention, 28–29, 66, 72–75, 88–89, 103,
    111–12, 113, 122, 128, 129, 130–31,
    132, 133–34, 135–36, 139, 156–57,
    237, 241, 245, 247–48, 251
attractiveness, 197, 251
attribution theory, 60–61
audience, 154, 169, 182–83, 184–85, 186–
    87, 196–200, 218, 288
auditions, 184, 186, 251–52
auditory processing, 78, 210, 244–45,
    250, 252
auditory system, 241–44, 242*f, See also* ear
aural modeling, 130–31, 132, 133–34,
    227–28. *See also* imitation

authenticity, 38, 114–15, 130, 276–77
automaticity, 66, 74–76, 102, 107, 132–33,
    157, 159, 210–11
autonomic nervous system, 171
autonomy, 51, 56–58, 58*f*, 222, 224, 232–
    33, 234, 278

Bach, 111–12, 128, 138
Bandura, Albert, 59
Beatles, 68, 69–70, 72–73
Beethoven, 9–10, 141–42, 145–46, 148,
    151, 154, 267–68, 275
beliefs, 48, 59, 179, 190
belonging, 39–40, 56, 199–200, 208, 272
beta blockers, 176–77
Big-C/little-c creativity, 141–42
biofeedback training, 176
Brahms, 148, 152
brain, 77, 78, 83–84, 159, 171–72, 243,
    260–61, 286
burnout, 46, 53

Carnegie Hall, 25, 66
catastrophe model, 172*f*, 174–75
catastrophizing, 174, 180, 182–83. *See also*
    catastrophe model
chaining, 87
chamber music, 43–44, 134, 184–85, 199–
    200, 204–5, 206–8, 219
chess, 96, 97–98, 98*f*
choice, 51–52, 258–59, 275, 278
choking, 174, 175*f, See also*
    catastrophe model
chunking, 86, 97, 103, 110, 111–12, 113.
    See also memory

classical music, 71, 101–2, 122, 135–36, 156, 183, 185, 199–200, 203, 205, 208–9, 215, 232–33, 265–68, 269–70, 271, 271*t*, 275
cognitive restructuring, 181–82, 190
cognitive skills, 67, 73, 80–82, 81*f*, 84–85, 102–4, 231, 250, *See also* goal imaging; motor production; self–monitoring
cohesion, 206, 208, 272, 274
Coltrane, 141–42
communication, 5, 6–7, 11–12, 13, 36, 63, 117, 122–23, 125–26, 129, 134–35, 160, 160*f*, 161, 180, 196, 202–3, 212–13, 224–25, 229, 230*t*
composers, 138, 164–65, 240, 267
    Beyond–Domain, 153, 154*t*
    inspirational type, 151–52
    working type, 151, 152–53
    Within–Domain, 153, 154*t*
composition, 138, 139, 148–55
concentration. *See* deliberate: thought
conducting, 228–31
confidence. *See* self–efficacy
conscious thought. *See* attention
conservatory culture, 130, 270–71
constraint of time, 111, 156–57, 159
Constructivism, 9
consumer behavior, 271*t*, 277–78
convergent thinking, 140–41, 145, 147, 148–49
conversion, 125–26, 133–34
coping, 46, 88, 272, 274, 283–84
Copland, Aaron, 246–47
creativity, 31, 138–39, 140
    defined, 140–42
    Ps of, 141
Csikszentmihalyi, Mihaly, 13, 149
cultural capital, 275–77
culture, 5–6, 9–12, 267, 272, 273*f*, *See also* enculturation
curriculum, 222–24

dance, 12
Davis, Miles, 155
deafness, 260–61
decision–making, 14, 39–40, 56, 59, 60–62, 117, 119–20, 127–28, 135–36, 138–39, 149–50, 153, 156–57, 159, 184–85, 207–8, 209, 223, 235*f*
depression, 179–80, 196
desensitization, 185–87
development, 21–44
dialogue, 153–55
disabilities, 31–33, 160–61, 260–61
divergent thinking, 140–41, 145, 147, 148–49
DJing, 78, 270–71
domain
    mastery, 143, 144–45, 147, 152 (*see also* expertise)
    specificity, 143–44
driving, 281
dropout. *See* quitting music
drugs, 147, 196, 282–83. *See also* beta blockers

ear
    learning by, 8
    physiology, 241–44, 242*f*
    playing by, 71, 82, 95, 101–3, 107–8, 113, 114–15, 158, 286
early childhood, 22–23, 36–37, 42–43, 48–49, 260. *See also* infant
Edison, Thomas, 150–51, 240
education, 6, 10–11, 28–29
ego–involved orientation, 52–53, 57*f*, 62–64, 180, 183
Ellington, Duke, 155
emergence, 161–62
emotion
    expression of, 12, 13
    regulation, 11, 256–57
    responses to music, 12–14, 240–41, 248*f*, 252–58, 254*f*, 263
emotional coding (of expression), 121–23
enculturation, 22, 56, 71, 158, 246, 259–60
enjoyment, 42, 48–50, 189–90. *See also* intrinsic motivation
entertainment, 5, 11, 196, 203, 248*f*, 265, 287
entrepreneurship, 215–16
environment, effect of, 27, 48–49
Ericsson, K. Anders, 68–70

evaluating music, 136–37, 150, 184,
205, 225, 228, 250–52, 262. *See also*
feedback
everyday life, 8, 11, 42–43, 49, 119–20,
141–245, 267, 280–82, 286–87
expectancy/expectation, 109, 110–11,
199*f*, 246, 247–50, 249*f*
expertise, 69, 70, 71*f*, 72–73, 75, 96–98,
113, 127–28, 236, 237
expressiveness, 111–12, 116–25, 202–
3, 227
eye
contact, 161, 197, 212–13, 229, 230*t*
fixations, 109–10
functioning of (*see* vision)
movement (*see* saccades)

facial expression, 195, 198–99, 204–5,
228–29, 230*t*
failure, 52–53, 60–61, 62–64, 88,
143, 183
fatigue, 69, 73–74, 80, 83–84, 90, 186
feedback, 39–40, 59, 64, 69, 134–35,
159–60, 160*f*, 169, 189, 222, 227–
31, 248*f*
fetal development. *See* prenatal
development
fixed mindset, 60, 61, 62
flow, 13, 51–52, 52*f*, 158, 160*f*, 161, 189
functions of music, 5–6, 11–12, 270–87

Gardner, Howard, 140, 142
geneplore model, 140–41
generative principles (of
expression), 120–21
generativity, 138–39
genetics, 26–27, 270
"genius," 23, 138, 141–42, 148, 150–51
Gestalt, 245
gesture, 195, 200, 203, 212–13, 228–29
Gladwell, Malcolm, 68
goal imaging, 79, 81, 81*f*, 82, 84–85, 89,
102–4, 112–13, 132, 133, 231, 232
orientation, 52–53, 62–63
setting, 62–63, 69, 72, 73, 82, 85–86, 88–
89, 90, 126, 182
Gould, Glenn, 125
group dynamics. *See* interpersonal
growth mindset, 60, 61

health, 196, 216–17, 283–84. *See also*
well being
Hugo, Victor, 116

identity, 267, 272–73
development, 39–41, 40*f*
musician, 41–42, 61–62
music teacher, 222, 236–37
idiosyncratic style (of expression), 124–25
illumination, 149, 150, 152
illusions, 244
imagery, 112, 131, 132–34, 226–27
imagination, 38, 131, 139, 144, 146, 147,
240, 248–49
imitation, 7–8, 71–72, 130–31, 133,
224, 227–28
imposter syndrome, 183
impression management, 139. *See also*
prestige
improvisation, 135–36, 138–40, 144, 156–
65, 165*f*, 185, 277
incubation, 139, 149–50, 153
independence, 42, 214–15, 235*f*
infant
directed speech, 36
musicality, 34–36, 35*f* (*see also* early
childhood)
informal music making, 7–181, 183, 190–
91, 199–200, 206–7, 213
injury, 196
innate talent. *See* talent
insight, 146, 147, 150, 152
inspiration, 150–51, 166
intelligence, 8, 25, 143, 284–85
interpersonal function, 12, 43–44, 71, 72,
161–62, 195, 196, 206–7, 208–10,
212. *See also* cohesion; relationship
interpretation, 117, 125–29, 135–36
intuition, 139

Jackson, Michael, 166
jazz, 71–72, 130, 144, 157–58, 161, 163–64,
183, 208–9, 259, 270, 286

knowledge, 73–75, 100, 101, 111,
113–14
declarative, 18, 29, 79–80, 97
procedural, 9, 18, 74–75, 79–80, 97
Kodály, Zoltán, 102–3, 108

language, 4, 6–8, 107, 110–11, 157–58, 252
leadership, 206–8, 234, 236–37
learning objectives, 222–24
lesson planning, 222–24, 226f, 263
letting go, 158–59
lifelong musicianship, 41–42, 233–35, 235f, 288–89
listening, 8, 144, 229–31, 240–63, 280–82
Liszt, 200, 201f

Maslow, Abraham, 13
McCartney, Paul, 119, 150
McPherson, Gary, 26, 104–5, 105f
meaningfulness, 95, 97–98, 98f, 100, 101, 111–12, 113–14, 119, 163, 245
memorization, 83, 96, 111–13. See also memory: encoding
memory, 79–80, 96, 104, 130–31
  consolidation, 80
  encoding, 95
  long-term, 99–101, 104, 133
  retrieval, 99–100, 99f, 110–12, 133
  sensory, 99, 99f
  short-term, 99–100, 99f
  working (see memory: short-term)
mental illness, 148, 160–61
mental practice. See practice: mental
mental representation, 73, 74, 75–76, 79, 83, 87, 111–12, 128, 132, 231, 250
Merriam, Alan, 5–6
metaphor. See imagery
mindset, 60–61
mood management, 11, 202–3, 249–50, 256–57, 278, 281–82. See also emotion regulation
motional patters (of expression), 123
motivation, 28, 46–63, 72–73, 189–90, 207–8, 233
  extrinsic, 53–58, 57f
  intrinsic, 47, 48, 49–50, 51–52
motor production, 81–82, 81f, 102–4, 231, 232
movement
  bodily, 196, 200–3 (see also dance; gesture)
  sociopolitical, 12, 273–75

Mozart, 16, 23–24, 138, 144, 148, 152, 197–98, 284–85
muscle memory, 79–80, 96. See also psychomotor skill
musician, defined 4
musicology, 127, 144, 268–69

neurology. See brain
neuroticism, 178, 214–15, 259, 283
notation, 87, 95, 101–2, 106–7, 111–13, 156, 204–5

one-to-one "private" lessons, 10, 71–72, 132, 213–14, 224, 228, 232, 234
openness to experience, 155, 214–16
open-earedness, 38

para-musical, 195
parental involvement, 27–28, 47, 48, 84–85, 88, 169
Parker, Charlie, 155, 157
participatory performance, 199–200, 218
passion, 50–51, 178–79, 232–33
pattern recognition. See chunking
peak experiences, 13, 49
peers, 47, 48, 55–56, 84–85, 88, 208–9, 275
perception, 78, 158, 196, 244–45, 286
perceptual span, 109–10
perfect pitch. See absolute pitch
perfectionism, 52–53, 62–63, 179–80, 181–83
PERMA model, 217
personality. See traits
person-focused approach, 267, 268–70, 287
philosophy, 5, 14–15, 41, 123, 125–26, 176, 255–56, 268–69, 274, 276
phrasing, 120–21, 126, 246–47
physiology, 26, 77–78, 171–77, 171t, 175f, 240–41, 256
Piaget, Jean, 22
planning, 85–86, 87, 90, 117, 124, 127–28, 129, 132
playing by ear. See ear: playing by
popular music, 11, 38–64, 114–15, 130, 144, 155, 166, 169–70, 183, 196, 203, 209, 258, 269–71, 271t, 275

practice, 29–30, 66–91, 170, 181, 187–
    88, 229–31
  defined, 66, 67–68
  deliberate, 29–30, 59, 67–70, 71f, 80, 96,
    113–14, 132, 214–15
  diary/journal/log, 70, 85–86, 90
  distributed, 80
  mental, 83–84, 185
  quality, 73, 84–90
  quantity, 66, 69–70
  strategy, 67, 80, 86–87, 89
praise, 27, 54, 64, 228
preference, 257–60, 275
prenatal development, 33–34,
    241–42
prestige, 197–98, 251, 277
psychology, 3–5, 14–16
psychomotor skill, 29, 78, 286. See also
    knowledge: procedural

quitting music, 46–47, 54, 61–62, 67, 79,
    207–8, 224–25, 233–34

reading, 82, 83
reflection, 87–88
rehearsal
  cognitive psychology, 100
  ensemble/group, 67, 206–9, 229–31
relatedness/relationship, 56–59, 58f, 222,
    224–25, 236
relaxation, 175–77, 186–87, 256–57
religion, 5, 10, 11–12, 23, 42, 259, 279–80
remix model, 145–46, 155
repertoire, 9–10, 51, 71, 83, 85, 127, 135–
    36, 160, 160f, 184, 189–90, 204–5,
    222, 223, 233
resilience, 61, 64, 143, 211
Rubinstein, Arthur, 169–70, 179

saccades, 109
savants, 32–33
Schuman, 138
science, 15–16, 116–17, 139
SDT. See self-determination theory
Seashore, Carl, 118
Segovia, Andrés, 49
self-determination theory, 56–59, 57f, 58f,
    61–62, 207–8, 233

self-efficacy, 59–60, 85–86, 88, 190
self-handicapping, 180–81
self-monitoring, 72, 81f, 82, 86, 231–32
self-regulation, 85, 86, 88, 113–14, 231
self-talk, 181–83
sex, 203, 251–52, 277, 282–83
sight–reading, 95, 108–11
Simonton, Dean Keith, 140, 142, 164–65
singing
  situational stress, 183–87
  skill acquisition, 4, 17–18, 26, 28–29,
    30–31, 47, 66, 68, 71–73, 74–76, 76f,
    89, 102, 237
Sloboda, John, 3, 70, 71–72
slowing, 87
social aspects, See culture; interpersonal
    functions
socialization. See enculturation
Songwriting, 138, 163, 167
specificity. See domain: specificity
speech, 7–8, 97, 107. See also language
spiral model of musical development. See
    Swanwick and Tillman spiral
    model
spirituality. See religion
sports, 25, 67, 134–35, 171–72, 174, 237,
    258, 273, 281–82
spreading activation theory, 145–46
stage presence, 183, 195, 196–97, 198–99,
    199f, 203–5, 251
Stravinsky, 141–42
Swanwick and Tillman spiral model, 31,
    32f, 37, 38, 41, 162
symbolic representation, 12, 273–74
symptoms (of performance anxiety),
    170, 171–78
synchronization, 208, 210–11
synesthesia, 261

tablature/TAB, 11, 106
talent, 17, 18, 22, 23–25, 27, 33, 60–61, 62.
    See also aptitude
task–involved orientation, 52–53, 62–64,
    180, 182–83, 187–88, 189–90
tastes, See also preference
teaching, 19–20, 44, 64, 91, 114–15, 136–
    37, 165f, 166, 191–92, 219, 221–39,
    262–63, 288–89

technique, 3, 29, 49–50, 63, 72, 83, 90,
    127–237
teenagers. *See* adolescence
threat, 170, 171, 177–78, 180, 183,
    189–90
tone deafness. *See* amusia
traits, 155, 177–78, 179, 181, 214–16, 222,
    225–26, 226*f*, 236, 241, 257–59
trance, 11

universals, 4, 6–7, 121–22, 130, 204, 240,
    252, 287
uses of music. *See* functions of music

values, 9, 10–11, 274–75, 287. *See also*
    culture
  of scientific psychology, 15
variations in sound, 13, 116, 117–20,
    131–32, 133, 134, 136–37, 227, 240–
    41, 253
verbalization, 133–34, 136–37, 225–
    27, 238–39

vernacular musicianship, 38–39, 49–
    50, 72, 95, 102–3, 104, 114–15,
    199–200, 208–9, 215, 250. *See also*
    popular music
vision, 109–11, 173
visual aspects (of performance), 195, 204–
    6, 205*f*

Wagner, 150
Waits, Tom, 162
Wallas stages of creativity, 141, 149–
    51, 152–53
well being, 6, 42, 196, 213–14, 216–17,
    232–33, 283–84
Werktreue, 127
Work–focused approach, 267–69
workplace, 278, 279*f*
writer's block, 147

Yerkes–Dodson, 172–73, 172*f*

zero history groups, 211–12